Handbook of Endovascular Peripheral Interventions

Christopher D. Owens
Yerem Yeghiazarians
(Editors)

Handbook of Endovascular Peripheral Interventions

Springer

Editors
Christopher D. Owens, M.D., M.Sc.
Division of Vascular Surgery
Department of Surgery
University of California –
San Francisco
San Francisco, CA
USA
christopher.owens@ucsfmedctr.org

Yerem Yeghiazarians, M.D.
Division of Interventional
Cardiology
Department of Medicine
University of California –
San Francisco
San Francisco, CA
USA
yeghiaza@medicine.ucsf.edu

ISBN 978-1-4614-0838-3 e-ISBN 978-1-4614-0839-0
DOI 10.1007/978-1-4614-0839-0
Springer New York Dordrecht Heidelberg London

Library of Congress Control Number: 2011943616

Printed on acid-free paper

Springer is part of Springer Science+Business Media (www.springer.com)

Foreword

Over the last decade, the field of peripheral vascular disease has seen a dramatic evolution – with an ever-expanding array of treatment options, and a growing interest among diverse medical practitioners as well as commercial entities. At the same time, the global scope of the problem continues to increase in magnitude. It is estimated that between 8 and 12 Americans harbor symptomatic or occult peripheral artery disease (PAD). While some risk factors, such as smoking and hyperlipidemia, have been targeted productively by education, public policy, and improved medications, others such as diabetes, obesity, and physical inactivity appear to be increasing in an ominous fashion. The continued aging of the population alone has major implications, as PAD prevalence is directly related to age and the disease affects as many as one in five individuals over age 65. The worldwide diabetes epidemic – recently estimated to afflict more than 23 million Americans and roughly 300 million worldwide – portends a growing burden of PAD on public health. For all vascular specialists, the treatment of PAD will dominate clinical practice demands for the foreseeable future.

Yet in no other area of vascular disease do we have such broad heterogeneity of treatment approaches, limited evidence to support practice guidelines, and lack of standardization in virtually all aspects of care – particularly interventional. The continued evolution of percutaneous revascularization techniques has allowed for a broader application of treatment to PAD patients with reduced invasiveness, with a concomitant explosive increase in the volume of procedures performed. Unfortunately, a bewildering and continuously changing array of devices, techniques, and expert opinions renders the field daunting, if not undecipherable, to the specialist-in-training or novice interventionalist. We vascular specialists practice in an era of rapid change, lack of consensus, and diverse sources of information of variable quality. Hence the need for a book like this.

The current treatment of peripheral vascular disease is optimized by a collaborative approach among practitioners with expertise in vascular medicine, vascular imaging, open surgery, and endovascular intervention. The editors have assembled a multidisciplinary group of expert authors to provide practical, focused chapters on the assessment and interventional management of peripheral vascular diseases. The goal is to provide the reader with a thoughtful review of the most current interventional approaches, key considerations in patient selection and optimization of outcomes, and technical tips to maximize success and avoid pitfalls. It is organized in a user-friendly, quick reference format that is ideal for use "in the trenches." I anticipate it will be used widely by students, residents, and fellows – as well as surgeons and interventionalists who are expanding their practice in these areas. I am grateful for their efforts and for the insight of the publishers in supporting this project, and congratulate them on producing a high-caliber reference that answers a major need in our field.

Michael S. Conte, MD
Professor of Surgery
Division of Vascular and Endovascular Surgery
University of California San Francisco
San Francisco, CA
USA

Preface

Why This Book?

Increasingly, peripheral vascular interventions are being performed by vascular surgeons, interventional cardiologists, and interventional radiologists. This handbook is meant to be a guide for the beginner and also for the more advanced interventionalist covering all aspects of percutaneous peripheral vascular interventions. Each chapter of this highly illustrated book provides brief background, etiology, clinical presentation, imaging, and percutaneous treatment of different vascular conditions. Importantly, "Tips of the trade" and "How I do it" sections in each chapter make this handbook very practical. These invaluable pearls are provided by the authors of each chapter who are experts in the field. This handbook is a collaborative effort between cardiologists, vascular surgeons, and radiologists as we strongly believe that each subspecialty brings unique expertise to the field of percutaneous peripheral vascular interventions.

This handbook was put together as many of our colleagues, fellows, residents, and medical students have expressed a need for an easily accessible book which will cover the essential principles and specific management issues with percutaneous peripheral vascular interventions.

How to Use This Book

This book starts with general concepts of vascular imaging, access sites issues, principles of sheaths/guides, diagnostic angiography, anti-platelet and anti-coagulation therapies, and ways to minimize contrast-induced nephropathy that all practitioners need to be familiar with. The second half of the book focuses on the different vascular territories and provides the reader an in-depth but concise review of the principles of percutaneous treatments of the specific peripheral vascular bed.

We envision trainees carrying this handbook in their white coat pockets so that before they scrub in for a case, they read the appropriate chapters and enhance their educational experience during the case. For the more experienced operator, this handbook provides more details about how the experts in the field do their cases by mentioning more specific use of different wires, guides, and techniques that they favor to overcome the challenges of percutaneous peripheral interventions. The selected references section located at the end of each chapter provides additional reading material that the author feels especially pertinent to the presented material.

Christopher D. Owens
Yerem, Yeghiazarians

Acknowledgments

First and foremost, we would like to deeply thank all the authors for their contributions. Their tolerance of our constant e-mails and calls and editing is much appreciated. A special thanks to Kevin Wright at Springer for his superb efforts in making this book possible.

We would also like to thank our families for their support while this book was being put together. Leon and Genia, Vartan, and Suzie Yeghiazarians, Nichole Kendall, and our children Sofia Yeghiazarians and Luke and Ellen Owens.

Contents

Contributors

Richard Bafford, M.D. Division of Vascular Surgery, University of Maryland School of Medicine, Baltimore, MD, USA

Joshua A. Beckman, M.D., MS Cardiovascular Division, Brigham and Women's Hospital, Harvard Medical School, Boston, MA, USA

Andrew J. Boyle, M.B.B.S., Ph.D. Division of Cardiology, Department of Medicine, University of California – San Francisco, San Francisco, CA, USA

Kerry C. Cho, M.D. Division of Nephrology, Department of Medicine, University of California – San Francisco, San Francisco, CA, USA

Mark A. Creager, M.D. Cardiovascular Division, Brigham and Women's Hospital, Harvard Medical School, Boston, MA, USA

Nihar R. Desai, M.D., MPH Cardiovascular Division, Brigham and Women's Hospital, Harvard Medical School, Boston, MA, USA

Muneer Eesa, M.D. Interventional Neuroradiology, Columbia University, College of Physicians and Surgeons, New York Presbyterian Hospitals, New York, NY, USA

Charles M. Eichler, M.D. Division of Vascular Surgery, Department of Surgery, University of California – San Francisco, San Francisco, CA, USA

Andrew C. Eisenhauer, M.D. Cardiovascular Division, Department of Medicine, Brigham and Women's Hospital, Harvard Medical School, Boston, MA, USA

Warren J. Gasper, M.D. Division of Endovascular and Vascular Surgery, Department of Surgery, University of California – San Francisco, San Francisco, CA, USA

Edwin C. Gravereaux, M.D. Department of Vascular Surgery, Brigham and Women's Hospital, Harvard Medical School, Boston, MA, USA

S. Marlene Grenon, MDCM, MMSc, FRCSC Division of Vascular Surgery, Department of Surgery, University of California – San Francisco, San Francisco, CA, USA

Randall T. Higashida, M.D. Interventional Neuroradiology, University of California – San Francisco, San Francisco, CA, USA

Robert K. Kerlan Jr., M.D. Interventional Radiology Division, Department of Radiology, University of California – San Francisco, San Francisco, CA, USA

Jeanne M. LaBerge, M.D. Interventional Radiology Division, Department of Radiology, University of California – San Francisco, San Francisco, CA, USA

David Lao, M.D. Department of Medicine, University of California – San Francisco, San Francisco, CA, USA

Andrew Lin, M.D. Division of Nephrology, Department of Medicine, University of California – San Francisco, San Francisco, CA, USA

Jong-Ping Lu, M.D. Department of Surgery, University of California – San Francisco, San Francisco, CA, USA

Matthew T. Menard, M.D. Division of Vascular and Endovascular Surgery, Brigham and Women's Hospital, Harvard Medical School, Boston, MA, USA

Philip M. Meyers, M.D. Interventional Neuroradiology, Columbia University, College of Physicians and Surgeons, New York Presbyterian Hospitals, New York, NY, USA

George V. Moukarbel, M.D. Cardiovascular Division, Brigham and Women's Hospital, Harvard Medical School, Boston, MA, USA

Sujal M. Nanavati, M.D. Interventional Radiology Division, Department of Radiology and Biomedical Imaging, University of California – San Francisco, San Francisco, CA, USA

Victor M. Ochoa, M.D. Division of Cardiology, Department of Medicine, University of California – San Francisco, San Francisco, CA, USA

Christopher D. Owens, M.D., M.Sc. Division of Vascular Surgery, Department of Surgery, University of California – San Francisco, San Francisco, CA, USA

Reena L. Pande, M.D. Cardiovascular Division, Brigham and Women's Hospital, Harvard Medical School, Boston, MA, USA

Punit S. Parasher, M.D. Division of Cardiology, Department of Medicine, University of California – San Francisco, San Francisco, CA, USA

Joseph Rapp, M.D. Division of Endovascular and Vascular Surgery, Department of Surgery, University of California – San Francisco, San Francisco, CA, USA

Lincoln Roland, M.D. Department of Vascular Surgery, University of Massachusetts Medical School, Worcester, MA, USA

Rajabrata Sarkar, M.D., Ph.D. Division of Vascular Surgery, Department of Surgery, University of Maryland, Baltimore, MD, USA

Rajiv Sawhney, M.D. Interventional Radiology Division, Department of Radiology and Biomedical Imaging, University of California – San Francisco and VA Medical Center, San Francisco, CA, USA

Andres Schanzer, M.D. Department of Vascular Surgery, University of Massachusetts Medical School, Worcester, MA, USA

Kendrick A. Shunk, M.D., Ph.D. Division of Cardiology, Department of Medicine, University of California – San Francisco and VA Medical Center, San Francisco, CA, USA

Piotr S. Sobieszczyk, M.D., R.V.T. Cardiovascular Division, Brigham and Women's Hospital, Harvard Medical School, Boston, MA, USA

Jeffrey M. Sparling, M.D. Cardiovascular Division, Brigham and Women's Hospital, Harvard Medical School, Boston, MA, USA

Kristian Ulloa, M.D. Division of Vascular Surgery, Department of Surgery, University of Maryland, Baltimore, MD, USA

Yerem Yeghiazarians, M.D. Division of Interventional Cardiology, Department of Medicine, University of California – San Francisco, San Francisco, CA, USA

Jeffrey Zimmet, M.D. Interventional Cardiology Division, Department of Medicine, University of California – San Francisco and VA Medical Center, San Francisco, CA, USA

Chapter 1
Vascular Access: Arterial, Venous, and Ultrasound Guidance

Punit S. Parasher and Andrew J. Boyle

Arterial Access

In this section, we will outline clinical pointers, tips, and "how we do it" in regards to obtaining access in the femoral, radial, brachial, and popliteal arteries and vascular grafts.

Femoral Artery Access

Retrograde Femoral Artery Puncture

Clinical Pointers

- Femoral puncture is the most common method of arterial access and the access of choice in the vast majority of endovascular interventions. The femoral artery is a large caliber vessel; it is superficial to the

P.S. Parasher • A.J. Boyle (✉)
Division of Cardiology, Department of Medicine, University of California – San Francisco, San Francisco, CA, USA
e-mail: aboyle@medicine.ucsf.edu

C.D. Owens and Y. Yeghiazarians (eds.), *Handbook of Endovascular Peripheral Interventions*, DOI 10.1007/978-1-4614-0839-0_1,

skin and therefore easy to access and it is compressible against the femoral head to achieve hemostasis.

- When obtaining access via femoral artery puncture, the common femoral artery (CFA) is the optimal site of entry and the vessel should be entered at the infra-inguinal level.
- If the vessel is punctured superior to the inguinal ligament, the risk of uncontrolled hemorrhage following sheath removal is higher due to the inability to maintain adequate external compression of the vessel against the femoral head.
- Lower punctures can lead to entry into the superficial femoral artery (SFA), which carries a higher risk of arteriovenous fistula and pseudoaneurysm formation due to manipulation of the smaller caliber vessel.[1–3]
- The true inguinal ligament lays 1–2 cm inferior to the imaginary line that runs between the anterior superior iliac spine and the pubic tubercle.
- In 97% of patients, the CFA lies on the medial third of the femoral head.[4,5]
- In obese patients, it is best to tape the protruding abdomen back to the chest wall with 3–4 in. tape, which is then secured to the sides of the table with tape. This will make the tissue overlying the CFA taut and prevent deflection of the needle away from the planned trajectory.

Tips of the Trade

- If available, it is helpful to review prior angiograms before gaining vascular access to determine if the patient has unusual anatomy (such as high femoral bifurcation or a severely calcified femoral artery).
- In the method described by Rupp et al.,[5] fluoroscopy is used to position the femoral head in the center of the frame and a 18-gauge or 19-gauge Seldinger

needle is targeted 1 cm lateral to the most medial aspect of the femoral head.

- Some practitioners endorse the use of a discreet 3–5 mm cut made at the skin surface overlying the CFA, followed by tissue dilation with a curved hemostat to decrease the resistance encountered when advancing the needle and sheath into the vessel. This might provide an outlet for bleeding from the puncture site and decrease the likelihood of formation of a post-procedure deep hematoma.
- Ensure that the dilator is "locked" into the sheath prior to insertion in order to avoid trauma to vessel.
- For peripheral interventions, many practitioners advocate the use of a 0.035 in. soft-tipped wire to secure entry into the iliac vessels and aorta due to the high incidence of unrecognized iliac artery disease in patients undergoing planned peripheral vascular interventions. Use of a J-tipped or straight wire may lead to dissections of the vessels in these instances.
- Avoid passing a coated wire through the needle, as the coating might be sheared off by the tip of the needle.
- In obese patients or in patients with severe peripheral vascular disease and poor peripheral pulses, a Doppler-guided SmartNeedle (Escalon Medical, New Berlin, WI) can be used to puncture the CFA. The SmartNeedle incorporates continuous Doppler ultrasound to provide auditory feedback regarding the proximity of the artery, providing a louder intensity signal when the artery is in close proximity.
- In patients with poor femoral pulses and heavily calcified vessels, the operator can often use fluoroscopy to visualize the outline of the vessel and direct the needle toward the common femoral artery.
- Ultrasound guidance can be used to assist in vascular access and this technique is described in detail below in Sect. "Ultrasound Guidance for Vascular Access".

- If the artery can be cannulated, but the wire does not easily advance, then the tip of the needle is likely adjacent to the contralateral wall of the vessel. In this case, the angle of the needle should be gently adjusted to allow the wire to exit the tip of the needle into the lumen of the vessel and not against the wall. Occasionally the J-tip guidewire can turn distally and therefore fluoroscopic confirmation that the tip of the wire is in the distal descending aorta is required.

How We Do It

- After the CFA is located by palpation of the artery and fluoroscopy of the forceps overlying the femoral head, the area is anesthetized with 10 cm^3 of 1–2% lidocaine or longer-acting bupivicaine. See Fig. 1.1.
- Once the right CFA is adequately palpated, the middle and index finger of the left hand are used to stabilize the vessel and an 18-gauge or 19-gauge Seldinger needle is used to cannulate the vessel.
- When obtaining left CFA access, the operator can choose to stand on either the left or right side, based on their individual comfort level, though it should be noted that left CFA access is associated with higher access-related complication rates.
- The needle should enter at an angle within a range of 30–45° to allow for easy passage of the J-tip guidewire.
- Once the needle tip is close to the vessel, the hub will begin to pulsate and further advancement along this trajectory will lead to arterial puncture.
- Once the guidewire has safely and easily passed into the vessel, the needle is removed while pressure is held proximal to the needle entry point to avoid excessive bleeding.

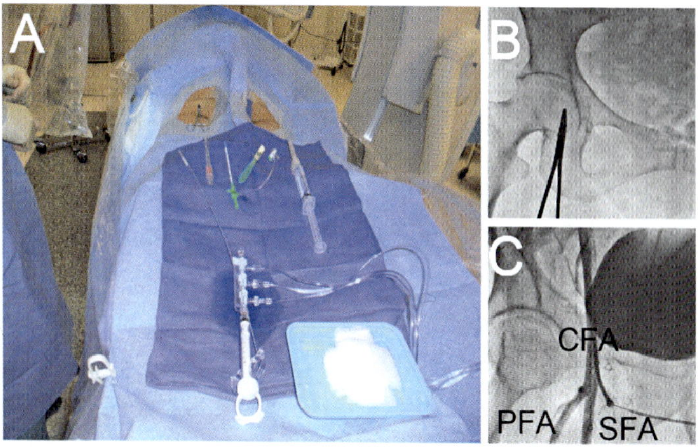

FIGURE 1.1 Femoral arterial access. Both groins are prepared and the equipment is ready (**a**), with arterial forceps in place to locate the optimal puncture site by x-ray (**b**). Angiography (**c**) reveals that the sheath is in the common femoral artery (*CFA*), above the bifurcation into the superficial femoral artery (*SFA*) and profunda femoris artery (*PFA*)

- Most commonly, a 0.035 in. J-tip steel guidewire is passed through the Seldinger needle after the vessel is punctured and pulsatile flow is noted.
- An introducer sheath with dilator is then advanced over the guidewire (modified Seldinger technique) and into the vascular lumen.
- The guidewire and dilator are then removed together, leaving the sheath in place to allow for easy endovascular access for the remaining procedure, whether interventional or diagnostic.
- For purely diagnostic catheterizations a 4–5 French introducer sheath may suffice, but for most interventions a 6–7 F (or higher size) introducer sheath will likely be required.

Equipment List

1. 1–2% Lidocaine, 10–20 mL
2. 18–19 gauge Seldinger needle
3. 0.035 in. J-tip steel guidewire
4. #10 blade surgical scalpel
5. 4–6 French standard arterial sheath with tissue dilator
6. 21 gauge micropuncture needle with 0.018 in. guidewire and 5 French introducer sheath with tissue dilator, "Micropuncture Kit" (*possible*)
7. Doppler-guided SmartNeedle (Escalon Medical, New Berlin, WI) [*possible*]

Antegrade Femoral Artery Puncture

Clinical Pointers

- Antegrade femoral puncture is more difficult and often requires greater experience to develop the appropriate skill set for mastery.[6]
- In order to puncture the CFA in an antegrade fashion, the skin-puncture site of the needle is often much higher than would be anticipated.
- Generally, right-handed operators tend to have an easier time in obtaining antegrade access to the right CFA by standing on the left-hand side of the patient and vice versa.
- Prior to beginning a peripheral intervention, it is extremely useful to review any prior angiograms or CT angiograms available to plan vascular access accordingly and based on known anatomy.
- Ultrasound guidance may also be a useful adjunct for vascular access (see Sect. "Ultrasound Guidance for Vascular Access") in these cases.
- In patients with severely calcified peripheral arteries, fluoroscopy guidance may be useful in directing the needle toward the SFA, when obtaining antegrade access.

- After initial puncture of the CFA with the Seldinger needle, radiocontrast may be injected through the needle to delineate the femoral bifurcation anatomy. At this point, the position of the needle may also be angulated to direct the guidewire more easily down the SFA.

Tips of the Trade

- For complicated access techniques such as this, we advocate the use of a 21-gauge micropuncture needle and advancement of the 0.018 in. guidewire provided in the micropuncture kit into the superficial femoral artery prior to advancing the 5 F micropuncture sheath.
- If the guidewire preferentially advances into the profunda femoral artery (PFA) instead of the SFA, the operator can use an angulated dilator with an opening 4 cm proximal to the tip, which can then direct the wire preferentially toward to the SFA. If the wire tends to advance laterally then it is likely in the PFA instead of the SFA, which tends to run in a straight caudal fashion.
- Once the small sheath has been advanced successfully, the 0.018 in. wire can be exchanged for a stiffer wire and the sheath size can be sequentially increased with serial dilations.[7,8]
- In patients with high bifurcations of the CFA, antegrade puncture can be technically difficult. In these cases it might be necessary to selectively cannulate the SFA to avoid a high arterial puncture of the CFA, which can then result in uncontrolled bleeding following sheath removal.
- To facilitate puncture of the SFA the thigh can be abducted and externally rotated, which allows a

more mediolateral puncture site in the CFA, which will then allow for easier passage of the wire into the SFA. Additionally, this maneuver will also allow for easier puncture of the SFA in rare cases of extremely high bifurcation of the CFA.[9]

Potential Pitfalls

- When using a single-wall needle with a beveled leading point, complications can arise when advancing the guidewire after obtaining pulsatile blood return. If the long bevel is partially placed within the vessel wall itself, adequate pulsatile blood return will still occur, but the guidewire will be inadvertently advanced into the vessel wall creating a subinitmal dissection. Subinitmal dissection should be suspected whenever smooth, easy intraluminal passage of the wire is impaired. Fluoroscopy can be used to further define the difficulty in wire passage and dissection should be suspected if the wire can be seen "curling" or "hitting a stop" shortly after exiting the needle. If this occurs, then removal of the wire and needle will likely be required and a new puncture will need to be attempted. Additionally, the sharp needle point can peel off the wire's plastic or hydrophilic coating when advanced guidewire through the Seldinger needle, therefore it is advisable to use an uncoated steel guidewire for initial entry.
- Severe peripheral arterial disease may result in occlusion of the aorta or iliac vessels and may prevent access via the femoral arteries
- Femoral artery hematoma, retroperitoneal bleeding, arterio-venous fistula, and pseudoaneurysm formation

are all recognized complications of femoral artery puncture.

- The clinician should have a high level of suspicion for retroperitoneal bleeding whenever hypotension, recurrent vasovagal events, and/or low hematocrit are encountered following femoral artery puncture.

Radial Artery Access

Clinical Pointers

- Radial artery access is associated with lower rates of bleeding complications, post-procedural blood transfusions, and vascular access site complications than femoral artery access.[10]
- However, the radial artery is smaller in caliber and can be tortuous, thereby limiting the size of sheaths used for interventions.[11]
- Prior to performing radial artery cannulation, the modified Allen or Barbeau test is performed to assess the adequacy of dual blood supply to the hand. A plethysmograph is placed on the patient's thumb on the side of the planned procedure. The radial artery is occluded and the presence of a waveform in the thumb confirms patency of the ulnar artery and the palmar arch vessels.
- Contraindications to this technique include severe radial artery spasm, small caliber vessels, anatomical anomalies, the requirement of large caliber sheaths, and inadequate collateral filling of the hand, such as an interrupted palmar arch (Barbeau type D – See Fig. 1.2).[12]
- Despite the large number of transradial procedures done worldwide, there have been few reports of hand ischemia resulting from radial artery occlusion,

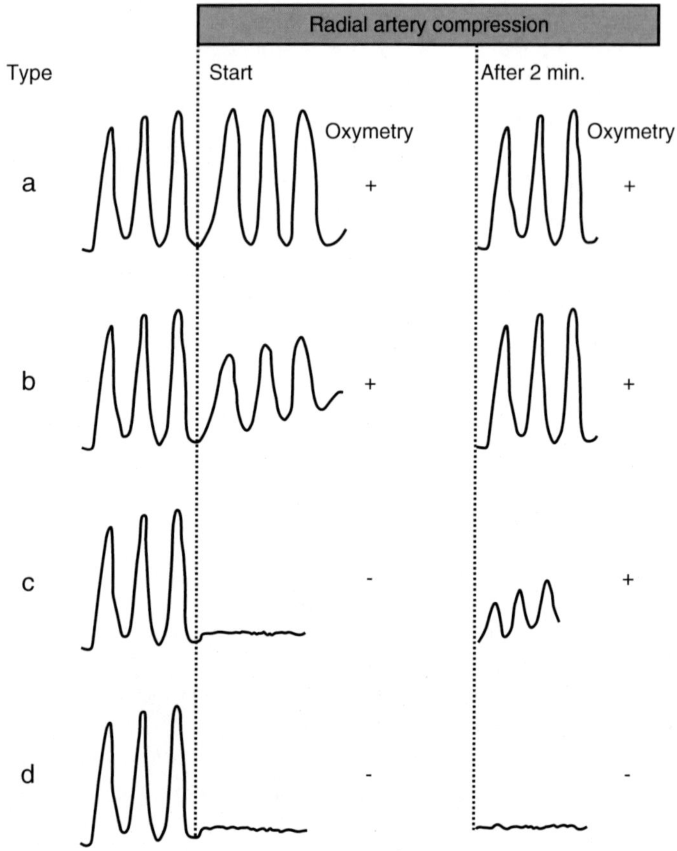

FIGURE 1.2 Barbeau classification. Schematic representation of the four types of ulnopalmar arch patency findings with plethysmography/oximetry. This is performed by placing the O_2 saturation monitor on the patients thumb and then simultaneously occluding both the radial and ulnar artery to ensure there is a loss of the pulse oximetry waveform. The ulnar artery is then released and the pulse oximeter is monitored to determine the amount of time required to regain a waveform (Reprinted with permission from *American Heart Journal*[12])

leading some to suggest that pre-procedure Allen or plethysmographic testing is not required.[13]

- Most operators would advocate refraining from transradial access in patients without evidence of dual blood supply to the hand unless there are compelling reasons to avoid femoral access.[14]

Tips of the Trade

- After securing placement of the introducer sheath in the radial artery, a solution of nitroglycerin and a calcium channel blocker (verapamil or nicardipine) is injected through the sheath to prevent spasm of the artery.
- Heparin reduces the risk of arterial occlusion after the procedure.
- Hydrophilic sheaths (e.g., Terumo Glidesheath) reduce the occurrence of radial artery spasm. Caution should be used if hydrophilic-*coated* sheaths (Cook brand) are being used, as they can result in a foreign body granulomatous reaction that is uncomfortable and unsightly.
- The arterial sheath can be removed immediately after the case is completed. A specially-made tourniquet, such as the Hemoband (TZ Medical), Radistop (Radi Medical Systems), or the Radstat (Wake Heart Associates), is applied at the radial puncture site for at least 30 min and the pressure in the tourniquet is then gradually released.
- After the pressure is completely released and hemostasis is achieved, a pressure bandage is applied to the site and the patient is instructed to restrict movement of the wrist for 6 h and to avoid lifting more than 5 lb for a week.

How We Do It

- The authors are comfortable performing this procedure on patients who rely upon their hands for professional purposes, given the low rate of ischemic complications associated with this procedure (see above), as long as the patient is able to follow the requisite limitations of hand usage following the procedure or unless there is a compelling reason to perform the procedure via transfemoral access.
- The arm is placed as close to the side of the body as possible on an arm-board and the wrist is hyperextended with a rolled gauze or small towel to facilitate arterial access. See Fig. 1.3.
- The site is anesthetized locally with 3–5 mL of 1–2% lidocaine and the artery is cannulated 2–3 cm proximal to the proximal palmar flexion crease of the wrist to avoid the flexor retinaculum and smaller superficial branches (which are present more distally). The styloid process of the radius is a palpable landmark that correlates with the proximal palmar flexion crease.
- A 4 cm 21-gauge micropuncture needle is used to puncture the radial artery at a 45° angle.
- Once pulsatile blood flow is noted, a 30–50 cm floppy-tip 0.018–0.025 in. straight or angled guidewire is inserted and advanced into the radial artery. We recommend fluoroscopic guidance of the passage of these micropuncture wires, as they can engage small vessels and easily perforate them. The guidewire should be advanced across the elbow to the brachial artery, so that recurrent radial loops can be detected at this early point in the case.
- We recommend using hydrophilic sheaths that taper onto the micropuncture wire (e.g., Terummo Glidesheath). After successful passage of the wire beyond the brachial artery, a 5 or 6 French hydrophilic sheaths can be advanced into the radial artery.
- After placement of the radial sheath, the authors will generally administer a combination of 200 mcg of intra-arterial nitroglycerin, 2.5–5 mg of intra-arterial verapamil, and 50–70 units/kg of intravenous heparin. If the patient is already bradycardic, then an equivalent dose of nicardipine can be substituted for verapamil.

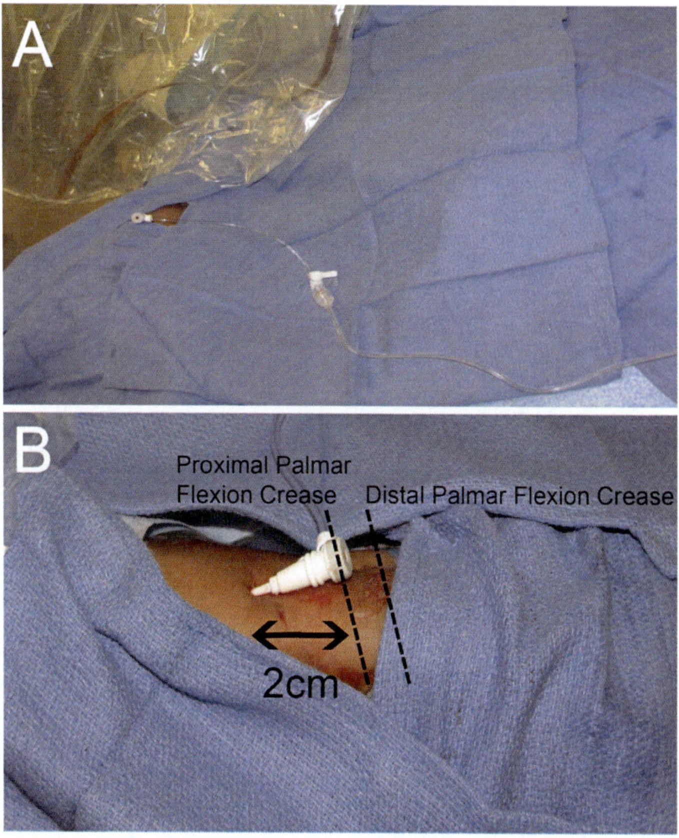

FIGURE 1.3 Radial artery access. The patients are prepared and draped with the right arm by their side on an arm board (**a**). The wrist is extended and taped to the arm board. The sheath is inserted into the radial artery 2 cm proximal to the proximal palmar flexion crease (**b**). Normally, the radial artery is relatively straight and is 2.0–2.5 mm in diameter (**c**). After the procedure, hemostasis is achieved at the radial arteriotomy with a compression device (**d**). Care must be taken not to compress the ulnar artery as well, or ischemia will develop in the hand. Continuous monitoring of plethysmography of the thumb is recommended during radial artery compression

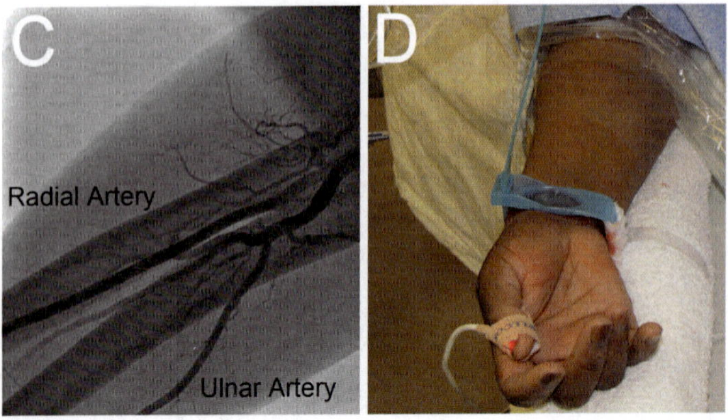

FIGURE 1.3 (continued)

Potential Pitfalls

- Radial artery occlusion occurs in approximately 4–10% of cases; this is virtually always asymptomatic and incidents of hand ischemia are exceedingly rare. The risk can be reduced by using smaller diameter sheaths and larger doses of heparin.
- Branches of the radial artery are easy to perforate, therefore 0.018 in. wires should always be advanced gently under fluoroscopic guidance.
- Anatomical anomalies, such as recurrent radial loop, recurrent brachial loop, severe tortuosity, and accessory radial arteries can prevent easy passage or wires and catheters in up to 5% of cases.
- Radial artery spasm is a complication best avoided. Once it occurs, it can be overcome with local administration of vasodilators, down-sizing the catheter, analgesia, and sedation. Sometimes alternate access is required.

Brachial Artery Access

Background

The brachial artery is generally superficial and fixed at (or directly above) the level of the antecubital fossa, therefore this is the preferred site of access when cannulating the brachial artery.[15] At this level, the artery can also be compressed against the humerus after sheath removal to provide adequate hemostasis. The authors no longer perform brachial artery cut-down (Sones technique).

The brachial artery is one of the preferred routes of access for performing complex peripheral vascular interventions of the downward sloping visceral and renal arteries and should be able to be utilized effectively by operators performing peripheral vascular interventions.

Clinical Pointers

- The method of obtaining access using the modified Seldinger technique is similar to that of femoral arterial access.
- 5–7 French sheaths are generally used for diagnostic or interventional angiography via this mode of vascular access.
- Pseudoaneurysm or large hematoma formation is unusual when using this mode of vascular access, however ecchymoses are frequently noted.

How We Do It

- After appropriate local anesthetic with 5–10 mL of 1–2% lidocaine is applied to the antecubital fossa, a micropuncture needle is used to cannulate the artery at a 30–45° angle.
- A micropuncture wire (0.018 in.) is advanced and a dilator inserted over it. A 0.035 in. guidewire is then passed into the brachial artery and advanced into the subclavian artery for support.

- The dilator is then removed over the wire while pressure is applied proximal to the entry point of the needle to prevent excess bleeding.
- An introducer sheath with dilator is then advanced into the vessel over the wire. After securing the sheath in place, the dilator and wire are removed together. The introducer sheath is then secured to the skin with sutures.
- Alternatively, a sheath with the dilator tapered onto the 0.018 in. wire can be used, similar to radial artery access.

Potential Pitfalls

- Care should be taken with the needle to avoid the bicipital aponeurosis, which is formed from fibers extending medially from the distal insertion of the biceps tendon passing obliquely to the ulnar side of the forearm across the hollow of the elbow, as this can be painful for the patient.
- Prolonged manual pressure should be used to obtain hemostasis because of the risk of hematoma formation at this site due to inadvertent bending of the elbow.

Popliteal Artery Access

Clinical Pointers

- Retrograde puncture of the popliteal artery is an infrequently employed, but useful alternative for treating ipsilateral iliofemoral lesions that are too close to employ CFA access or to treat complete SFA occlusions in a retrograde manner.
- In addition, chronic total occlusions (CTO) of the SFA may be easier to approach in a retrograde fashion via the popliteal artery, as there is theoretically softer plaque found at the distal end of a CTO.

- Requirements for this type of access include absence of obesity or a large lower extremity, and a reasonably sized popliteal vessel (greater than 4 mm).

How We Do It

- The patient is initially laid supine and retrograde femoral arterial access is obtained and a 5-French sheath is placed under modified Seldinger technique and sutured into place.
- Radiocontrast is then injected through the sideport of the femoral arterial sheath in order to visualize the popliteal artery, which is then centered under fluoroscopy.
- The popliteal artery is then punctured using fluoroscopic guidance and a 4- to 7-French sheath (pending on which intervention is to be performed) is then placed in the popliteal artery using modified Seldinger technique.
- Given the technical difficulty of this procedure, Micropuncture technique (described previously in this chapter) is frequently employed by the operator.

Vascular Grafts

Clinical Pointers

- Percutaneous puncture of synthetic grafts older than 6 months may be performed for vascular access.
- The operator should note that passage through the synthetic tissue may be difficult when inserting the sheath due to the nature of the graft material.
- Puncture of vascular grafts can be technically difficult and may result in uncontrollable bleeding due to the non-vascular nature of the graft, may cause disruption of the anastomotic suture lines in the graft, in addition to the risk of developing thromboembolism or graft infection.
- To avoid puncture of the anastamosis, it is best to puncture at the proximal end of the inguinal incision or as close to the inguinal ligament as possible.

- The angle of needle entry should still be 30–45° to the long axis of the graft, but serial dilations with successively larger tissue dilators may be required prior to sheath insertion.
- If the native artery is inadvertently punctured the operator will find that the guidewire may not advance, as the native artery may be occluded. The bypass graft will likely be lateral to the native vessel and will have a stronger pulsation than the native vessel.[9,13]
- Some operators consider low level anti-coagulation with unfractionated heparin (2,000–3,000 units) after obtaining vascular graft access

How We Do It

- We routinely use ultrasound guidance to determine the optimal site of entry.
- Cannulation of the bypass graft is performed in similar fashion to the technique described earlier for femoral arterial access; however a stiff wire (e.g., Amplatz Superstiff) can be passed through the needle to provide more support when advancing the sheath through the synthetic graft material.

Venous Access

Femoral Vein Puncture

Clinical Pointers

- The femoral veins are large caliber veins through which large guide catheters can be advanced.
- If the ipsilateral femoral artery and vein are to be accessed, then it is preferable to first cannulate the femoral vein followed by the femoral artery.
- After the femoral vein is cannulated first, the J-wire is usually left in place in the femoral vein for 1–2 min while arterial access is obtained in order to avoid

distortion of the femoral artery by placement of a large sheath in the femoral vein.

- After arterial access is obtained, the venous sheath with tissue dilator is then advanced over the J-wire and then the J-wire and dilator are removed simultaneously.
- In cases where the CFA cannot easily be palpated due to significant peripheral vascular disease, micropuncture technique should be used to cannulate the femoral vein. If the SFA or Profunda femoral arteries are inadvertently cannulated, then the micropuncture needle may be withdrawn and pressure can be held over the arterial puncture site for 5–10 min with appropriate hemostasis and minimal complications.
- Ultrasound guidance can also be used effectively as an adjunct to obtaining femoral venous access in patients with poor peripheral pulses or bypass grafts (see Sect. "Ultrasound Guidance for Vascular Access").
- Fluoroscopy can also be used to guide femoral venous access. The femoral vein usually traverses the outer medial border of the mid-femoral head.

How We Do It

- In order to cannulate the femoral vein, topical anesthetic with 10–20 mL of 1–2% lidocaine is first applied in the same fashion as when obtaining arterial access.
- When obtaining venous and arterial access, more lidocaine will be required to appropriately anesthetize both the venous and arterial access points.
- When puncturing the femoral vein, we advocate the use of a 5 cm^3. "slip-tip" syringe partially filled with normal saline attached to an 18–19 gauge Seldinger needle. See Fig. 1.4.
- The common femoral artery at the medial third of the femoral head is palpated with the left hand and, with the right hand, the Seldinger needle is inserted 1–3 cm medial and inferior to the arterial pulsation at a 45° angle, while applying gentle suction with the syringe in order to obtain venous blood return.

- When dark red blood indicative of venous blood return is noted in the syringe, the needle is stabilized with the left hand and the syringe is removed with the right. Non-pulsatile, dark red blood return should be noted from the needle hub after removal of the syringe.
- A 0.035 in. J wire is then advanced through the Seldinger needle, and small nick at the needle entry point is made with a 10-blade scalpel.

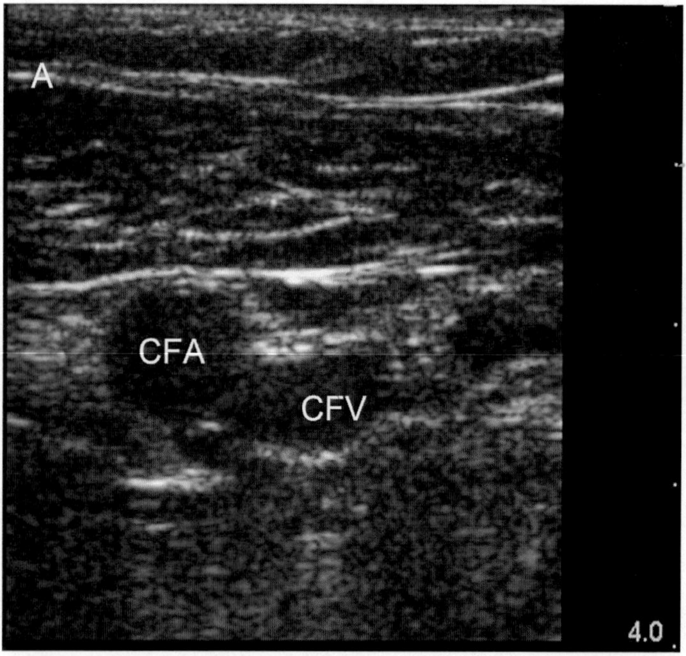

FIGURE 1.4 Femoral vein access. Ultrasound demonstrates that the common femoral vein (*CFV*) lies deep and medial to the common femoral artery (*CFA*) in most patients (**a**), but sometimes the vein may lie directly underneath the artery. Whilst palpating the artery with the left hand and maintaining gentle suction on the syringe with the right hand (**b**), the physician inserts the needle into the common femoral vein 1–3 cm inferior and medial to the common femoral artery (**c**)

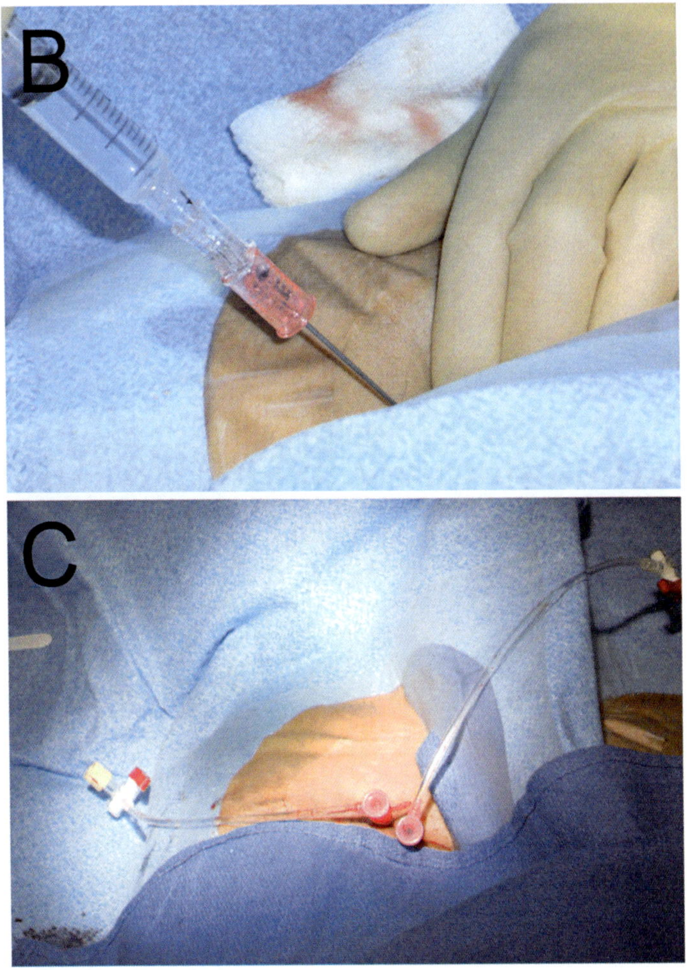

FIGURE 1.4 (continued)

- The needle is subsequently withdrawn over the wire, and a 6–7 French sheath with tissue dilator is advanced over the wire.
- The wire and tissue dilator are then removed together and the venous sheath remains in place.

Potential Pitfalls

- The femoral veins lie medial and deep to the femoral artery. Sometimes, the femoral vein lies directly behind the femoral artery during parts of its course. If the femoral vein is not easily accessed, we recommend ultrasound guidance to determine the relationship of the femoral artery to the femoral vein.
- The left iliac vein is sometimes compressed at the level of the pelvic brim by the right common iliac artery; this is known as May-Thurner syndrome. It results from the high-pressure, often calcified, right iliac artery as it arises from the aorta and crosses from the left to the right causing external compression of the lower-pressure left iliac vein as it approaches the inferior vena cava crossing from left to right. If difficulty is encountered passing a J-wire from the left iliac vein, venography should be performed. If compression of the left iliac vein is found, an alternate access site may be used, or the vein may be stented.

Internal Jugular Vein Access

Background

The internal jugular vein (IJ) lies superficial and lateral to the carotid artery and medial to the external jugular vein. The best point of access to the IJ is high in the anterior triangle toward the apex, in order to avoid puncturing the lung apices and causing a pneumothorax. The anterior triangle is formed by the two heads of the sternocleidomastoid muscle (SCM), medial and lateral, and the clavicle, which forms the base. The apex of the triangle is where the two heads of the SCM meet. The IJ usually courses just lateral to the outer edge of the medial head of the SCM.

Clinical Pointers

- In obese patients, the borders of the anterior triangle may be difficult to define. In these cases, a finger can be placed in the suprasternal recess and then moved laterally. As the finger is moved laterally the first elevation palpated will be the medial head of the SCM. Ultrasound can also help in this situation.
- Patients with low venous pressures may be placed in Trendelenburg position, or simply have their legs elevated, to facilitate venous blood return as the needle is advanced into the IJ.
- If the carotid artery is inadvertently punctured then the needle should be removed and pressure should be applied to the site for 10–15 min to achieve adequate hemostasis before another attempt is made. If a sheath is inadvertently placed in the carotid artery, consultation with vascular surgery should be made prior to removing the sheath. Surgical removal in the OR is probably the safest way to remove a large sheath from the carotid artery.
- Due to the inability to apply adequate manual pressure to the carotid artery in some patients because of a strong vagal response, we advocate the use of micropuncture technique to limit the size of the arteriotomy should the carotid artery be inadvertently punctured.

How We Do It

- The patient is asked to lie flat without the use of a pillow in order to better define the borders of the anterior triangle. See Fig. 1.5.
- The patient's head is then turned 30° away from the side of access (if performing a right IJ cannulation the patient should be asked to turn his head to the left.)
- Topical anesthetic is then applied in the form of 4–5% lidocaine over the desired IJ access site in advance. During the procedure, subcutaneous 1–2% lidocaine 5–10 mL is used.

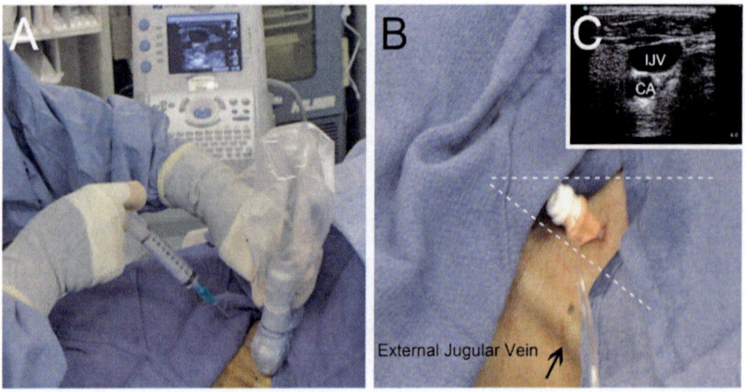

FIGURE 1.5 Jugular vein access. We routinely use real-time ultrasound guidance to locate the jugular vein (**a**). The sheath should be inserted through the apical portion of the triangle bounded by the medial and lateral heads of sternomastoid and the clavicle. In (**b**), the dotted lines indicate the heads of sternomastoid. Note the close proximity of the internal jugular vein (*IJV*) to the carotid artery (*CA*), which usually lies medial and deep to the vein (**c**)

- A 5 cm^3 syringe filled with normal saline is attached to the needle.
- We now routinely use real-time ultrasound-guidance and a micropuncture kit to cannulate the IJ. Because of the proximity of the carotid artery to the IJ, ultrasound reduces the risk of accidental carotid artery puncture, or puncturing too low in the anterior triangle which would increase the risk of developing a pneumothorax.
- With the right hand, the IJ is cannulated by advancing the needle at a 30–45° angle lateral and caudally, with the needle pointed toward the ipsilateral nipple, high in the anterior triangle while applying gentle suction on the syringe.
- When non-pulsatile, dark red blood return is noted, the left hand is used to stabilize the needle and the right hand is used to remove the syringe in order to confirm the return of low-pressure venous blood return.
- If using a micropuncture kit, the wire should be advanced under fluoroscopic guidance; this is not usually required for 0.035-in. J wires.

- The needle is then removed over the wire and a 6–7 French sheath with tissue dilator is then advanced over the wire.
- After securing the sheath in place, the J wire and tissue dilator are then removed simultaneously.

Subclavian and Upper Extremity Veins

Clinical Pointers

- Because subclavian venous punctures tend to carry a higher risk of pneumothorax and inadvertent arterial puncture, and due to the difficulty in compressing the subclavian vein to avoid hematoma formation, ultrasound-guided axillary vein puncture has gained wider favor.
- In addition, when performing a subclavian vein puncture on the left side, it is important to note that the thoracic duct drains into the subclavian vein at usual site of puncture and inadvertent injury to this vessel may cause a chylothorax.
- The axillary vein courses approximately 3–4 cm below the coracoid process and just lateral to the lateral border of the pectoralis minor.
- When puncturing the axillary vein, the needle is aimed toward the junction of the lateral and middle third of the clavicle. The insertion of a 6-French catheter is performed in the same Seldinger technique as that described above for the insertion of an IJ venous catheter.
- The cephalic vein is the major tributary into the axillary vein and can be imaged on ultrasound, as well.

How We Do It

- When performing subclavian venous puncture it is advisable to position the patient in 10–15° Trendelenburg to reduce the risk of air embolus.
- To identify landmarks, a finger can be inserted into the subclavian groove and passed medially until resistance is felt, which will be the lateral edge of the subclavius muscle.

- After appropriate application of topical anesthetic with 1–2% lidocaine, an 18–19 gauge Seldinger needle with a 5 cm^3 syringe filled with normal saline attached to the hub is inserted at this point, which should also correspond to the junction of the medial and middle third of the clavicle.
- The needle will be inserted infraclavicularly at this point with the leading edge aimed toward the sternoclavicular joint and the suprasternal notch, while maintaining suction on the syringe.
- Once adequate venous blood return is noted, the needle is stabilized with one hand and the syringe is removed with the other.
- A 0.035 or 0.025 in. guidewire is then advanced through the needle to secure access to the subclavian vein. The needle is then removed while maintaining gentle pressure at the skin surface to avoid excess blood loss, and a 6-French sheath with tissue dilator is advanced over the wire and secured in place. The tissue dilator and guidewire are then removed simultaneously.
- Upper limb venous access can be achieved with a standard 20 gauge IV cannula. After the tourniquet is removed, a micropuncture wire (0.018 in.) can be advanced via the IV cannula under sterile conditions using fluoroscopic guidance. The cannula is then removed and a sheath is inserted over the wire. We prefer a tapered introducer (e.g., Terumo Glidesheath) to facilitate atraumatic entry. A 5–7 French sheath can be used in most patients.

Potential Pitfalls

- Subclavian vein access is associated with increased risk of pneumothorax, accidental arterial puncture, and blood loss due to inability to compress the vein. We rarely use this site now, preferring the internal jugular vein.

- Upper extremity venous access should be used for procedures only, not for longer-term access due to movement of centrally placed catheters when the arm is moved.
- Venous spasm is a problem in the peripheral venous system in approximately 5–10% of patients. It can sometimes be overcome with vasodilators.

Ultrasound Guidance for Vascular Access

- The increased availability and reduced cost of portable ultrasound machines has led to their widespread use.
- Many operators advocate the use of ultrasound-guidance when obtaining venous access, particularly with IJ cannulation.
- Knowledge of arterial and venous anatomy is the key to successful vascular access. Ultrasound is only as good as the operator's anatomic knowledge.

How We Do It

- As with all sterile procedures, the gel is applied to the surface of the ultrasound probe, which is then placed into a sterile sleeve. Sterile ultrasound gel is then applied to the skin surface of the patient as well and gray-scale 2D imaging can be performed.
- For IJ cannulation, the probe is placed high in the anterior triangle and the vessels are imaged in short axis. The carotid artery will appear thick-walled, pulsatile, and noncompressible, while the IJ will appear thin walled, nonpulsatile, and entirely compressible.
- The vessels can be imaged in real-time as the needle is advanced to ensure correct trajectory toward the IJ and not the carotid artery. Once the IJ has been punctured and venous blood return is confirmed, the probe can be removed.
- When accessing the femoral artery, ultrasound guidance can be very helpful. We scan up the common femoral artery

until the vessel "dives into the pelvis," and then down until the bifurcation into the profunda femoris and superficial femoral arteries is seen. This delineates the common femoral artery. We choose a point away from branches and free of significant atherosclerosis to puncture.

Bibliography

1. Hessel SJ, Adams DS, Avrams HL: Complications of angiography. *Radiology* 1981; 138:273–281
2. Illescas FF, Baker ME, McCann, et al: CT evaluation of retroperitoneal hemorrhage associated with femoral arteriography. *AJR* 1996;146:1289–1292.
   → *This was a case series of six patients that examined the factors that predispose to bleeding complications during femoral arterial puncture and provides clues and techniques to diagnose retroperitoneal hematomas rapidly.*
3. Altin RS, Flicker S, Naidech HJ: Pseudoaneurysm and arteriovenous fistula after femoral artery catheterization: Association with lower femoral punctures. *AJR* 1989; 152:629–631.
   → *This retrospective study included 11 patients who had undergone cardiac catheterization with subsequent development of a pseudoaneurysm or AVF and through femoral arteriography it was determined that the overwhelming majority of these complications resulted when the site of the femoral artery puncture was below the level of the femoral head.*
4. Grier D, Hartnell G. Percutaneous femoral artery puncture: Practice and Anatomy. *Br J Radiol* 1990; 63:602–604.
   → *This paper compared operator preference for femoral arterial puncture (inguinal crease vs. maximal femoral pulse vs. fluoroscopy guided) and found that the most accurate predictor of CFA puncture was use of the maximal femoral pulse to guide the arterial puncture.*
5. Rupp SB, Vegelzang RI, Nemcek AA, et al: Relationship of the inguinal ligament to pelvic radiographic landmarks: Anatomic correlation and its role in femoral arteriography. *JVIR* 1993;4:409–413.
   → *This was a case series of ten cadavers that underwent radiographic and manual determination of the inguinal ligament, followed by dissection and inspection of the gross*

anatomical specimen to determine accuracy, with results showing that the midportion of the femoral head will most often provide the best anatomical landmark for puncture of the CFA.

6. Criado FJ, Twena M, Halsted M, Abul-Khoudoud, O: Percutaneous femoral puncture for endovascular treatment of arterial occlusive lesions. *Am J Surg* 1998;176:119–121.
7. Khoury M, Batra S, Berg R, et al. Influence of arterial access sites and interventional procedures on vascular complications after cardiac catheterizations. *Am J Surg* 1992;164(3):205–209.
8. Kiemeneij F, Laarman GJ, Odekerken D, et al. A randomized comparison of percutaneous transluminal coronary angioplasty by the radial, brachial and femoral approaches: the access study. *J Am Coll Cardiol* 1997;29(6):1269–1275.
   → *This was a randomized comparison between transradial, transbrachial, and transfemoral approaches to PTCA with primary endpoints being access site difficulty (requiring the need for an alternative access site) and access-site complications, which found that vascular complications were significantly more frequent after transbrachial and transfemoral approaches.*
9. Grossman M: How to miss the profunda femoris. *Radiology* 125:379–382, 1977.
10. Agostoni P, Biondi-Zoccai GG, de Benedictis ML *et al.* Radial versus femoral approach for percutaneous coronary diagnostic and interventional procedures; Systematic overview and meta-analysis of randomized trials. *J Am Coll Cardiol* 2004; 44(2): 349–56.
   → *This is a meta-analysis of 12 randomized trials examining procedural complications related to transradial vs. transfemoral approaches for vascular access and demonstrates significant decrease in local vascular complications with transradial vascular access.*
11. Kiemeneij F, Fraser D, Slagboom T, Laarman G, van der Wieken R. Hydrophilic coating aids radial sheath withdrawal and reduces patient discomfort following transradial coronary intervention: a randomized doubleblind comparison of coated and uncoated sheaths. *Catheter Cardiovasc Interv* 2003; 59(2): 161–4.
   → *This is a double-blind randomized comparison of hydrophilic-coated or uncoated sheaths in preventing radial artery spasm following transradial access, but also demonstrates that use of a vasodilator cocktail after sheath placement reduces the incidence of radial artery spasm.*

12. Barbeau GR, Arsenault F, Dugas L, Simard S, Lariviere MM. Evaluation of the ulnopalmar arterial arches with pulse oximetry and plethysmography: Comparison with the Allen's test in 1010 patients. *Am Heart J* 2004; 147:489–93.
13. Ghuran A, Dixon G, Holmberg S, et al. Transradial coronary intervention without prescreening for a dual palmar blood supply. Int J Cardiol 2007;121:320–322.
14. Rhyne D and Mann, T. Hand ischemia resulting from a transradial intervention: Successful management with radial artery angioplasty. *Cath and Cardiovasc Interv* 2010;76:383–386.
    → *This is a case report describing a patient who developed radial occlusion leading to hand ischemia following transradial access despite having a pre-procedural plethysmograph showing dual blood supply.*
15. Kamada RO, Fergusson DJ, Itagaki RK. Percutaneous entry of the brachial artery for transluminal coronary angioplasty. *Cathet Cardiovasc Diagn* 1988;15:132–133.

Chapter 2
Access Site Hemostasis

Jeffrey Zimmet

To Close or Not to Close?

The majority of arterial access procedures use the femoral route, with its attendant risks and lengthy periods of immobility. The traditional method for closure is manual compression, either with pressure through the operator's hands or with an external compression device. Multiple vascular closure devices (VCDs) have been developed over the years with the idea of speeding the process of hemostasis and potentially reducing the incidence of vascular complications, which can include hematoma, pseudoaneurysm, AV fistula, retroperitoneal hematoma, need for surgical repair, and infection. VCDs have been successful on multiple fronts, most notably in shortening the time needed to achieve hemostasis and the time to ambulation, and thus can significantly impact patient comfort. The ability to close the access site at the end of a procedure means not only that the patient spends a shorter period of time laying supine, but also that fewer human resources need to be expended in caring for

J. Zimmet
Interventional Cardiology Division, Department of Medicine,
University of California – San Francisco and VA Medical Center,
San Francisco, CA, USA
e-mail: jeffrey.zimmet@va.gov

C.D. Owens and Y. Yeghiazarians (eds.),
Handbook of Endovascular Peripheral Interventions,
DOI 10.1007/978-1-4614-0839-0_2,

patients with arterial sheaths, in manually pulling those sheaths, and in subsequent recovery. The data on complications of these devices when compared with manual compression is mixed and is difficult to interpret. For the most part, VCDs seem to have a comparable safety profile to manual compression, with some notable exceptions (e.g., the Vasoseal device, which appeared in some studies to have an increased rate of complications and has since been removed from the market). This is based on registry data, small studies, and meta-analyses, all of which have significant flaws. At least one large registry, as well as data from the ACUITY trial, has suggested that VCDs actually lower the risk of bleeding. In the end, the decision to use or not use VCDs must be made by each operator based on their own experience and institutional resources, and on the needs and vascular anatomy of each particular patient.

The following is the recommendations of the American Heart Association regarding the use of arteriotomy closure devices (AHA 2010) (see references):

1. Patients considered for deployment of arteriotomy closure devices at the femoral artery site should undergo a femoral angiogram with identification of sheath insertion site and other features (atherosclerosis, calcification, etc.) to ensure anatomical suitability for their use (Class I – Level of Evidence C).
2. Facilities with standard manual compression regimens should aim to achieve the reported low vascular complication rates (<1%), in patients undergoing uncomplicated 5 Fr diagnostic angiography (Class I – Level of Evidence C).
3. Use of arteriotomy closure devices is reasonable following invasive cardiovascular procedures performed via the femoral artery to achieve faster hemostasis, shorter duration of bed rest, and possibly improved patient comfort. The use of these devices should be weighed against the risk of increased complications in certain patient subsets and also take into account body habitus, location of arteriotomy, size and condition of the parent vessel, sheath size, and presence or absence of systemic disease in the patient

(Class IIa – Level of Evidence B). This recommendation is based on a meta-analysis and several small scale trials. However, in these studies there are trends toward higher rates of complications.

4. Arteriotomy closure devices should not be used routinely for the specific purpose of reducing vascular complications in patients undergoing invasive cardiovascular procedures via the femoral artery approach (Class III, Level of Evidence B). This recommendation is based on the aggregate of three meta-analyses, registry data, and moderate-size randomized controlled trials of suboptimal quality. It should be noted that there is significant heterogeneity among the reported effects of the different devices deployed. The writing committee did not feel there was sufficient evidence to warrant a separate recommendation at this time for specific arteriotomy closure devices, or active versus passive closure devices.
5. Complications encountered during or following deployment of arteriotomy closure devices should be collected systematically either as part of local quality efforts or national registries (such as the ACC-NCDR) and systematically reported to the FDA (Class I – Level of Evidence C).

Manual Compression

Manual compression has long been the gold standard for obtaining access site hemostasis. Although compression is straightforward and simple, success requires good preparation and technique.

Preparation

- Have a sphygmomanometer attached to the patient, and take a blood pressure directly prior to sheath removal. In the case of a single operator, set an automatic monitor to take the blood pressure every 2–4 min and make certain that someone is immediately available to assist in case of problems.
- Make sure there is a working peripheral IV, with isotonic fluid (e.g., NS or RL) attached and ready to go if needed.

- Have atropine ready in case of vasovagal episode.
- Although usually not necessary, re-instillation of lidocaine may be useful in case the sheath has been indwelling for a prolonged period.
- Assess the peripheral pulses and examine the access site for hematoma prior to sheath removal.
- Position the patient near to the side of the bed. Set the bed at an appropriate height, such that the operator can extend the arms fully and use upper body weight to apply pressure.

Technique

- For a right femoral sheath, place the middle three fingers of the hand such that pressure will be exerted proximally from the sheath site. Remember that the arteriotomy will in most cases be 2–3 cm proximal to the skin entry site.
- If both arterial and venous sheaths were used, remove the arterial sheath first and confirm good hemostasis before proceeding. We generally remove the venous sheath once only 5–10 min are remaining for the arterial site (see below for appropriate "hold times"), and complete the hold with pressure over both sites.
- Remove the sheath slowly at the same angle at which it was inserted.
- Apply firm pressure over the arteriotomy site once the sheath has been removed. Initial pressure should be occlusive, but should be decreased gradually after the first 5 min such that distal pulses can be felt.

What Is the Target ACT for Sheath Removal?

We generally wait until the ACT has fallen below 170 s before removing the sheaths. Recognize, however, that there is little objective evidence supporting the traditional thresholds of 150–180 s. In fact, several recent trials have removed sheaths using a much higher ACT threshold of <250 s, reportedly without a significant increase in bleeding complications. For patients with normal to moderately reduced renal function anticoagulated with bivalirudin, arterial sheaths can be removed safely 2 h after discontinuation of the medication, without checking the ACT. For patients given bivalirudin with severe renal dysfunction or who are on hemodialysis, we use an ACT threshold of 170 s to guide manual sheath removal.

How Long Do I Need to Hold Pressure?

The easy answer is to hold until hemostasis is attained. Protocols will differ from institution to institution. A good starting place is to hold pressure for approximately 3 min per French size – that is, 15 min for a 5-Fr sheath, 18 min for a 6-Fr sheath, and so on.

How Long Should the Patient Be Immobile After Sheath Removal?

This is another area where very little data exists. Many labs including ours routinely keep patients in bed for 1 h per sheath French size. For example, patients are kept supine for 6 h following removal of a 6-Fr sheath. Raising the head of the bed up to 30° after the first 1–2 h improves patient comfort without appreciably increasing the risk of bleeding.

When Can Anti-coagulation Be Restarted After Sheath Removal?

Anti-coagulation following femoral access site hemostasis is a tricky subject. Of course, coumadin may be restarted immediately after a procedure, since it will not take effect for several days. However, heparin and low molecular weight heparins given soon after femoral arterial sheath removal will significantly increase the risk of rebleeding and of the development of pseudoaneurysm. Just how soon heparin may be restarted is a matter of clinical judgment, balancing the indication for anticoagulation with the risk of bleeding. In our lab, we wait at least until the end of the bedrest period (6 h for a 6-Fr sheath) before starting heparin, and then do so without a bolus. Because it cannot be readily reversed, LMWH should be given cautiously.

What About Vascular Grafts?

In the PAD population, femoral access adjacent to or even through vascular grafts is sometimes necessary. Manual compression is the method of choice for sheath removal, and should be performed by an experienced operator. Although the technique is similar to that used with native femoral vessels, the risk of graft thrombosis from over-compression must be considered. The principle here is to achieve hemostasis at the site while maintaining flow down the graft by avoiding full occlusive compression. Because of the relatively fine control required, we tend to avoid mechanical devices such as the FemoStop and C-clamp in these patients. Initial holding times are similar to those used for native vessels, but can vary widely. Because of the increased risk of complications, we do not use any of the available arteriotomy closure devices with grafts.

Potential Pitfalls

Effective early control is essential. However, do not start with full pressure until the sheath is removed, so as to avoid stripping off any thrombi. Consider allowing blood to flow for one to two heartbeats to allow any thrombus to be flushed out before applying pressure.

Active Closure Devices

Angio-Seal

The Angio-Seal (St. Jude Medical, St. Paul, MN) device is currently the most widely used VCD, primarily because of its ease of use, short-learning curve, and high initial success rate. The device sandwiches the arteriotomy between a resorbable anchor inside the vessel and a collagen plug outside, with the two joined by a self-tightening suture. The device comes in separate 6 and 8 Fr sizes, and is currently manufactured in three configurations: the STS-Plus, the VIP, and the Evolution. The Evolution is the most recent iteration of the device, and improves on previous versions by including a self-tamping mechanism that standardizes the pressure used to deploy and tamp the collagen plug.

Technique

- Perform an angiogram to confirm that the vessel and sheath placement are suitable for the device. Specifically, the sheath must be in the common femoral artery with a vessel size ≥5 mm and less than 40% stenosis near the entry site. This device should not be used if entry point is at or below the femoral bifurcation, or at or above the inferior epigastric artery.
- Flush the procedure sheath, re-prep and drape the access site, and don new sterile gloves.
- Prepare the Angio-Seal sheath by inserting the arteriotomy locator (the green dilator) into the sheath, confirming that the two snap together firmly.
- Insert the included guidewire into the procedural sheath and remove the sheath, leaving the wire in place in the artery.
- Place the Angio-Seal sheath/arteriotomy locator onto the wire with the arrow on the sheath pointing upward, and advance the sheath into the artery until blood drips from the back of the locator. To avoid over-insertion into the artery, the manufacturer recommends withdrawing the

sheath until blood flow stops, and then slowly re-advancing it until blood again drips from the locator.

- Holding the sheath securely with one hand, remove the wire and locator by flexing the base of the arteriotomy locator upward and withdrawing both from the sheath.
- Pick up the Angio-Seal device by grasping it just behind the bypass tube, and insert it into the sheath with the reference indicator facing upward. Advance the device all the way into the sheath until you hear a click. Holding the sheath securely in place, grasp the handle of the device and gently pull back until you hear another click.
- Holding two fingers against the puncture site to provide support pull back on the device handle along the same angle as the sheath tract.
  - For the Evolution device, simply pull back until the green compaction marker is revealed. Then depress the Suture Release button and pull back until the suture is exposed, and cut the suture below the skin surface.
  - For the VIP device, pull back on the handle until the green compaction tube appears and the suture has stopped spooling. Keeping firm backward tension on the device, advance the compaction tube until resistance is felt and (in most cases) the black compaction marker is revealed. Cut the suture to remove the device, and then cut the suture again below the skin surface.

Advantages

- One of the easiest devices to learn and use.
- Has a very high initial success rate.
- The collagen plug in the tract also acts to reduce oozing from the site.
- The retained components of the device are completely resorbed over the course of weeks to months after insertion.

Disadvantages

- The intravascular anchor has the potential to further obstruct a heavily diseased vessel.
- Although extremely rare, embolization of the intravascular anchor is a possibility.

- Repeat access of the same vessel within 90 days of device deployment should be avoided using the same puncture site to avoid disrupting the plug; the manufacturer recommends puncture 1 cm proximal to the initial site. Depending on the location of the initial site, going 1 cm above is not always possible.
- As with all devices with retained components, this device is a potential nidus for infection. Cutting the suture below the skin surface is important for minimizing this risk.

How We Use It

The Angio-Seal is a dependable and easy-to-use device. We tend to employ it in suitably large and relatively disease-free common femoral arteries when the sheath is well clear of the femoral bifurcation and of significant branch vessels. We tend not to use it when we predict possible need for re-access within 3 months, for the reasons stated above.

Starclose

The Starclose (Fig. 2.1; Abbott Vascular, Menlo Park, CA) device employs a nitinol clip that grasps the outside of the vessel to appose the arteriotomy and achieve closure. It is therefore an active (rather than passive) closure device that leaves nothing inside the vessel. The Starclose is approved for closure of 5 and 6 Fr sheaths.

Technique (for the Starclose SE Platform)

- Perform an angiogram to confirm that the vessel and sheath placement are suitable for the device. The device requires a vessel size of 5 mm or greater to allow the vessel locator to be withdrawn to the arteriotomy.
- Make sure that the sheath has a dermotomy of 5–7 mm, and perform blunt dissection to ensure smooth delivery of the clip down to the artery. In our hands, an inadequate tract, leading to inability to fully advance the delivery tube, is the most common reason for device failure. To minimize oozing, consider making the incision and blunt dissection

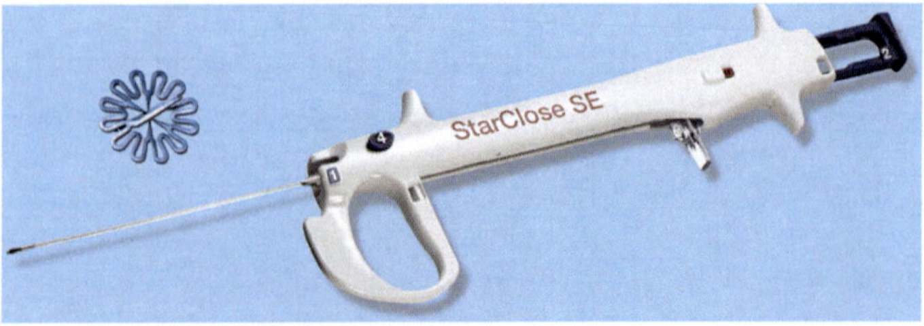

FIGURE 2.1 Starclose device

at the beginning of the procedure prior to the administration of anticoagulants.

- Flush the procedure sheath, re-prep and drape the access site, and don new sterile gloves.
- Using the supplied guidewire, exchange the procedural sheath for the Starclose sheath.
- Insert the tip of the Starclose device into the sheath and advance the device into the sheath, taking care not to bend the shaft of the device.
- Advance the device until it clicks securely in place in the hub of the sheath (labeled #1 on the device). This usually requires that the sheath be withdrawn slightly from the skin surface.
- Stabilize the device by holding it securely with the left hand by the Stabilizer finger loop. Retract the device 3–4 cm out of the tissue tract (be careful not to retract too far).
- Using the right hand, depress the plunger (labeled #2) fully until a click is heard and the number "2" is fully seen in the number window. This expands the locator wings within the artery and begins the splitting of the sheath, which can be seen above the skin surface.
- Gently retract the device with the right hand along the angle of sheath insertion until resistance is felt, indicating that the vessel locator wings are in contact with the inner surface of the arteriotomy. Again stabilize the finger loop with the left hand.

- Using the right hand, depress the thumb advancer (#3) all the way down, until a click is heard and the number "3" is seen completely within the number window.
- Raise the body of the device to a 70° angle.
- Apply gentle downward pressure on the device to seat the delivery tube against the artery.
- Using the thumb of the right hand, depress the deployment button (#4) until a click is heard. Maintain downward pressure on the device for another 3 s.
- With the left hand providing counter traction, remove the device and apply moderate pressure with the left hand.
- Although not always necessary, we generally apply several minutes of pressure to minimize oozing from the tract.

Advantages

- The Starclose device deploys on the outside of the artery, leaving nothing in the lumen.
- The external nature of the device means that it may be appropriate for use in situations in which other devices are unsuitable, including vessels with moderate disease at the access site or with the arteriotomy near the femoral bifurcation.
- Note that while the manufacturer advises against using the Starclose when the arteriotomy is below the femoral bifurcation, the device is being used in practice to close the SFA when the vessel is sufficiently large (>5 mm).
- Re-puncture through a deployed Starclose clip may in general be performed safely at any time. Note again that the manufacturer cautions that the safety of repeat puncture and closure has not been fully established, despite two successful bench studies in a porcine aorta model.

Disadvantages

- The ability to deliver the Starclose clip depends on having an adequate dermotomy and a patent tract to allow passage of the relatively bulky delivery system. This generally results in more post-closure oozing from the site compared with other devices.

- Although the device is deployed on the external surface of the artery, remember that the vessel locator portion of the device is inserted into the artery and is drawn back after deploying the wings until it reaches the arteriotomy. This has the potential to disrupt intravascular plaque, similar to other VCDs.
- The Starclose is designed for closure of 5 and 6 Fr arteriotomies only. Although closure of 7 Fr and even 8 Fr sheath sites has been reported, the risk of device failure with these larger sheaths is higher, as is the likelihood of hematoma formation during deployment due to leakage around the 6 Fr Starclose sheath.

How We Use It

The Starclose has become one of the workhorse VCDs in our lab for routine closure of 5 and 6 Fr sheaths. It allows secure closure of vessels that were previously un-closeable, including relatively diseased vessels and arteriotomies near the femoral bifurcation. We routinely re-puncture and re-close the same access site using this device.

Perclose

The Perclose (Abbott Vascular, Menlo Park, CA) is the prototype of the suture-based VCD, and has gone through several iterations since its inception. Since the first Perclose device was introduced in 1994, several advances have made the device simpler to use. The precursor of the currently available devices, the Closer, delivered polyester suture to the vessel. The knots were hand-tied and advanced to the arteriotomy to effect closure. In 2002, Abbott Vascular (which acquired the Perclose company in 1999) introduced the Perclose A-T (auto-tie), which greatly simplified the procedure through use of a pre-tied knot, allowing faster deployment with a single operator. Although the A-T is still available, most labs have adopted the more recent Proglide version (Fig. 2.2), which replaced the braided polyester suture

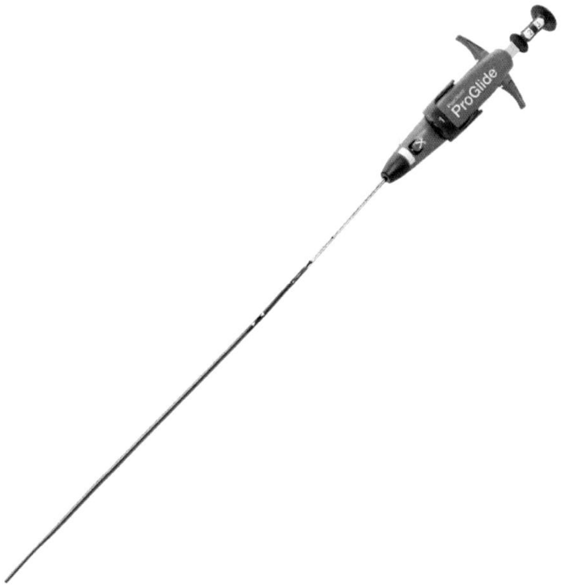

FIGURE 2.2 ProGlide device

with a polypropylene monofilament for easier knot advancement, and added a suture-cutting mechanism on the device. The Proglide is approved for closure with sheath sizes between 5 and 8 Fr.

Technique (for Closure at the End of a Procedure)

- Perform an angiogram to confirm that the vessel and sheath placement are suitable for the device. The Proglide requires a vessel size of >5 mm, and should not be used if the puncture site is at or below the femoral bifurcation.
- Flush the marker lumen of the device with saline to confirm lumen patency.
- Flush the procedural sheath, place a 0.035 or 0.038 in. guidewire into the artery, and remove the sheath. Note that the device does not come packaged with a guidewire. Any standard 0.035 or 0.038 in. guidewire can be used.

We generally clean and save the J wire used to deploy the sheath at the beginning of the case.

- Backload the Proglide device onto the guidewire, and advance it into the artery until the guidewire port reaches the skin surface. Remove the guidewire.
- Continue to advance the device into the artery until a continuous flow of blood is seen through the marker lumen.
- Deploy the foot process inside the vessel by lifting the level marked #1.
- Gently retract the device until resistance is felt, positioning the foot process against the inside of the vessel wall. Blood flow through the marker lumen should be reduced or stopped altogether.
- Push firmly on the plunger marker in the direction marked #2 to deploy the needles.
- Stabilizing the device firmly with the left hand, remove the plunger and needles by pulling back on the plunger in the direction marked #3. The plunger should be attached to one suture limb. Pull gently until the suture is taut.
- Cut the suture, either by using the Quickcut mechanism on the body of the device or using a scissors or scalpel.
- Push the lever (marked #4) down.
- Stabilizing the access site with the left hand, withdraw the Proglide device until the guidewire port (marked on each side by a white arrow) is visible above the skin.
- Harvest the sutures by pulling the suture ends from the device. You should have one blue (rail) suture end and one white (non-rail, knot-tightening) suture end.
- If you wish to retain wire access, then re-insert the guidewire through the wire lumen.
- Load the blue rail limb of the suture onto the snared knot pusher, and wrap the end around the index finger of your left hand. Keep the white non-rail limb out of the way by weighting it down with wet sterile gauze.
- Remove the Proglide device, and advance the knot to the arteriotomy by pulling gently on the blue rail limb.
- If the site is hemostatic, then remove the guidewire and proceed with advancement and tightening of the knot as

described below. (If no hemostasis was achieved, then a sheath may be advanced over the guidewire to re-secure the access site.)

- Keeping tension on the blue end, advance the knot pusher to complete advancement of the knot. Make sure that the knot pusher is going all the way to the arteriotomy, and is not getting caught up in the tissue tract.
- Keeping the knot pusher in place, pull on the white limb of the suture to tighten the knot.
- Remove the knot pusher from the tract. Hemostasis may be checked at this point by asking the patient to cough or bend the leg. Continued bleeding should be managed by further knot advancement, followed again by again securing the knot through tension on the white non-rail suture end.
- Once hemostasis has been achieved, remove the knot pusher completely.
- Load both ends of the suture onto the suture trimmer device and advance down to the arteriotomy. Pull back on the red trimming level to cut the sutures, and remove the device and suture ends from the wound.
- Hold gentle pressure until oozing is controlled.

Advantages

- Guidewire access is maintained until at least partial hemostasis is confirmed. This advantage is important in situations where device failure may have serious consequences.
- May be used to "preclose" the vessel (see discussion below) for procedures requiring very large sheaths.
- Effective use results in effective closure with only suture in the wall of the vessel, with no bulky or thrombogenic material in the lumen.
- A single device closes arteriotomies in the 5–8 Fr range.
- Re-access of the vessel has no restrictions.
- The device needles enter the artery from above (in contrast to the Prostar devices), thus minimizing the risk of getting the needles stuck if the device fails.

Disadvantages

- Somewhat more difficult to learn than some of the other devices.
- Difficult to use in calcified vessels, as the needles may fail to penetrate the arterial wall, causing the device to fail.

How We Use It

I prefer the Perclose Proglide in appropriate vessels when I cannot afford to have the device fail, since access with a guidewire can be maintained until at least partial success is confirmed. We use the Proglide preferentially for the preclose technique. We avoid the Proglide in very heavily calcified vessels or with sheath entry in the superficial femoral artery or profunda, as the foot process can catch on the femoral bifurcation and result in inappropriate deployment of the suture.

Prostar XL

The Prostar (Fig. 2.3; Abbott Vascular, Menlo Park, CA) is one of the original suture-based devices. It results in the deployment of two sutures at right angles to one another, via four suture needles. Of the several Prostar devices that have been manufactured over the years, only the Prostar XL 10 Fr device is still sold in the US. The suture is polyester and requires manual knot tying, and is therefore more challenging to use compared with the Perclose Proglide. Also in contrast to the Perclose Proglide and A-T, the Prostar needles are deployed from the inside of the vessel outward. This brings up the possibility of getting the device stuck in the event of improper use. For these reasons the Prostar is labeled by Abbott as a Percutaneous Vascular Surgical device (as opposed to the Suture Mediated Closure label applied to the Proglide) and is marketed primarily to vascular surgeons.

Advantages

- Deploys two sutures with a single device, making it a natural device for use in "preclosure" of large access sites.
- No restrictions on re-access of the vessel.

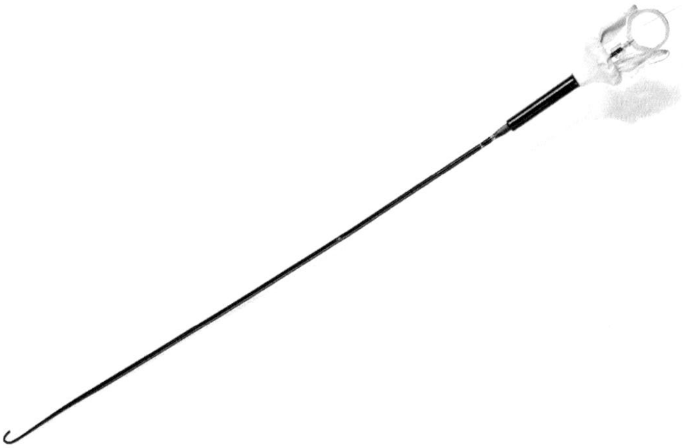

FIGURE 2.3 ProStar XL device

Disadvantages

- Relatively difficult to learn and use.

Passive Closure Devices

Mynx

The Mynx (Fig. 2.4; AccessClosure, Inc., Mountainview, CA) is a more recent device that effects closure by depositing a polyethylene glycol (PEG) sealant in the tissue tract, through the procedural sheath. Because it does not anchor to the artery itself, it is often referred to as a passive, rather than an active, closure device. The device is manufactured in a 5 Fr version and a separate 6Fr/7 Fr version.

Advantages

- Because it is placed directly through the procedural sheath and uses a synthetic sealing agent, the Mynx theoretically has low infection potential.
- Causes very little discomfort during deployment, in comparison to other devices.

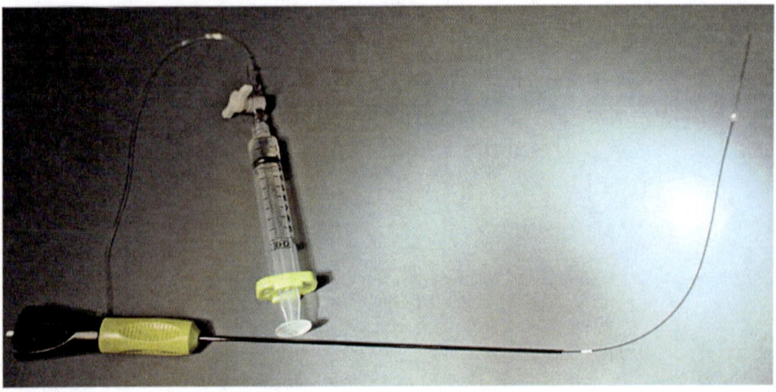

FIGURE 2.4 Mynx

- The device places the sealant entirely external to the artery, and therefore does not compromise the lumen.
- Use of multiple Mynx devices to close larger-bore access sites has been reported.

Disadvantages

- Because this is a passive device, closure is potentially less secure than with active devices. Testing the device (by having the patient cough or lift the leg) is actually contraindicated.

Technique

- Remove the Mynx device from its tray.
- Fill the locking syringe with 3 mL of saline.
- Attach the syringe to the stopcock on the device, and draw vacuum to prep the balloon.
- Inflate the balloon until the black mark on the inflation indicator is visible.
- Deflate the balloon completely and leave the syringe neutral. Submerge the tip of the shuttle tube in sterile saline for 5 s.
- Insert the device into the sheath and advance until it reaches the white marker. Inflate the balloon until the black inflation mark is visible, and turn the stopcock.
- Holding the device by the handle, draw back at an angle parallel to sheath insertion. Resistance will first be felt

when the balloon abuts the tip of the sheath. Continue withdrawing until the balloon reaches the arteriotomy.

- Confirm that the balloon is against the arteriotomy by opening the stopcock on the procedural sheath. Brisk flow of blood would indicate that the balloon is not adequately against the arteriotomy and needs to be repositioned.
- While maintaining light backward pressure on the handle with the right hand, grasp the shuttle with the left hand and advance down through the procedural sheath until resistance against the balloon is felt. A quiet "click" should be heard.
- Now grasp the procedural sheath and withdraw it until the sheath, shuttle, and handle all come together.
- While continuing to maintain backward tension on the handle, grasp the advancer tube at skin level and advance two markers.
- Lay the device down and allow at least 10 s for the device to swell in the tract. Wait longer (at least 60 s) for anti-coagulated patients.
- With the left hand, grasp the advancer tube at the skin to stabilize it. Pull back on the syringe until it locks, and open the stopcock to deflate the balloon. Wait until all fluid and air bubbles have stopped moving through the tubing to be certain that the balloon is completely deflated.
- Maintaining light forward pressure on the advancer tube, slowly withdraw the balloon catheter through the advancer tube lumen.
- Remove the advancer tube and apply light pressure for 2 min.

Tips of the Trade

In situations where it may be more difficult to determine by feel whether the balloon is all the way back against the arteriotomy (e.g., iliac tortuosity or disease, scar tissue at the access site), fill the syringe with a 50:50 contrast/saline mix and use fluoroscopy to guide.

> In patients with iliac tortuosity that prevents tracking of the device up the iliac, first placing a 0.035-in. wire as a "buddy" can facilitate the initial device insertion.

How We Use It

Because of its essentially painless deployment process, the Mynx is my go-to device for patients who are sensitive to groin pressure or who may have a vagal response to full manual pressure. It is a good alternative as a completely external-to-the-artery device when a passive device is suitable.

Cardiva Catalyst

The Cardiva Catalyst (Cardiva Medical, Sunnyvale, CA) device is the successor to the Boomerang Wire. These devices are intended to assist with arteriotomy closure while leaving nothing behind either in the artery or the tract. The concept is simple: replace the 5, 6, or 7 Fr sheath with a wire that has a collapsible biconcave disc near the distal end that can be retracted against the inner surface of the arteriotomy to achieve temporary hemostasis. During a dwell time of between 15 min and several hours, the natural recoil of the vessel wall around the arteriotomy results in a smaller arterial defect and more efficient manual closure. The Catalyst II device improves on the earlier Boomerang by incorporating a biocompatible coating (containing kaolin and chitosan) that aids hemostasis. The Catalyst III is intended for use in heparinized patients, and incorporates protamine sulfate into the coating to locally neutralize heparin.

Advantages

- The Catalyst leaves no foreign body behind in the vessel. Theoretically, this should translate into a lower risk for infection and lower potential for adverse reactions.
- Because nothing is left in the artery, vascular disease at the access site has less effect on the ability to use the device.

- Manual compression time is significantly shorter than without the device.
- With anti-coagulated patients, the time to hemostasis is significantly shorter than when using manual compression without the device.

Disadvantages

- Manual compression is still required.

Potential Pitfalls – Common to All Closure Devices…

- Risk of infection. Caution in certain groins, with long-dwelling sheaths, etc. Consider antibiotics in certain cases.
- Always perform an angiogram prior to insertion. Look for problems including calcification or tortuosity, severe luminal disease.
- Do not deploy devices with intravascular components at or below the femoral bifurcation.
- If the sheath is at or above the inguinal ligament, use caution! The vessel turns posteriorly here, and most devices will not deploy properly. Unrecognized device failure can lead to severe retroperitoneal hemorrhage.

Mechanical Devices That Assist with Manual Compression

FemoStop

The FemoStop device (Fig. 2.5; St. Jude Medical) consists of a rigid frame that holds a clear pneumatic dome that can be inflated to provide pressure over the femoral artery. The frame is held in place by a wide adjustable belt that is placed under the patient's hips. The dome pressure is controlled

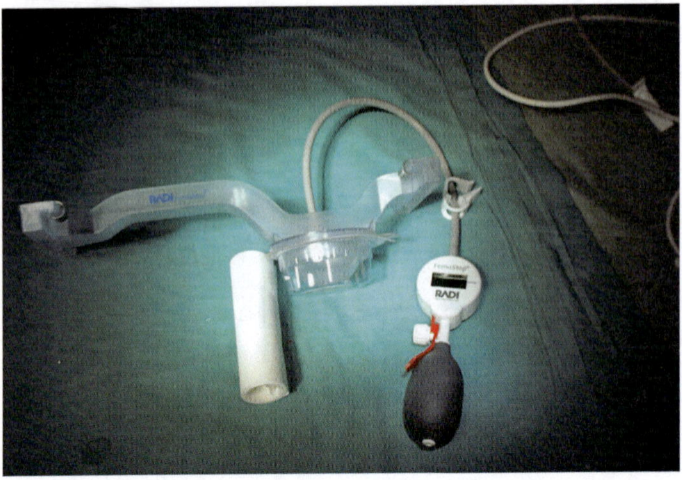

FIGURE 2.5 FemoStop device

precisely by way of a pump with a manometer, very similar to that used with blood pressure cuffs.

- The FemoStop can be used to replace manual compression, by placing the device before sheath removal. For this indication, pressurize the device to 60–80 mmHg for sheath removal, then increase the pressure to just above the systolic pressure for approximately 3 min. Then reduced the pressure in the dome to just above the diastolic blood pressure and confirm return of distal pulses. Retain the device at this pressure for at least 15 min. Then reduce the pressure by 10–20 mmHg every few minutes until all the pressure is released.
- Another option is to remove the sheath manually, and then apply to FemoStop device. When this is the intention, be sure to place the belt in good position under the patient's hips BEFORE removing the sheath, so that the device is ready to apply.
- The FemoStop can be a good option for manual compression when very long compression times are anticipated, or when a hematoma has developed prior to sheath removal, making compression with the hands challenging.

- The FemoStop device may remain in place at low pressure (30 mmHg or less) during bedrest. This is especially useful for patients on gpIIb/IIIa inhibitors or for whom re-bleeding is otherwise considered likely.

Clinical Pointers

- The FemoStop can be an effective device for treating a femoral pseudoaneurysm, and is formally indicated for this purpose.
- Compression of a pseudoaneurysm can be uncomfortable. Consider giving local anesthesia and systemic pain medication prior to starting.
- Examine the site by duplex ultrasound in order to locate the artery, vein, pseudoaneurysm, and tract. Mark the skin over the site to be compressed with an "X."
- Position the FemoStop over the marked site and inflate. Do not keep at occlusive pressure for more than 3 min. Maintain a constant pressure for 20 min, making sure that distal pulses are palpable during compression.
- Release pressure and repeat ultrasound, looking for flow in the pseudoaneurysm and tract.
- If abnormal flow persists, then repeat 20 min of compression.
- Bedrest with low-pressure (30 mmHg or less) compression. Repeat ultrasound to confirm resolution.

C-Clamp

Several "c-clamp" devices are manufactured, marketed as the CompressAR (Advanced Vascular Dynamics) and ClampEase (ClampEase, Portland, OR). These devices are comprised of a stand with an arm that applies direct pressure to a disc situated over the artery. In skilled hands, these devices can be very effective for applying manual compression. They are not meant to be used unmonitored, however. Once placed, they need to be evaluated frequently for bleeding, misalignment, or excessive pressure leading to limb ischemia.

Safeguard

The Safeguard device (Maquet Cardiac Assist, Mahwah, NJ) is a large sterile dressing with an integrated inflatable bulb that adheres over the access site and assists with pre- and post-hemostasis management.

- When placed prior to sheath removal (the "manual assist" technique), the Safeguard reduces active compression time. Because pressure is exerted through the bulb of the device, the application of pressure can be more comfortable than using the hands alone.
- As a post-hemostasis management device, the Safeguard can be applied once hemostasis is achieved to stabilize the site. This can decrease the rate of recurrent post-procedure bleeding, especially with patients who are heavily anti-coagulated or who are non-compliant with the restrictions on mobility post-procedure.
- The clear window on the device allows monitoring of the site while it is in place. This offers an advantage to the traditional "pressure dressing" made of tape and gauze, which usually obscures the site.
- The device relies on adhesive to hold it in place. In our experience the Safeguard can be expected to fit poorly on certain patients, such as those with a large abdominal pannus.

Potential Pitfalls

- Each of the mechanical compression devices needs to be placed by a trained operator, and must be monitored closely.

- Minimize the amount of time that full occlusive pressure is applied. Full occlusive pressure does not speed hemostasis, can be painful, and can cause complications.
- The FemoStop and C-clamp devices can be very uncomfortable for the patient. Beware of vagal episodes when using these.
- Be aware that use of these devices generally compresses the adjacent vein as well as the artery, and therefore carries a small risk of deep venous thrombosis. Make sure that the device does not stay in place longer than is necessary.

Topical Hemostasis Aids

A variety of topical patches, pads, bandages, and powders is available for use to assist with hemostasis with manual compression. The idea is that these devices accelerate the clotting process and thus accelerate hemostasis, potentially allowing for shorter compression times and lower incidence of re-bleeding. Approximately 10 such products are currently approved by the FDA for use.

- Most of these agents have been approved based on studies showing that they improve time to hemostasis and time to ambulation, versus unassisted manual compression.
- Topical agents leave no foreign body behind, and act by accelerating natural hemostasis.
- Topical agents still require manual compression.

The Preclose Technique

The suture-based devices, Perclose Proglide and Prostar XL, rule in the arena of closure of large-bore access sites. That is because these devices may be used to place sutures in the arteriotomy at the beginning of a case with small-bore access (5–8 Fr with the Proglide, or 10 Fr with the Prostar) and lay the suture ends aside. The arteriotomy may then be dilated up to the desired size, up to 25 Fr in some series. At the end of the procedure, the large sheath is removed, and the sutures are tightened down to effect hemostasis. The technique is known as Preclose because the devices are deployed at the beginning rather than at the end of the case. If the Proglide is used, two devices are deployed resulting in two separate sutures at the puncture site. The Prostar only requires a single device, since it is designed to place two sutures at right angles to one another.

How I Do It

- Safe closure starts with good access. Use fluoroscopy and a 4-Fr micropuncture kit to access the common femoral artery. Confirm appropriate positioning by a contrast injection before proceeding.
- Dilate the puncture site with a 6 Fr sheath. Remove the sheath, leaving a 0.035-in. guidewire in the artery.
- Place a Proglide over the wire and advance into the vessel. Rotate the device counterclockwise to the 10 o'clock position, and deploy.
- Harvest the suture ends from this first device, tag them with a small hemostat, and lay them aside. Maintain guidewire access.
- Insert a second Proglide device, rotate clockwise to the 2 o'clock position, and deploy.
- Harvest the suture ends from the second device and tag them with another small hemostat. Again replace the guidewire before removing the device.
- Make sure to save the knot pusher and suture trimmer for later.
- Now serially dilate the access site over a stiff guidewire and place the procedural sheath. Proceed with the planned intervention.
- Once the procedure is complete, replace the stiff 0.035-in. guidewire and slowly remove the large sheath while applying manual pressure to the site.
- Use the knot pusher to cinch down both of the previously placed sutures. Release manual pressure to assess the site.

If hemostasis has been achieved, then remove the guidewire and further tighten and lock the knots.

Tips of the Trade

- If pulsatile flow is still seen after both sutures are secured, a third Proglide device can sometimes be deployed successfully. If this does not work, then reinsert an appropriate-size sheath to regain hemostasis and consider surgical repair of the artery.

Radial Access Closure

Radial access for interventional vascular procedures continues to gain traction due to its overall excellent safety profile. Multiple hemostasis devices are now on the market, each essentially providing local pressure over the access site. The simplest of these is the Hemoband (HemoBand Corporation, Portland, OR), which is essentially an adjustable plastic compression strap. The RadAR device (Advanced Vascular Dynamics, Portland, OR) is similar, but adds an adjustable screw for more fine control of wrist pressure. Vascular Solutions manufactures a version that incorporates its D-stat hemostasis pad into a compression band. The TR band (Terumo Medical Corp., Somerset, NJ) uses dual compression balloons, inflated with air by a syringe, to accomplish hemostasis. The RadiStop (St. Jude Medical) incorporates a compression pad and straps onto a support plate that holds the hand, wrist, and forearm.

How hemostasis is achieved can have a significant impact on the rate of subsequent radial artery occlusion.

- The hemostasis device should not remain in place too long. On average, the device should be able to be removed after 2–3 h.
- Use the "patent hemostasis" approach:
  - Place the compression device with the least pressure necessary to achieve hemostasis.

- Place a pulse oximetry probe on the thumb or index finger of the involved hand.
- Occlude the ipsilateral ulnar artery with manual compression. If oximeter signal is present, then the radial artery is patent and you have achieved "patent hemostasis."
- If no signal is present, gradually loosen the compression device until either signal returns or bleeding occurs. Note that we are not able to achieve patent hemostasis in every patient.
- Devices allowing for more fine control over radial artery pressure, such as the TR band and RadAR device, are somewhat easier to use for this purpose.

Bibliography

Manesh R. Patel, Hani Jneid, Colin P. Derdeyn, Lloyd W. Klein, Glenn N. Levine, Robert Lookstein, Christopher White, Yerem Yeghiazarians MD, and Kenneth Rosenfield. **Arteriotomy Closure Devices for Cardiovascular Procedures – A Scientific Statement from the American Heart Association** From the American Heart Association Council on Clinical Cardiology and the Diagnostic and Interventional Cardiac Catheterization Committee, Council on Cardiovascular Radiology and Intervention, and the Interdisciplinary Working Group on Atherosclerotic Peripheral Vascular Disease. Circulation. 2010 Nov 2; 122(18): 1882–1893.

→ *This is an excellent review of arteriotomy closure devices which includes the scientific statement from the American Heart Association.*

Dangas G, Mehran R, Kokolis S, et al. Vascular complications after percutaneous coronary interventions following hemostasis with manual compression versus arteriotomy closure devices. Journal of the American College of Cardiology. Sep 2001;38(3):638–641.

→ *This is one of the earlier studies that reported increased rates of hematoma, hematocrit drop, and vascular surgical repair with VCDs compared with manual compression. Notably, the use of VCDs was by operator preference, and was only used in 8% of the population studied.*

Sanborn TA, Ebrahimi R, Manoukian SV, et al. Impact of femoral vascular closure devices and antithrombotic therapy on access site bleeding in acute coronary syndromes: The Acute Catheterization and Urgent Intervention Triage Strategy (ACUITY) trial. Circ Cardiovasc Interv. 2010;3:57–62.

→ *A more recent post-hoc analysis of the ACUITY trial reported a decrease in access site-related bleeding with VCD use.*

Narins CR, Zareba W, Rocco V, McNitt S. A prospective, randomized trial of topical hemostasis patch use following percutaneous coronary and peripheral intervention. J Invasive Cardiol. 2008 Nov;20(11):579–84.

→ *One of many trials of a topical hemostasis aid, this study used an ACT cutoff of ≤250 for sheath removal and ambulated patients after only 2 h, without a reported increase in complications.*

Dauerman HL, Applegate RJ, Cohen DJ. Vascular closure devices: the second decade. Journal of the American College of Cardiology. Oct 23 2007;50(17):1617–1626.

→ *A well-written review of closure devices.*

Kahlert P, Eggebrecht H, Erbel R, Sack S. A modified "preclosure" technique after percutaneous aortic valve replacement. Catheterization & Cardiovascular Interventions. Nov 15 2008;72(6):877–884.

→ *One of many good articles describing the use of the Perclose Proglide for preclosure of large-bore arteriotomy sites.*

Koreny M, Riedmuller E, Nikfardjam M, Siostrzonek P, Mullner M. Arterial puncture closing devices compared with standard manual compression after cardiac catheterization: systematic review and meta-analysis. JAMA. Jan 21 2004;291(3):350–357.

→ *A meta-analysis of 30 VCD randomized trials. Although no significant difference in complications between manual compression and VCDs was found, this analysis noted the limited methodological quality inherent in many VCD studies.*

Arora N, Matheny ME, Sepke C, Resnic FS. A propensity analysis of the risk of vascular complications after cardiac catheterization procedures with the use of vascular closure devices. American Heart Journal. Apr 2007;153(4):606–611.

→ *A prospective registry reporting a lower risk of access site complications with VCDs compared with manual compression.*

Chapter 3
Sheaths, Guides, and Catheters

Kendrick A. Shunk

"If you can't list at least four ways to get into trouble with something, you have no business using it in a patient."
– David Thiemann, M.D. (The John Hopkins Hospital)

Introduction

When planning a case, thoughtful development of a strategy for sheaths, guides, and catheters is arguably the most important contributor to a successful outcome free of complications, yet these comparatively unglamorous considerations are frequently given inadequate attention.

General Considerations

- Generally there are more degrees of freedom (and therefore more pitfalls) in sheath/guide/catheter selection for peripheral interventions than for certain other procedures that operators may have in their background.

K.A. Shunk
Division of Cardiology, Department of Medicine, University of California – San Francisco and VA Medical Center, San Francisco, CA, USA
e-mail: kendrick.shunk@va.gov

C.D. Owens and Y. Yeghiazarians (eds.), *Handbook of Endovascular Peripheral Interventions*, DOI 10.1007/978-1-4614-0839-0_3,

- One main goal is to secure a base of operations closer to the lesion or in some cases at both the antegrade and retrograde approaches to a lesion.
- Type of hemostasis mechanism.
  - Traditional side arm versus rotating hemostatic valve (Touhy-Borst adapter) is largely a matter of preference for smaller access (~4–10 F).
  - Side-arm sheaths in larger sizes (up to 24 F) are often not truly hemostatic and may require a smaller "sheath in sheath" technique between steps to minimize blood loss.
  - Keller-Timmermans hemostatic system is another option for large access cases (e.g., AAA).
- Manifold with continuous pressure monitoring is generally optional, but can be quite useful in assessing severity and/or result by measuring gradients.

Purpose

The main objective of sheath and guide selection is to move the "base of operations" closer to the lesion and optimize operator control. Collectively these devices provide a supportive hemostatic conduit through which one may pass equipment to the intended site of treatment while minimizing the potentially hazardous interaction with features along the way such as atherosclerotic plaque, excessive tortuosity or angulation, ectasia or frank aneurysms. By pairing these devices in a telescoping coaxial configuration – or a trio of them into a triaxial arrangement – additional control can be achieved, usually at a small cost to total case complexity.

Sheath, Guide, Catheter Selection

- Plan backward, starting with, for example, the anticipated stent size required, including contingencies such as potential need for covered stents, snares, and occlusion balloons.

- Check minimum inner lumen diameter (ID) requirements for all devices you anticipate potentially needing to use.
- Think about catheter length for all potential devices.
- Choose access strategy, sheath, guide, or combination to ensure that selected devices are compatible with minimum ID and catheter length requirements for the case and any contingencies.
- Always remember to have your team "readback" each item as it is passed into the sterile field and if ever in doubt, read the sizing on the package label yourself before accepting an item. In some cases, it may be desirable to "test-fit" any questionable tolerances on the back table before attempting it in the patient.

Knowing when to increase the complexity and when to keep it simpler is no easy task*. Staying abreast of sheath, guide, and catheter options as they evolve is an important component of the lifelong learning commitment that one makes to mastery of endovascular procedures.

How I Do It

Talk through the case backward and select length and diameter of sheath and/or guide strategy based on the requirements of the intended device(s), taking into account potential contingencies.

Sizing Considerations and Conventions

Scenario: You have just accessed the artery with an 18G needle, a 0.035-in. wire, and a 23-cm 6 F sheath through which you will advance a 7 mm × 4 cm balloon. Congratulations! You have just managed to use four different sizing systems in a single sentence. But why do we do this? The answer is partly history lesson and not as illogical as it may sound at first.

---

*"Everything should be made as simple as possible, but not simpler." (Albert Einstein)

The Most Common Source of Confusion About Sizing of Sheaths vs. Guides and How to Avoid It

- Guides and sheaths are not sized the same way! What? Why not?!!
- Remember that sheaths are relatively recent inventions. In the days of the giants, all catheterization was performed "sheathless" by operators with left hypothenar hypertrophy, a result of their practice of holding pressure on the artery with half of the left hand while performing catheter exchanges with the other half.
- When sheaths were introduced (pun intended), in order to avoid confusion about which size to use with a given catheter, a convention developed that is unique to sheaths: they are described in F ("French") according not to their size, but to the *size of the catheter they will admit.* Thus, while a typical "6 F" sheath actually has an outer diameter (OD) of approximately 7 F, and even its ID is not 6 F, but in fact a little bit larger to allow for clearance, it is *labeled* as "6 F" in order to indicate that it will allow passage of a 6 F-guide catheter or other device.
- Example: A 6 F Flexor (Cook) sheath has an ID of 0.087 in.. A 6 F guide that will be passed through it has a "true" OD of 6 F = 2 mm = 0.079 in. The sheath lumen incorporates ~0.008–in. clearance to permit catheter movement and rotation within the sheath.
- Bottom line: a device that can easily pass through a 6 F-sheath may require a 7 F or 8 F guide. Double-checking clearances is highly advisable!

Which Units Should One Expect Will Be Used in Particular Situations?

- When describing the size of the hemostatic access conduit required for passage of a catheter (ID of the

sheath, or arteriotomy size for "sheathless" catheter introduction), expect to be "talking French";
- When describing the diameter of a wire or the clearance required inside a guide or other catheter, expect thousandths of an inch;
- When describing how much a vessel lumen is being stretched, or how long a lesion is, expect metric (mm or cm).

Situations will arise in which conversions become necessary or at least expedient. So it is important to understand what each system means and which devices are traditionally described with which system and in addition to understand how they can all be converted one to the other with the aid of a table or a little math (Table 3.1).

Platforms

The wires over which devices will travel are standardized into major "platforms." Simple cases can usually be completed using a single platform, but certain situations require facility with techniques to exchange platforms without forfeiting wire/catheter position. In general, smaller platforms require smaller access and may be less traumatic, but offer less support. The wires themselves are all available in a variety of lengths. See Table 3.2.

Sheaths

Traditional workhorse sidearm sheaths are available in a variety of diameters and lengths. There is a color-coding scheme to which many manufacturers adhere that signifies the size. The middle panel of Fig. 3.1 shows fairly typical 4, 6, 7, 8, 12,

TABLE 3.1 Size conversion

Sheaths				Guides and other			Needles		
Labeled size[a]	Typical color code[b]	Typical ID (in.)[b]	Estimated OD(F)[b]	OD (F)	OD (in.)	OD (mm)	Stubs needle gauge	OD (in.)	ID (in.)[c]
				3	0.039	1.00			
4	Red		~5	4	0.052	1.33			
5	Grey	0.07	~6	5	0.066	1.67	10	0.134	0.106
6	Green	0.09	~7	6	0.079	2.00	11	0.120	0.094
7	Orange	0.10	~8	7	0.092	2.33	12	0.109	0.085
8	Blue	0.11	~9	8	0.105	2.67	13	0.095	0.071
9	Black	0.13	~10	9	0.118	3.00	14	0.083	0.063
10	Black	0.13	~12	10	0.131	3.33	15	0.072	0.054
11		>0.144	~13	11	0.144	3.67	16	0.065	0.047
12		>0.157	~14	12	0.157	4.00	17	0.058	0.042
13		>0.171	~15	13	0.171	4.33	18	0.050	0.033
14		>0.184	~16	14	0.184	4.67	19	0.042	0.027

15	>0.197	~17	15	0.197	5.00	20	0.036	0.024
16	>0.210	~18	16	0.210	5.33	21	0.032	0.020
17	>0.223	~20	17	0.223	5.67	22	0.028	0.016
18	>0.236	~21	18	0.236	6.00	23	0.025	0.013
19	>0.249	~22	22	0.289	7.33	24	0.022	0.012
20	>0.262	~23	20	0.262	6.67	25	0.020	0.010
22	>0.289	~25	22	0.289	7.33	26	0.018	0.010
24	>0.315	~27	24	0.315	8.00	27	0.016	0.008
						28	0.014	0.007

[a]Black stripe on top of background color indicates additional 0.5 F
[b]May vary by manufacturer and specific-sheath design
[c]Thin-walled access needles (same OD, larger ID) are available

TABLE 3.2 Common wire platforms

Main wire platforms	Typical uses
0.014″	Smaller vessels (e.g., coronary, renal, carotid, tibials)
0.018″	Multipurpose mid-range, most cases
0.035″	Larger vessels (e.g., iliac, subclavian, aorta)

and 16 F sheaths of various manufacturers. The top panel shows the fundamental difference between these and the other major option for hemostatic control and delivery: the guide catheter with an adjustable Touhy-Borst adapter (a.k.a. rotating hemostatic valve, O-ring). The lower panel shows a longer armored sheath (Arrow) which is thicker-walled and kink-resistant, which can be beneficial at the expense of a slightly larger OD and potential for over-straightening of a tortuous vessel and subsequent obstruction of flow.

Guides

Guiding catheters (aka Guides, Guiders) typically are placed coaxially through a sheath to optimize control. This allows manipulation of the guide catheter without direct interaction with the endothelial surface of the access vessel, which can be important in minimizing spasm, particularly for radial access cases. Guides are not typically supplied with a tapered dilator to aid in penetrating the skin and arteriotomy but they can be used in a sheathless mode if necessary (off-label). Working with a guide through a sheath will afford the operator the maximal potential availability of tip shapes but does nominally increase expense compared to using a workhorse sheath alone. Also, a "same size" guide provides a conduit of smaller size compared to a sheath due to differences in sizing conventions (see sheath vs. guides sizing box). Guides are available in

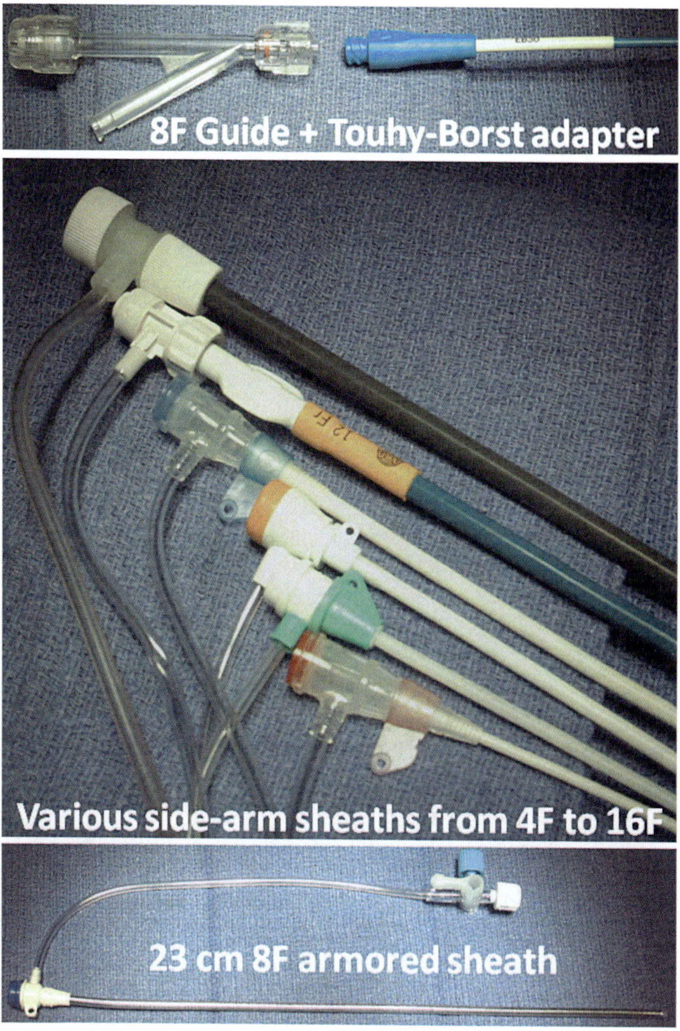

FIGURE 3.1 Examples of side-arm sheaths compared with guide + Touhy-Borst option

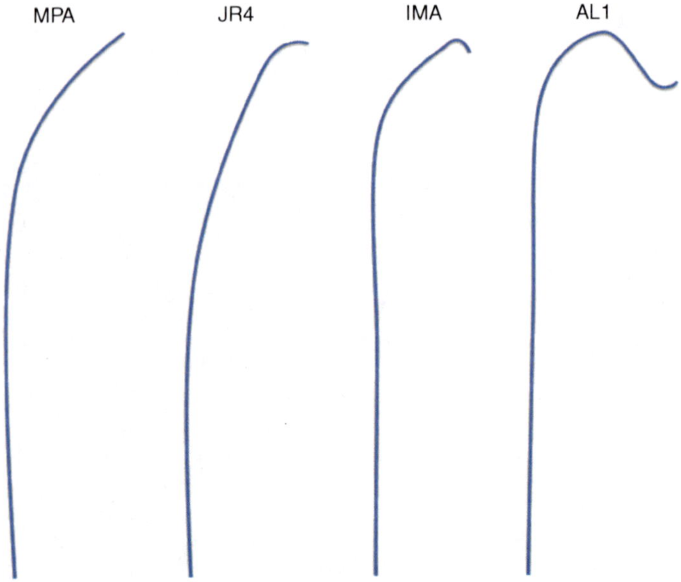

FIGURE 3.2 Guide tip shape examples

a variety of lengths and the important consideration is that the guide must be longer than the sheath and protrude enough to allow the shaped portion to exit the guide, and they must be short enough for the balloons and other equipment to pass through them (plus the hemostasis valve) and still have enough additional length to reach the intended treatment site beyond the guide tip. Shown below are four examples of available guide shapes (Fig. 3.2). Operators should become familiar and facile with the use of a wide range of shapes.

Combo Guide/Sheaths

No longer can every sheath be described as a simple straight conduit with a side-arm hemostatic valve on the proximal end. The field has enjoyed significant cross-over with incorporation of many of the features of guide catheters into sheath design.

The "guidesheath" represents a merged device that is available with a choice of hemostasis valve and a reasonable variety of guide-like shapes at the distal end to facilitate engagement of and support within the target vessel. The main advantage of this device over the use of a sheath with a separate guide is a smaller access site arteriotomy requirement for the same size ID. A line of combination guidesheaths which are on the horizon for radial cases will have the same OD as a 6 F sheath, but an ID comparable to a 7 F-guide catheter.

Catheters

Balloons, stents, other therapeutic devices are discussed in detail in Chapter 4.

Here are discussed mainly catheters used to provide access to and/or control of a base of operations proximal and/or distal to an area of intended treatment once that position is initially established by a wire or other device (i.e., to eliminate the need to "give up wire position") during wire exchanges or other maneuvers.

Equipment List

This is a partial list as a variety of equipment can be successfully utilized.

Sheaths

Workhorse standard short (10–15 cm) sheaths with side-arm hemostasis valve in variety of sizes from 4 to 12 F

- Cordis
- Terumo
- St. Jude
- Many others reasonable

6, 7, 8 F long (23 cm) sheath for tortuous iliac anatomy

- Cordis Brite Tip
- Arrow "armored" sheath (caution: any long sheath, but especially the armored sheath, can sometimes straighten the vessel excessively with production of kinking and pseudo-lesions, which, despite their name, can produce real effects in terms of downstream ischemia and/or vessel thrombosis. It is advisable to monitor patency angiographically and/or by distal pulse checks to avoid this.)

Larger and longer sheaths in 45–90 cm

- Flexor (Cook) 5–12 F
- Destination (Terumo) 6, 7, 8 F
- Curved variants- Raabe, Balkin, etc.

Specialty Sheaths

- Morph- sheath version (BioCardia) see below.
- SoloPath (Onset Medical). This sheath system is inserted as a low-profile device created by "wrapping" a larger sheath over a smaller dilator which has its own integrated high-pressure balloon. This allows the 5.3 F dilator tip/low profile sheath to be delivered through an unfavorable iliac artery to the distal aorta before the sheath itself is expanded to full size by inflation of the balloon/dilator. Available in 19, 20, and 21 F I.D. (22, 23, 24 F O.D., respectively) All of the cautions listed above for armored sheaths apply, and the operator should be prepared to treat the Iliac artery if needed "on the way out" and should be experienced with managing large sheath removal.

Guiding Catheters

5–8 F guiding catheters with varying shapes, in standard 95 or 100 cm lengths; the following catheters are useful in numerous cases

- JR4
- IMA
- Multipurpose

- Sos Omni
- Amplatz left (AL1, AL2)

Dedicated renal guiding catheters with varying shapes, in shorter lengths are useful but not essential if longer equipment is available

- RDC
- JR4
- IMA
- Hockeystick (HS1, HS2)
- PK-1

Actively shape-controlled guide/sheath

- Morph catheter (BioCardia)

"Mother and child" coaxial guide accessory:

- GuideLiner 5-in.-6, 6-in.-7, or 7-in.-8 F (Vascular Solutions)

Guidesheaths

Many sheaths, straight or curve-tipped, can be ordered with a choice of standard side-arm hemostasis valve or rotating hemostasis valve (Touhy-Borst type)

- Destination (Terumo)
- Flexor (Cook)
- Others

Accessory Catheters

A good variety of 4 F angiographic (diagnostic) catheters in 100 and 120 cm length can be quite useful for gaining access to a lesion, 0.035-in. wire exchanges, platform switches, and other maneuvers

- JR4
- IMA
- AL1
- MPA2

In addition, there has been a proliferation of dedicated exchange catheters, crossing catheters, and related delivery catheters

- QuickCross 0.035 in., 0.018 in., and 0.014 in. (Spectranetics)
- CXI 0.035 in. and 0.018 in. straight or angled (Cook)
- Specifically for smaller wire platform crossing/exchanges, a variety of catheters are available from the cardiac and neuro interventional arenas for the 0.014-in. platform:
  - Transit (Cordis)
  - Finecross (Terumo)
  - Excelsior (Boston Scientific)
  - Corsair (Abbott)
  - Minnie, SuperCross (Vascular Solutions)
- Finally, specialty 0.014-in. platform catheters are available that are designed with a threaded tip for advancement by manual rotation:
  - Tournis (Abbott)
  - Gopher (Vascular Solutions)

  Or for "second wire" placement
  - TwinPass (Vascular Solutions)

  Or with an actively deflectable tip for directional steering
  - Venture (St. Jude Medical)

Potential Pitfalls

* Remember that sheaths and guides are sized differently

- It is critically important to plan ahead and be familiar with available inventory and resources.
- Consider potential need for bail out strategies (occlusion balloons, snares, covered stents) and whether sheath or guide diameter and length are adequate for them.
- "Stuck" situations (and remedies):

- Balloon catheter or other device will not reach through a long sheath, guide catheter, or combination (requires switch to longer balloon catheters and/or shorter sheaths/guides)
- Wire is across lesion but catheter will not advance beyond lesion and wire is too short to exchange for a different catheter. (Doc the wire if possible, or exchange catheter by hydraulic technique, only consider intentionally forfeiting wire position if it is safe to do so. Consider using longer wires and/or doc-able systems)

Summary/Conclusions

- Plan – think backward from final intended therapy and the sizing, tolerance, length delivery support, and other requirements. Consider contingencies and potential disasters and bail out strategies and all of the same considerations for those (length, delivery support, ID requirements, etc.). Think about other steps prior to final Tx such as the balloon pre-treatment, ultrasound, need for atherectomy, or other requirements of the case and all of the requirements for those individual devices. Typically it is the largest, bulkiest, and/or stiffest device that the operator potentially plans to use for the case that will drive the choices about delivery support, ID, and length requirements of the sheath and/or guide.
- Remain aware of options.
- Develop protocols for the more common procedures, but never stop learning and do not be afraid to modify or deviate from your own protocols in a rational way.
- Learn from every case, especially from any "mistakes."
- Brief and de-brief with a colleague, partner, fellow, chief technician, or other appropriate team member(s) on a regular basis, especially as you are expanding your endovascular repertoire. Talk it through!

Bibliography

1. Endovascular Today annual product reviews (http://bmctoday.net/evtoday/buyersguide/2010/).
   → *Extremely useful resource with comparative notes, supplier information, and archives that extend back several years.*
2. Annual catalogues and websites of individual suppliers. (see #1 for lists).
   → *These are replete with technical data, charts, diagrams, and descriptions of available option. Instructions for use (IFU) or Directions for use (DFU) documents can generally be found on individual vendor websites.*

Chapter 4
Angioplasty Balloon, Stents, and Stent Grafts

S. Marlene Grenon

Basic Concepts in Angioplasty and Stenting

- Angioplasty in brief:
  - Angioplasty is a controlled dissection created by exerting a dilating force on the internal surface of a vessel. It also leads to compression of an atherosclerotic lesion and stretching of the elastic components of the arterial wall.
  - A biological response takes place with platelet and fibrin deposition at the area where the subendothelial surface is exposed. This is followed by an inflammatory response comprised of smooth muscle cell migration and proliferation and secretion of extracellular matrix. Following that, there is re-endothelialization and organization of the extracellular matrix and remodeling of the vessel with lumen preservation. However in many cases the inflammatory response is pernicious and results in lumen compromise.
  - Angioplasty can be done in a transluminal or subintimal fashion.

S.M. Grenon
Division of Vascular Surgery, Department of Surgery, University of California – San Francisco, San Francisco, CA, USA
e-mail: marlene.grenon@ucsfmedctr.org

C.D. Owens and Y. Yeghiazarians (eds.), *Handbook of Endovascular Peripheral Interventions*, DOI 10.1007/978-1-4614-0839-0_4,

  - Typical indications:
    - Stenosis
    - Re-stenosis
    - Occlusion
  - Etiology of arterial stenosis includes atherosclerosis, intimal hyperplasia, fibromuscular dysplasia, and vasculitis. Atherosclerotic occlusive disease is by far the most common.
- Stenting in brief:
  - A stent is a device that acts as scaffolding to hold open diseased vessels. Stenting prevents elastic recoil after balloon angioplasty
  - Stents may be covered (stent graft) with ePTFE or Polyester, or uncovered
  - Important concepts:
    - Primary stenting: Placing a stent at the site of intervention without first performing a balloon angioplasty. This is best for lesions such as recurrent lesions, and occlusions. It is controversial whether orifice lesions should be treated with primary or secondary stenting
    - Secondary stenting: Starting with angioplasty and placing a stent if the result is not satisfactory (residual stenosis, persistent pressure gradient, significant, or flow-limiting dissection)
  - Indications for stents:
    - Post-angioplasty dissection
    - Residual or recurrent stenosis after angioplasty
    - Pressure gradient
    - Occlusion
    - Embolizing lesions
    - Arterial rupture
    - Aneurysms or pseudoaneurysms
    - Recoil
  - Downside of using a stent is an increased risk of thrombosis and intimal hyperplasia
  - Persistent foreign body irritation resulting in inflammation and accumulation of fibrin and platelets on the stent surface followed by recruitment of inflammatory

cells. There is subsequently smooth muscle migration leading to intimal hyperplasia and restenosis.

- What is a hemodynamically significant lesion?
  - Lesion likely to compromise blood flow and which is involved in patient's symptoms
  - To evaluate the hemodynamic significance, you may use pressure gradients with or without reactive hyperemia
    - A baseline gradient can be measured proximal and distal to the lesion, followed by a gradient with reactive hyperemia [after injecting papaverine (30 mg IV) or nitroglycerin (100–200 mcg IV) in the vessel]. The gradient is measured simultaneously or after pull-back by using a 4-Fr end hole catheter such as a hydrophilic glide catheter.
    - You can use the mean pressure or the systolic pressure
    - A difference of more than 5–10 mmHg is considered significant
  - Other modalities to evaluate the significance of a lesion: intravascular ultrasound (IVUS), computed tomography angiography (CTA), and magnetic resonance angiography (MRA).

Important Characteristics of the Devices

Important concepts

- General classification of devices (Fig. 4.1)

Basic Definitions and Characteristics

- *Balloon Diameter*: This is the nominal inflated balloon diameter measured at a specified pressure.
- *Balloon Length*: This refers to the working length or the length of the straight body section, corresponding to the distance between the radio-opaque markers.
- *Shoulder*: This is the distance from the radio-opaque marker, where the balloon is filled out to its specified diameter, to the actual end of the balloon.
- *Shaft Length*: This is the working distance between the operator and the angioplasty site.

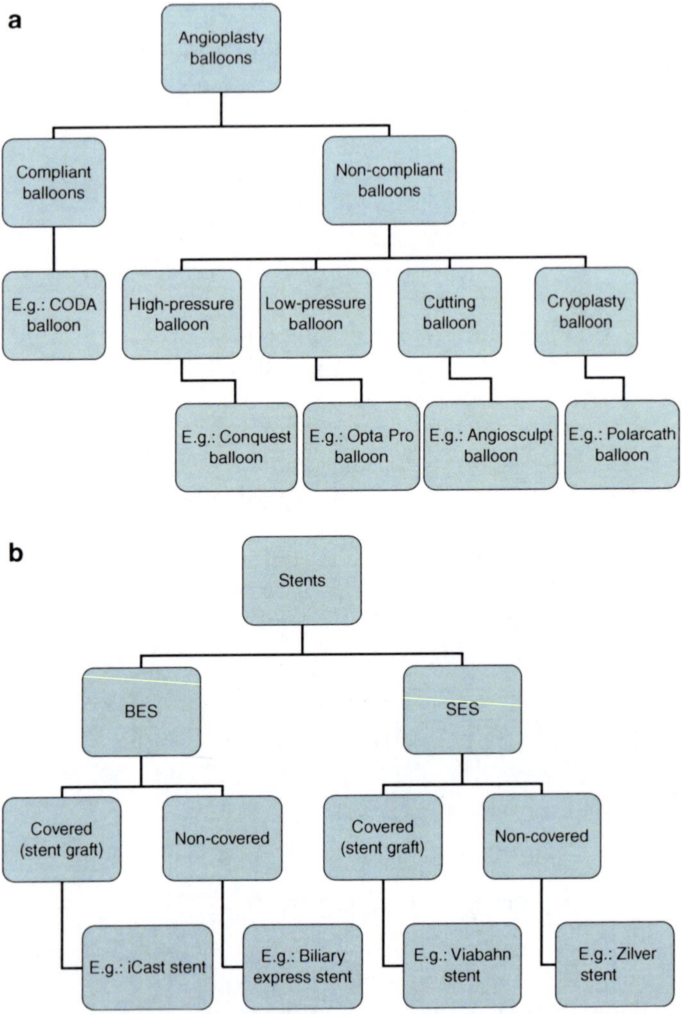

FIGURE 4.1 General Classification of angioplasty balloons (**a**) and Stents (**b**). *BES* Balloon-expandible stent, *SES* Self-expandible stent

- *Nominal Pressure*: This represents the pressure needed to inflate the balloon to a pre-determined diameter.
- *Burst Pressure*: This is the average pressure required to rupture a balloon; usually measured at body temperature.

- *Rated Burst Pressure* (*RBP*): This corresponds to the maximum recommended pressure for safe use of a balloon, ensuring that 99.5% of the tested balloons will not fail at RBP with a 95% confidence.
- *Balloon Profile*: This is the maximum diameter of the balloon when mounted on a catheter in its deflated and wrapped condition, or the smallest hole through which the deflated wrapped balloon catheter can pass.
- *Balloon Compliance*: This is the change in balloon diameter as a function of inflation pressure.
- *Pushability:* The ability to advance a balloon or catheter through the vessel.
- *Trackability:* The ability of the balloon or catheter to follow or "track" the guidewire.

Angioplasty Balloons

- Balloons can be compliant, non-compliant, or semi-compliant (Fig. 4.1)
  - Compliant balloon will increase their diameter with increasing pressure. They are typically made of silicone and thermoplastic elastomers, polyethylene, or polyolefin polymers.
    - Example: CODA balloon (Cook)
  - Non-compliant balloons remain at a pre-selected nominal maximum diameter even when the internal balloon pressure is increased beyond what is required to fully inflate the balloon, which facilitates high-pressure inflation. They are made of polyethylene terephthalate or polyamides.
    - Example: Fox Plus (Abbott Vascular), Conquest (Bard Peripheral Vascular), Synergy (Boston Scientific)
  - Semi-compliant balloons are an intermediate class of compliance between the compliant and non-compliant balloon. These balloons are usually made of nylon.
- Inflation Pressures: Pressures for inflation vary from 4 to 16 atm, but can be as high as 30 atm.
  - The ability for the balloon not to break or rupture is dependent on the material the balloon is made of as well as the presence of calcifications in the lesion being treated.

- Higher pressures are usually used for relatively stiff venous stenosis or dialysis fistula.
  - Example: Conquest balloon (Bard Peripheral Vascular), Dorado balloon (Bard Peripheral Vascular).
- Cutting Balloons
  - These are balloons with extra mechanical portion such as small blades or external metal wires that is advocated for the treatment of resistant or complex atherosclerotic lesions. The blades allow to "score" the lesion which purportedly facilitates a controlled dilatation.
    - Resistant renal artery in-stent restenosis
    - Resistant high-grade dialysis graft stenosis
  - Examples: Angiosculpt (Angioscore), VascuTrak2 (Bard Peripheral Vascular)
- Cryoplasty Balloons
  - These balloons allow simultaneous dilation and cooling of the plaque and vessel wall in the area of treatment. The cooling theoretically induces apoptosis of the smooth muscle cells and thereby prevents restenosis. However this has not been borne out in clinical trials. It is advocated for suboptimal angioplasty balloon or for in-stent restenosis.
  - Example: PolarCath (Boston Scientific)
- Drug-Eluding Balloons
  - Mostly uses dry-state paclitaxel, the active ingredient of Taxol, which has been approved by the US Food and Drug Administration and is widely used in oncological therapy
  - By not using stents, follow-up treatment options (re-PTA, anastomosis site for surgical bypass) are preserved.
  - Example: Freeway peripheral balloon (Eurocor)

Stents and Stent grafts

- Stents can be balloon-expandable or self-expandable, covered (i.e., stent-graft) or not covered (Fig. 4.1)
- Self-expandable stents
  - Used in the treatment of long lesions and tortuous vessels

TABLE 4.1 Comparison of balloon expandable vs. self-expanding stents

Characteristic	Balloon expandable	Self-expandable
Method of deployment	Balloon inflation	Unsheathing
Length	Shorter	Longer available
Precision of landing	↑	↓
Foreshortening	↓	↑
Flexibility	↓	↑
Ability to withstand crushing by external pressure	↑	↓
Radial strength	↑	↓
Ability to be recaptured or repositioned prior to complete deployment	↓	↑
Radioopacity	↑	↓

- Made of Elgiloy or NiTiNOL (Nickel Titanium Naval Ordinance Laboratory) (takes a heat-treated shape above a transition temperature depending on the composition of the alloy)
- Deployed by retracting a restraining sheath with the final diameter based on stent geometry, hoop strength, and vessel size
- In general, self-expanding stents should be oversized by 1–2 mm (or 10–20%) relative to the largest diameter of the normal vessel (see below)
- The advantages (Table 4.1)
  - Come in longer lengths than BES
  - Ability to expand after delivery can accommodate adjacent vessels of different sizes
  - More flexible but will recoil if compressive force is added
- The disadvantages
  - Less radial force
  - More difficult to visualize (less radio-opaque)
  - Less accurate deployment

TABLE 4.2 Types of stents for the vascular bed

Vascular bed	Type of stent
Abdominal aorta	Balloon expandable
Aortic bifurcation	Balloon expandable
Common iliac artery	Balloon expandable
External iliac artery	Balloon expandable or self expandable
Superficial femoral artery	Self expandable
Popliteal artery	Self expandable
Tibial artery	Recommend against stenting
Infrainguinal graft	Self-expandable
Renal artery	Balloon-expandable or self-expandable
Subclavian artery	Balloon-expandable

  - Typical areas where they are deployed: external iliac artery, SFA, and popliteal artery (Table 4.2).
  - Examples: Zilver (Cook), Lifestent (Bard Peripheral Vascular), Complete SE stent (Medtronic), Protege (EV3), Sentinol Self-Expanding stent (Boston Scientific).
- Balloon-expandible stents (BES)
  - Used in the treatment of orificial, calcified or resistant lesions
  - Made of stainless steel (or a cobalt alloy)
  - Mounted on a balloon and deployed when balloon inflated
  - Can be expanded beyond its predetermined diameter
  - More rigid and associated with a shorter time to complete endothelialization
  - Higher degree of crush resistance compared to self-expanding ones
  - Best for short-segment lesions
  - Typical areas where they are deployed: aorta, common iliac artery, renal artery, and subclavian artery
  - Advantages (Table 4.1)
    - Stronger radial force
    - More precise
    - Easier to see (more radio-opaque)

- Disadvantages
  - Shorter
  - More rigid
- Examples: Biliary Express (Boston Scientific), VisiPro (EV3), Paramount (EV3).

- Stent-Grafts
  - They are stents (stainless steel or nitinol) covered with fabric (ePTFE or polyester fabric). They can be balloon-expandible (e.g., iCast from Atrium Medical Corporation) or self-expandible (e.g., Viabahn from Gore)
  - Used for:
    - Traumatic vascular lesions (arterial disruption, arteriovenous fistulas)
    - Iliac or femoral occlusive disease
    - Popliteal aneurysms
    - Abdominal aortic aneurysms
- Palmaz Stents
  - Palmaz stents are hand-mounted on a balloon to be deployed.
  - For deployment, a sheath is usually advanced carefully to the area of deployment. The Palmaz stent, after being crimpled on balloon such as a Maxi LD or Coda balloon, is advanced to the deployment site. The sheath is retracted then the Palmaz deployed.
  - Additional foreshortening is to be expected if stent diameter is pushed up beyond its recommended limit
- Drug-eluting stent
  - Local release of a drug to prevent restenosis
    - i.e., sirolimus, paclitaxel
  - Examples: Cypher stent (Cordis), Taxus (Boston Scientific), Endeavour (Medtronic), and Xience V (Abbott), Promus (Boston Scientific)

Sizing of the Device

- There are three important numbers for sizing of a device:
  1. Diameter of device (Table 4.3)
     - Balloons: do not oversize.

TABLE 4.3 Balloon sizing based on vascular bed

Vascular bed	Balloon diameter (mm)	Typical balloon length (cm)
Abdominal aorta	8–18	2–4
Aortic bifurcation	6–10	2–4
Common iliac artery	6–10	2–4
External iliac artery	6–8	2–4
Superficial femoral artery	4–7	2–10
Popliteal artery	3–6	2–4
Tibial artery	2–4	2–4
Infrainguinal graft	2–5	2–4
Renal artery	4–7	2
Subclavian artery	5–8	2–4
Common carotid artery	6–8	2–4
Internal carotid artery	4–6	2
Dialysis graft	4–6	2–4

Adapted from Rutherford Textbook of Vascular Surgery, 7th Edition, Table 85.4.

- ◦ Stents and stent-grafts: oversize 10–20%. One caveat to this is that the Viabahn stent graft should not be oversized. In fact, oversizing these stent grafts has led to fabric impingement and premature restenosis. Recent Viabahn proximal graft design modifications have resulted in a contoured edge that have resulted in improved flow dynamics and improved wall apposition.

2. Device length (Table 4.3)
3. Catheter length

- To determine sizing, look at:
  - Diameter of device:
    - ◦ Pre-op imaging (CTA, MRA)
    - ◦ Intra-op imaging measurement (quantitative angiography)

    - IVUS
    - Optical Coherence Tomography (OCT) (mostly experimental at this time)
    - Eyeball
  - Device Length:
    - Pre-op imaging (CTA, MRA)
    - Intra-op imaging with techniques such as "pull-back" or "glow-and-tell" tape, calibrated marking catheter
    - Using markers on certain of the wires to make an estimate
    - IVUS (and potentially OCT in the future)
    - Eyeball
    - Note: balloon should be long enough to dilate the lesion with a short overhang on both ends
    - A balloon that is too long can traumatize adjacent "normal" endothelium. If it is too short, which may "squirt" "water balloon" out of position during inflation.
  - Length of catheter:
    - Think of the area that needs to be treated in relation to the access (so *lesion location* and *access site*)
      Femoropopliteal from ipsilateral femoral: 75 cm
      Femoropoliteal from contralateral femoral: 75–110 cm
      Infrapopliteal from ipsilateral: 75–90 cm
      Infrapopliteal from contralateral: 90–120 cm
      Iliac from ipsilateral femoral: 40–75 cm
      Iliac from contralateral femoral: 75 cm
      Renal from femoral: 75–90 cm
      Carotid from femoral: 110–130 cm
- Other important baseline concepts for devices:
  - Coaxial or monorail
    - Coaxial: over the wire system
    - Monorail: also referred to as "rapid-exchange" when only the distal portion of the balloon catheter tracks in a co-axial fashion over the guidewire
  - System size: go over 0.014 in., 0.018 in., or 0.035 in. wires

Clinical Pointers

Follow this simple three-step process:

1. **EVALUATE:** In your decision to treat the patient, always think of the following (Fig. 4.2)
   - Clinical state patient with respect to (1) symptoms, (2) comorbidities
   - Lesion [Trans-Atlantic Inter-Society Consensus (TASC) classification and recommendations]
   - Indications for treatment (look at evolving literature on subject, etc.)
   - Consider alternatives (open surgery, hybrid, no treatment)
2. **DISCUSS:** Before offering an endovascular treatment, review complications of the procedures and discuss them with the patient in obtaining consent (Table 4.4)
3. **TREAT:** Decide on treatment strategy and make your plan

Patient	Lesions
Symptoms Co-morbidities Tissue loss Presence of vein For alternate option (i.e.by pass)	TASC classification Length Stenosis/occlusion
Indication	**Alternatives**
Is there an indication? CLI vs claudication	No treatment Open surgery Hybrid

FIGURE 4.2 Factors to consider prior to endovascular treatment

TABLE 4.4 Complications of percutaneous transluminal angioplasty for lower extremity ischemia

Location	Type	Incidence (%)
Puncture site		4
	Bleeding	3.4
	False aneurysm	0.5
	Arteriovenous fistula	0.1
Angioplasty site		3.5
	Thrombosis	3.2
	Rupture	0.3
Distal vessel		2.7
	Dissection	0.4
	Embolization	2.3
Systemic		0.4
	Renal failure	0.2
	Myocardial infarction	0.2
Consequence		
Surgical repair		2
Limb loss		0.2
Mortality		0.2

Adapted from Rutherford Textbook of Vascular Surgery, 6th Edition, Table 84.10.

Equipment List

- Access needle and guidewire
  - 18-gauge hollow bore introducer needle (Cook)
  - Micropuncture set if calcified vessel, scarred groin, or brachial approach
  - Ultrasound
  - Smart needle (Doppler ultrasound-guided vascular access needle) can be considered for difficult vascular

access cases (Peripheral Systems Group, Mountain View, Calif)

- Sheath and its dilator
  - Choose sheath size depending on size of balloon or stents that you will be using for angioplasty
- Contrast
  - Usually a mixture of saline and contrast (50–50 mix) is used for angiogram as well as for balloon inflation. For larger aortic balloons, a 20–30% contrast solution may help decrease the viscosity and inflate/deflate more rapidly.
- Heparinized saline
- Selective guidewire
  - The glidewire (Terumo) is a very useful and versatile wire.
  - Length depends on your target vessel and access size
    - 50–80 cm: catheterization of dialysis access
    - 145–150 cm for: aortoiliac interventions, antegrade approach to infra-inguinal disease
    - 180–210 cm for: arch/carotid angiography, subclavian interventions, renal/visceral interventions, contralateral infrainguinal
    - 200–300 cm: carotid interventions
- Selective catheter
  - The catheter to be used will depend on your target vessel
- Inflation device
- Balloon
  - Refer to Table 4.5 for selection
- Stent
  - Refer to Table 4.5 for selection

How I Do It

- STEP #1: Plan your case
  - It is really important to plan your case and know the material you will need in advance to make sure it is on the shelves
  - You can plan your case from backward looking at the access you will need for treatment or alternatively, you can start with a smaller access and upgrade your sheath

TABLE 4.5 Commonly used balloons and stents and size sheaths needed

Task	**Recommend (my favourite)**	**Size sheath needed**
Common iliac stenting	Biliary express	6 Fr
External iliac stenting	As above or	6 Fr
	Smart stent (Cordis)	
SFA BA	Opta Pro (Cordis)	5–7 Fr
SFA stenting	Short lesion: Smart (Cordis)	6 Fr
	Long lesion: Viabahn (Gore)	7–8 Fr
Popliteal BA	Opta Pro (Cordis)	5–7 Fr
Tibials BA	Savvy (Cordis)	4–5 Fr
	Nanocross	4 Fr
Carotid stenting	Emboshield protection device	
	Stent X–Act	
Renal artery stenting	Biliary express	6 Fr
Dialysis fistula BA	Blue Max	6–9 Fr

size as needed. The smallest sheath adequate for the device to be used is the best.

- STEP #2: Get access
  - Obtain access with access needle, sheath, and guidewire through the ipsilateral or contralateral femoral, brachial, or other site. This is usually done with lidocaine 1% local + IV sedation
  - To help you with access, consider using ultra-sound guidance or landmarks (such as the femoral head) on fluoroscopy. You may also start with a micropuncture set.
  - Once access is gained, heparin IV is given (50–100 IU/kg)
- STEP #3: Get close and evaluate the lesion
  - You will have to travel with a wire and catheter to get to the lesion
  - Having the shortest distance that provides adequate working room is best

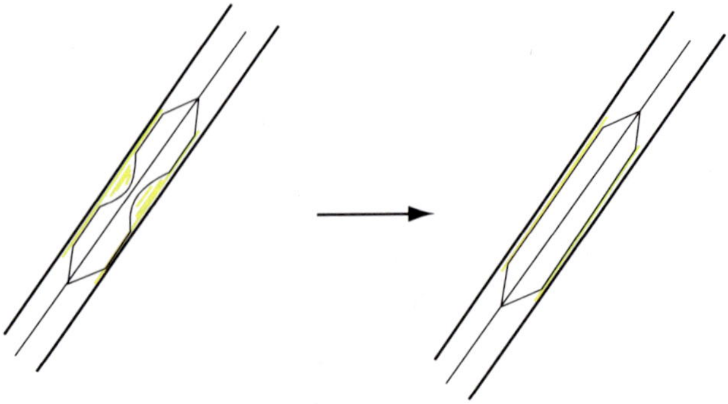

FIGURE 4.3 Appearance of a significant lesion with "waist" on angioplasty balloon, then successfully treated

  - Identify the lesion through an angiogram: site, extent, run-off
    - Anatomic confirmation
    - Hemodynamic confirmation (mean gradient ≥10 mmHg)
- STEP #4: Get across the lesion
  - Get wire across the lesion and *do not loose access*
  - Confirm your treatment strategy
  - Mark the lesion by one or several means such as
    - Roadmapping
    - External markers on the field or on the screen
    - Body landmarks
- STEP #5: Treat lesion
  - Treat lesion: always do this under fluoroscopic guidance
  - Balloon or stent is positioned with radio-opaque marker at each end to see position
  - Check for waist on balloon (Fig. 4.3)
  - Careful with branch vessels
  - About treatment times for angioplasty: different strategies exist:
    - Inflate and "crack the plaque" then deflate.
    - Keep the balloon up for 30–60 s or even 2 min. May repeat inflation
    - Find what works for you, keeping in mind that longer inflation times will probably be needed for intimal

TABLE 4.6 Methods to evaluate results of balloon angioplasty and stenting

May use	Consider
Completion angiogram	Should always be done. May add oblique views, magnified views
Pressure gradient	May add vasodilator challenge
Intravascular U/S	If available: very useful
Clinical evaluation – Appearance – Symptoms – ABI – Toe pressure	Should always be done after an intervention and repeated in the post-op course

TABLE 4.7 Causes of poor visualization of outflow vessels

Cause	Consider
Poor technique	Repeat with more contrast and greater strength of injection
Low flow	Optimize hemodynamics of patient
Thrombosis	Ensure appropriate anticoagulation, treat as required
Embolization	Ensure appropriate anticoagulation, consider aspiration cath (Export Catheter), treat as required
Dissection	Consider repeat angioplasty and stenting
Spasm	Vasodilator: papaverine, NTG

hyperplasia, recurrent lesions, residual lesions, and sometimes heavily calcified lesions

- STEP #6: Check your result (Table 4.6)
  - Post-angiogram in which you need to visualize the outflow vessels, the inflow vessels, and the primary site of treatment (Table 4.7)

- Treat complications if any
- Keep guidewire in position across lesion until the evaluation of the lesion is satisfactory

Tips of the Trade

- Most important concept to remember:
  - Once you have access, never lose it!
- Crossing the lesion
  - Make sure you have appropriate support with sheath close to your work area
  - Get comfortable with two or three wires that will become your favorite wires.
  - Try combinations: straight-tip catheter with an angled wire or an angle catheter with a straight wire. This should help you cross lesions.
  - Make use of the magnified view for precise navigation and deployment of your device
  - Consider using a smaller wire to cross (e.g., Roadrunner, 0.014 system) followed by a smaller profile catheter (e.g., Quick Cross), then upgrading your wire to an 0.035 system. Twirling the wire between your fingers like a "fish in the sea" will help going across.
  - If a pre-occlusive stenosis cannot be crossed with an appropriately sized balloon, a lower-profile balloon can be used first
  - If the balloon does not track over the guidewire, consider a stiffer wire or a longer sheath to improve your pushability and support
  - Always try to go transluminal first. If not successful, consider subintimal.
  - Refer to Table 4.8 for more trouble-shooting
- The subintimal technique
  - If wire passage is subintimal (usually in the setting of an occlusion), certain steps are important to ensure re-entry into the vessel lumen.

- This can be done by:
  - Spinning the wire and observing free rotation of the angled tip
  - Inspection of the course of the wire in several projections
  - Advancing a small catheter (e.g., Quick-cross) over the guide wire into the re-entered vessel followed by injection of a small amount of contrast to ensure that there is no extra-vasation.
- If you realize that the wire is not back into the vessel lumen, try crossing again in through another location or consider other options (e.g., re-entry devices such as Outback LTD reentry catheter from Cordis or Pioneer device from Medtronic). Remember that you can always abandon the procedure and consider open strategy.

- Slow-to-deflate balloon
  - If having problem removing contrast having problem removing contrast from the balloon, apply high negative pressure by withdrawing the plunger from the syringe and locking it in place. This creates a vacuum and should help deflating the balloon
- Should you treat proximal or distal lesions first?
  - If a proximal stenosis will not allow passage of balloon angioplasty catheter for distal treatment, treat proximal first
  - If wire and balloon can be passed easily distally, treat distal first
- The "jumpy" self-expandible stents
  - Self-expandible stents have a tendency to jump. When deploying, use the "dog-on-a-leash" trick: imagine you are walking a dog and just keep enough tension on the leash (i.e., device) to keep it straight.
- Kissing balloon/stent technique
  - When atherosclerotic plaques are at a bifurcation such as aortic bifurcation, dilation of only one

branch vessel can lead to a fracture of the plaque and possible dissection, occlusion, or embolization.

– For these instances, the best technique is called a "kissing balloon" or "kissing stent" technique, where both vessels common iliac arteries are dilated/stented simultaneously using bilateral groin access.

TABLE 4.8 Trouble-shooting during angioplasty

Problem	Consider
Balloon not tracking	Stiffer guidewire, place a long sheath
Balloon not going through lesion	Pre-dilate, lower profile balloon
Cannot dilate residual atherosclerotic lesion	Non-compliant balloon, cutting balloon, covered stent
Balloon rupturing on calcified lesion	Thicker balloon, place stent
Balloon keeps popping off lesion	Hold sufficient tension on catheter
Balloon won't empty	Withdraw plunger from syringe to form a vacuum; as a last resort, and performed by experienced operators, one can use the stiff back-end of a 0.014-in. wire and rupture the balloon

Potential Pitfalls, Complications, and Bail-Outs

- Repeat key point: NEVER LOSE ACCESS! Anything can happen but if you keep your access, you can treat most complications
- Overall, the risk of major complications after procedures vary between 2.5% for lower extremity ischemia and 6% for aortoiliac interventions (Table 4.4)

- If you have a non-satisfactory result, consider re-angioplasty, cutting balloon, or stenting
- Access site complications
  - Hemorrhage, hematoma formation, pseudoaneurysm
- Pain
  - Present with stretching of the adventitia
  - Ensure no rupture or dissection
- Dissections
  - More likely at branch points, close to bulky plaque, in arteries with longitudinal plaque
  - Treat with repeat angioplasty and if no improvement, stenting
- Arterial rupture
  - Usually an immediate event, although subacute presentations occur
  - Often caused by overdilation of the artery
  - Other factors: calcific artery, steroid therapy, fibromuscular dysplasia, infection of the wall
  - Management
    - Never loose wire access
    - Recognize the problem (pain, hypotension)
    - Reinflate the balloon
    - Resuscitate the patient
    - Definitive treatment: endovascular stent graft
- Embolization
  - 3–7% of patients
  - Try to prevent by: optimal anticoagulation, careful passage of devices, minimal manipulation of the lesion
  - At risk: occlusions, highly irregular or ulcerated, fresh thrombus, aneurysmal, complex located in infrarenal abdominal aorta.
  - See a filling defect
  - May decrease risk by primary stenting iliac lesion
  - Treatment options (p. 235, 236)
    - Local thrombolytic therapy
    - Percutaneous aspiration thrombectomy
    - Open embolectomy

- Stent-related complications
  - Rare: failure to deploy, misplacement
  - Stent infection
    - Treat aggressively: antibiotics, often requires resection of infected segment and bypass

Bibliography

Books and Book Chapters

Mastering Endovascular Techniques: A Guide to Excellence. Peter Lanzer. Lippincott Williams & Wilkins; 1 edition (September 1, 2006).

→ *Good description of endovascular skills and principles.*

Endovascular Therapy: Principles of Peripheral Interventions. Alan B. Lumsden Peter H. Lin, Ruth L. Bush, Changyi Chen, Michael E. DeBakey (Foreword). Wiley-Blackwell; 1 edition (February 17, 2006).

→ *Good description of endovascular skills and principles.*

Endovascular Skills: Guidewire and Catheter Skills for Endovascular Surgery, Third Edition, Peter Schneider, Informa HealthCare; 3 edition (December 18, 2008).

→ *Very complete, step-by-step description of endovascular techniques.*

Rutherford's Vascular Surgery, Cronenwett and Johnson (Eds). Saunders; 7 edition (March 9, 2010). Chapter 85: Technique: Endovascular Therapeutic (Makoto Sumi and Taka Ohki).

→ *Well-written chapter on endovascular principles.*

Consensus Documents

Inter-Society Consensus for the Management of Peripheral Arterial Disease (TASC II). Norgren L, Hiatt WR, Dormandy JA, Nehler MR, Harris KA, Fowkes FG; TASC II Working Group. J Vasc Surg. 2007 Jan;45 Suppl S:S5-67.

→ *Up-to-date principles in endovascular management of peripheral lesions.*

Society of Interventional Radiology Standards of Practice Committee. Guidelines for percutaneous transluminal angioplasty. J Vasc Interv. Radiol 2003;14:S209-17.

→ *Good description of standards to aim for in clinical practice.*

Important Trials

Randomised comparison of primary stent placement versus primary angioplasty followed by selective stent placement in patients with iliac-artery occlusive disease. Dutch Iliac Stent Trial Study Group. Tetteroo E, van der Graaf Y, Bosch JL, van Engelen AD, Hunink MG, Eikelboom BC, et al. Lancet 1998:18;351:1153–9.

→ *Classical trial for primary vs. secondary stenting for iliac disease.*

Dutch iliac stent trial: long-term results in patients randomized for primary or selective stent placement. Klein WM, van der Graaf Y, Seegers J, Spithoven JH, Buskens E, van Baal JG, et al. Radiology 2006; 238:734–44.

→ *Long-term results of DUTCH trial.*

BASIL trial participants. Bypass versus angioplasty in severe ischaemia of the leg (BASIL): multicentre, randomised controlled trial. Adam AJ, Beard JD, Cleveland T, Bell J, Bradbury AW, Forbes JF, et al. Lancet 2005;366:1925–34.

→ *Classical trial for endo vs open in infra-inguinal disease.*

Bypass versus Angioplasty in Severe Ischaemia of the Leg (BASIL) trial: An intention-to-treat analysis of amputation-free and overall survival in patients randomized to a bypass surgery-first or a balloon angioplasty-first revascularization strategy. Bradbury AW, Adam DJ, Bell J, Forbes JF, Fowkes FG, Gillespie I, Ruckley CV, Raab GM; BASIL trial Participants. J Vasc Surg. 2010 May;51(5 Suppl):5S-17S.

→ *Long-term results of BASIL trial.*

Sirolimus eluting vs bare Nitinol stents for obstructive superficial femoral artery disease. The SIROCCO II trial. Duda SH, Bosier SM, Lammer J, Scheinert D, Zeller T, Tielbeek A, et al. J Vasc Interv Radiol 2005;16:331–8.

→ *Important trial for drug-eluding stents in SFA disease.*

Randomised comparison of percutaneous Viabahn stent grafts vs prosthetic femoro-popliteal bypass in the treatment of superficial femoral arterial occlusive disease. Kedora J, Hohmann S, Garrett W, Munschaur C, Theune B, Gable D. J Vasc Surg 2007;45:10–6.

→ *Important trial for stent-graft in SFA.*

Chapter 5
Embolic Protection Devices

George V. Moukarbel and Piotr S. Sobieszczyk

Introduction

1. Distal embolic protection devices have been developed to reduce the rates of periprocedural complications in arterial interventions.
   (a) Disruption of occlusive plaque or thrombus during arterial intervention can lead to downstream embolization and microvascular obstruction.
   (b) Embolic debris usually consists of platelets, red blood cells, inflammatory cells, extracellular matrix, and cholesterol.
   (c) Clinical consequences of distal embolization depend on the affected tissue and include cerebral and myocardial injury, renal failure, and acute limb ischemia.
2. First developed for myocardial protection during saphenous vein graft interventions, embolic protection devices

G.V. Moukarbel • P.S. Sobieszczyk (✉)
Cardiovascular Division, Brigham and Women's Hospital, Harvard Medical School, Boston, MA, USA
e-mail: psobieszczyk@partners.org

C.D. Owens and Y. Yeghiazarians (eds.),
Handbook of Endovascular Peripheral Interventions,
DOI 10.1007/978-1-4614-0839-0_5,

available today span a wide spectrum of sizes and designs (Table 5.1) with features specific for a wide range of vascular applications (Table 5.2). These devices can be divided into two major groups:

(a) Distal embolic protections devices:
   - The need to cross the lesion to deploy the device inherently poses the risk of distal embolization

(b) Proximal protection devices:
   - Deployment proximal to the lesion may reduce the risk of embolization at the price of increased complexity and caliber of the device.

3. Each embolic protection device has a specific "landing zone" requirement which defines the length of a vessel segment free of disease and branch points where the device can be deployed (Fig. 5.1). The suitability of a device for a particular lesion and vessel configuration is particularly defined by the length of the device and by how close the tip of balloon or stent catheter can approach the filter hoop. These distances determine whether there is enough space to place the device before tortuous segment or bifurcation and still deploy a balloon or stent to adequately treat the lesion. To allow greater versatility, distal embolic protection devices available today have progressively shortened the length of the landing zone to an average of 20 mm.

Types of Embolic Protection Devices

Distal Protection Devices

Balloon Occlusion of the Vessel Distal to the Lesion

This form of distal protection relies on inflation of an atraumatic balloon in the vessel beyond the lesion, arrest of antegrade flow, capture of debris in a stagnant column of blood between the site of intervention and balloon and its

TABLE 5.1 Embolic protection devices and their specific characteristics

Device	Device type	Crossing profile	Available device size (mm)	Device position	Sheath compatibility	Pore size	Approved indication	Company
FilterWire EZ	Fixed wire polyurethane bag with nitinol loop	3.2 Fr	2.25–3.5 3.5–5.5	Distal	5 Fr sheath or 6 Fr guide	110 μm	Carotid and coronary SVG	Boston Scientific Corporation
Accunet Rx	Fixed wire nitinol filter with polyurethane membrane	3.5–3.7 Fr	4.5, 5.5, 6.5, 7.5	Distal	6 Fr sheath or 8 Fr guide	≤150 μm	Carotid	Abbot Vascular
Emboshield NAV6	Nylon filter with nitinol frame delivered over independent proprietary wire	2.8 Fr 3.2 Fr	Small: 5.0 for vessel size 2.5–4.8 Large:7.2 for vessel size 4.0–7.0	Distal	5 Fr sheath or 6 Fr guide	120 μm	Carotid	Abbot Vascular
Spider FX	Braided nitinol filter delivered over any 0.014–0.018" wire	3.2 Fr	3.0 , 4.0, 5.0, 6.0 7.0	Distal	5 Fr sheath or 6 Fr guide	Variable	Carotid and coronary SVG	eV3

(continued)

TABLE 5.1 (continued)

Device	Device type	Crossing profile	Available device size (mm)	Device position	Sheath compatibility	Pore size	Approved indication	Company
FiberNet EP	Dacron fiber based filter	1.7–2.9 Fr	3.5–5 5–6 6–7	Distal	5 Fr sheath or 6 Fr guide	40 μm	Carotid	Lumen Biomedical
Angioguard XP and RX (Fig. 5.2g)	Fixed wire polyurethane filter	3.2–3.9 Fr	4.0, 5.0, 6.0, 7.0,8.0	Distal	6 Fr sheath	100 μm	Carotid	Cordis Corporation
GuardWire	Temporary distal occlusion and aspiration system	2.1 Fr 2.7 Fr	2.5–5.0 3.0–6.0	Distal	6 Fr guide	NA	Coronary SVG	Medtronic
Proxis	Proximal balloon occlusion with a working lumen	NA, proximal device	Vessel size 3.0–5.0	Proximal	7 Fr guide	NA	Coronary SVG	St. Jude Medical
Gore Flow Reversal System	Proximal vessel occlusion and flow reversal	NA, proximal device	Vessel size 6–12 mm	Proximal	9 Fr access sheath	NA	Carotid	W.L Gore & Associates
MoMa Ultra Proximal Cerebral Protection Device	Balloon occlusion and temporary flow interruption	NA proximal device	Maximum vessel size 13 mm	Proximal	8 Fr and 9 Fr access sheath	NA	Carotid	Invatec, Inc.; Medtronic, Inc.

TABLE 5.2 Advantages and disadvantages of embolic protection devices

Device Type	Advantages	Disadvantages
Filter DEP	Antegrade flow preserved	No protection during lesion crossing
	Lesion and vessel optimally visualized during intervention	Protection limited by pore size
	Easy to use	Vessel tortuosity hinders delivery and apposition of filter hoop
	Small sheath compatibility	May cause spasm or dissection at landing zone
	Choice of crossing wire in wire-independent devices	Landing zone requirement may limit applications
		Interventional wire dictated by the device in wire-dependent devices
Distal occlusion balloon	Lowest crossing profile	Cessation of target organ perfusion
	Complete protection independent of particle size	No protection during device deployment
	Excellent delivery in tortuous anatomy	More complicated deployment
		May cause spasm or dissection at landing zone
		Vessel and lesion visualization may be suboptimal during intervention
		Interventional wire dictated by the device

(continued)

TABLE 5.2 (continued)

Device Type	Advantages	Disadvantages
Proximal balloon occlusion	Embolic protection before lesion crossing	Complicated and time consuming set up and deployment.
	Complete protection independent of particle size	Large caliber vascular access
	Not limited by vessel tortuosity	Cessation of target organ perfusion
		Potential vessel injury at balloon occlusion site
		Suboptimal lesion visualization during intervention
		Cannot be used for ostial lesions

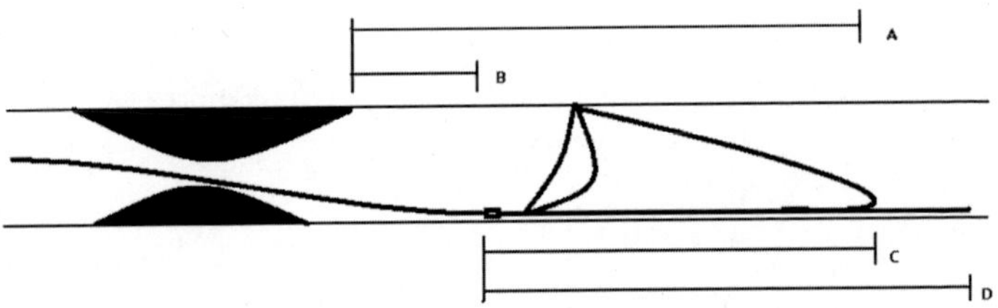

FIGURE 5.1 This schematic drawing illustrates landing-zone distances for distal embolic protection devices. Distance A defines the vessel segment from the distal aspect of the lesion to the apex of the filter. This is the minimum distance required to "land" and deploy the DEP. Distance B is the length from the distal lesion edge to proximal attachment point of the DEP. This distance determines how close the tip of a stent or balloon catheter can approach the DEP. Distance C specifies the longitudinal dimension of the DEP device while distance D includes the length of the attached guidewire

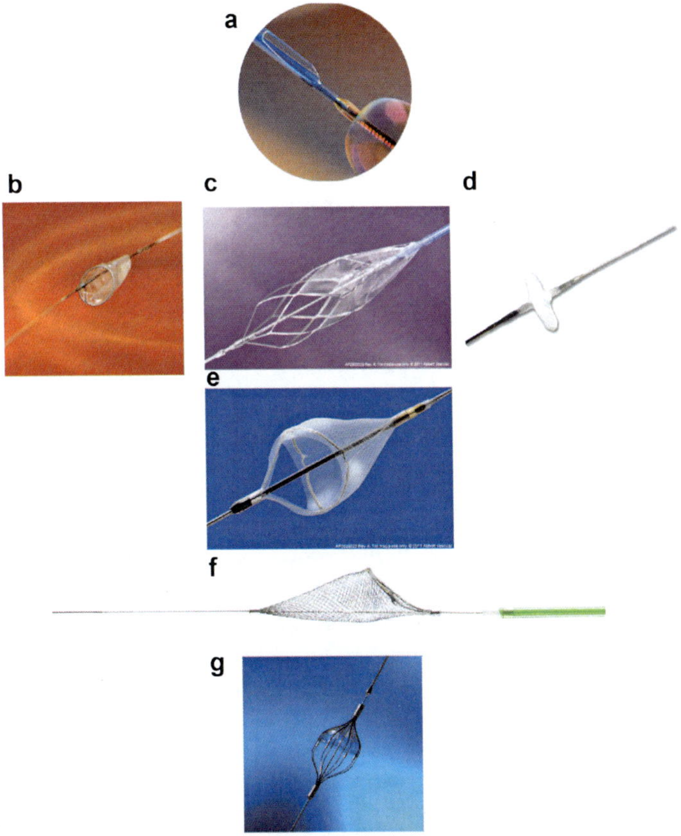

FIGURE 5.2 Types of embolic protection devices. (**a**) GuardWire (Image Courtesy Medtronic). (**b**) Filterwire (Image Courtesy of Boston Scientific. ©2011). (**c**) Accunet (Image Courtesy of Abbott Vascular. ©2011 Abbott Laboratories. All Rights Reserved). (**d**) FiberNet (Image Courtesy Biolumen. (**e**) Emboshield (Image Courtesy of Abbott Vascular. ©2011 Abbott Laboratories. All Rights Reserved). (**f**) SpiderFX (Image Courtesy of ev3 inc.). (**g**) Angioguard (©Cordis Corporation 2011)

subsequent aspiration prior to balloon deflation. GuardWire (Fig. 5.2a; Medtronic, Minneapolis, MN) was the first embolic protection system ever developed and to this day it offers the lowest crossing profile of any DEP. The balloon is mounted on a 0.014-in. wire which after balloon inflation serves as the working wire. It was approved for and previously used extensively in saphenous vein graft interventions. It has also been used in carotid interventions without contralateral vessel occlusion. Obligatory arrest of distal flow and short period of distal ischemia limited clinical applications of this system and led to subsequent development of filter-based devices.

Distal Filter Systems

The windsock-shaped filter basket deployed distal to the lesion allows perfusion of the target tissue while capturing embolic particles. The smaller the size of filter pores, the higher protective efficacy of the device, a characteristic which must be balanced to avoid stagnation of blood flow and filter occlusion. Most of the currently available devices are capable of capturing particles of 100 μm in size. The filter systems utilize 0.014-in. guidewires and small caliber catheters for delivery and recovery of the basket. Filter delivery methods allow them to be divided into two general categories:

- Wire-dependent system: The filter is attached to the 0.014-in. wire and the two are advanced as a unit. The filter is constrained in a micro catheter with a short floppy end of the wire leading the way. The disadvantage of this design is limited steerability when crossing tortuous vessels or severe stenosis. The fixed relationship between the wire and the filter basket requires meticulous handling of the wire when the basket is deployed to avoid its movement in the distal artery. The FilterWire (Fig. 5.2b, Boston Scientific, Natick, MA) was the first filter system designed and approved for use in SVG interventions, followed by the Accunet (Fig. 5.2c, Abbot Vascular, Abbot Park, IL) designed specifically for carotid interventions. The FiberNet device (Fig. 5.2d, Lumen

Biomedical) is a novel fixed-wire system. A cylinder of Dacron fibers fixed to a 0.014-in. wire is stretched to provide a low crossing wire and becomes a porous, debris-trapping plug in the vessel when the stretching tension is released.

- Wire-independent system: the second generation of distal filters allowed crossing of the lesion with an independent 0.014-in. guidewire before advancing the filter constrained in a monorail catheter. Devices, such as Emboshield (Fig. 5.2e, Abbot Vascular, Abbot Park, IL) require a proprietary wire and are more forgiving of wire movement during the procedures as the filter rests on a hypotube constrained by a distal wire bead. Other devices (Spider FX, Fig. 5.2f, eV3, Minneapolis, MN) allow deployment of the filter over any available wire but once deployed the filter becomes a fixed-wire system.

Proximal Protection Devices

Balloon Occlusion Proximal to the Lesion

This form of distal embolic protection assures that the lesion is never crossed before embolic protection is in place. The flow in the artery is arrested by inflating a balloon at the tip of the interventional guide or sheath thus trapping embolic particles in a stagnant column of blood. Aspiration before balloon deflation removes any debris before flow is restored. The success of such device depends on the absence of collateral run-off from the target vessel. The Proxis system (St. Jude Medical) was developed for SVG interventions and uses a guide with a circumferential balloon at its tip which can occlude up to a 5-mm vessel. The Proxis system requires that a brief period of ischemia is well tolerated and is limited by a small internal diameter of its catheter. The MoMa system (Fig. 5.3, Invatec/Medtronic, Minneapolis, MN) consists of two integrated balloons and a working lumen specifically designed to arrest flow in the common and external carotid arteries during CAS to avoid retrograde collateral flow from the external to the internal carotid artery.

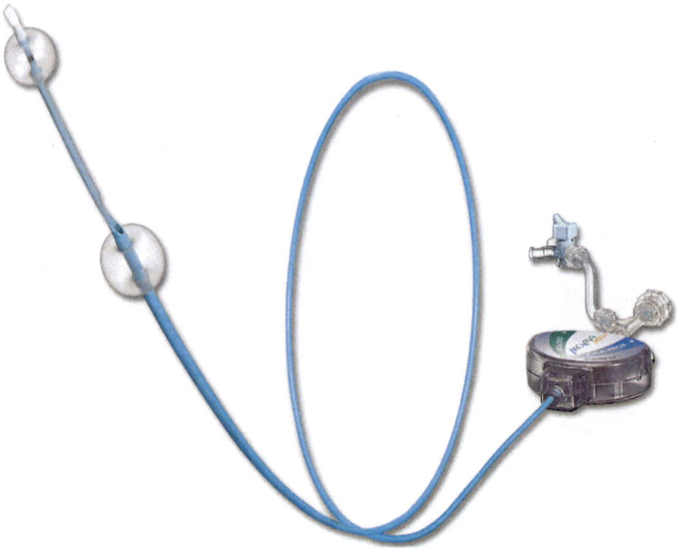

FIGURE 5.3 Proximal protection device. MoMa (Image Courtesy Medtronic)

Proximal Balloon Occlusion Device with Reversal of Flow

The GORE Flow Reversal System functions by balloon occlusion of the external and common carotid arteries proximal to the internal carotid stenosis. It allows backflow of blood through the sheath lumen and an external filter into the low pressure femoral venous system. This reversal of flow via a temporary arteriovenous shunt adds another level of protection from particulate debris but, in the initial trials, 2.4% of patients did not tolerate occlusion and flow reversal in the cerebral circulation.

Clinical Applications of Embolic Protection Devices

Cerebrovascular Interventions

- There are no large-scale randomized comparisons of internal carotid artery interventions with and without embolic protection. Few recent small trials appear to suggest that the rates of periprocedural cerebrovascular events are not lowered by DEP. However, multiple registries have repeatedly shown a 50% decrease in the risk of periprocedural stroke with the use of these devices. They are now the standard of care for any internal carotid intervention.
- There is no evidence to suggest clinical difference between filter- and occlusion-type devices.
- Embolic protection has not been specifically studied in interventions of ostial or proximal lesions of the common carotid arteries, but its use appears justified by experience from ICA interventions. Treatment of ostial lesions may be challenging with the support offered by DEP and their 0.014-in. wires.
- Embolic protection devices have not been widely studied in vertebral artery interventions and are usually avoided in these spasm-prone vessels.

Renovascular Interventions

- Undetected atheroembolization may be responsible for lack of improvement or worsening of renal function in patient undergoing renovascular interventions. The clinical impact and incidence of periprocedural embolization are difficult to gauge using currently available crude determinants of renal injury.

- Small registry series show that embolic debris can be retrieved in 44–100% of patients undergoing renal stenting with distal embolic protection.
- Short renal artery and early branching limit utility of distal protection devices while ostial nature of renovascular lesions prevents the use of proximal devices.
- The only randomized evaluation in a small RESIST (3) trial did not show clinical benefit among patients undergoing renal artery stenting with or without a distal embolic device. Improved renal function was noted only in patients treated simultaneously with embolic protection and glycoprotein IIb/IIIa inhibitors.
- Current evidence does not support routine use of these devices in atherosclerotic renal interventions. Lesion and patient-specific characteristics (such as solitary kidney, ulcerated plaque) may warrant embolic protection in complex procedures. The NIH-sponsored CORAL trial comparing medical therapy to renal artery stenting in patients with hypertension and renovascular disease initially required the use of embolic protection. Technical complications during the roll-in phase, however, led to elimination of this requirement.

Peripheral Artery Interventions

- The straight course of femoral and tibial vessels allows effortless deployment of DEP devices.
- Small series suggest that while distal embolization is common in lower extremity interventions, it is rarely clinically significant.
- Distal embolization may occur more frequently during laser atherectomy and atherectomy with the SilverHawk device.
- DEP should be considered when treating lesions where substantial amount of thrombus is suspected: acute or subacute arterial occlusion, stent thrombosis, or arterial

complications related to femoral access and vascular closure devices. DEP may be of benefit in suprapopliteal interventions when single vessel tibial run-off is encountered and tibial artery embolization may lead to acute limb ischemia.

- Available data, however, does not support routine use of these devices in treatment of atherosclerotic occlusive lesions.

Other Applications

- In authors' experience, wire-independent filter devices can be used as embolectomy devices in infrainguinal arteries. Filter deployed just beyond the embolic lesion can be a traumatically "dragged" back to capture the embolic material and then captured just above the occlusion using a 5 or 6 Fr multipurpose guide.

Complications Associated with Embolic Protection Devices

Vessel Injury

Although rare, injury at the site of deployment may occur with any device type. Balloon occlusive devices may be less traumatic than more rigid filter hoops. Vessel injury is more likely to occur when vessel tortuosity is present at the deployment site and during back and forth movement of a deployed filter caused by poor technique or difficulty advancing stent and balloons.

- Optimal filter size exceeds vessel diameter by 1 mm. Oversizing of the filter or occlusive balloon may increase the risk of vessel injury
- Vessel spasm is best treated by removal of distal embolic protection device and watchful waiting, especially in cere-

brovascular interventions. Intra-arterial vasodilators (papaverine, nitroglycerine) can be safely administered in noncerebral arterial beds. Nitroglycerine should be used judiciously if at all when treating carotid artery spasm as excessive dilation of the cerebrovascular bed increases the risk of hyperperfusion syndrome.
- Dissection at the landing zone may be best treated with anticoagulation if it is not flow limiting and occurs distal in the arterial bed.

Target Organ Embolization

Incomplete protection occurs as a function of filter pore size, malapposition of the filter or balloon at vessel bend, or undersizing of the device.

Complications During Retrieval

- Difficulty advancing filter retrieval sheath may be caused by stent-induced changes in the geometry of the vessel, protrouding stent struts, tortuosity in the stent. Commonly employed solutions include additional stent postdilation, curved retrieval sheath (available for FilterWire DEP), use of nonproprietary catheters to traverse the stent, and collapse the filter or careful advancement of the working sheath closer to the filter.
- Stent entrapment. Retrieval of partly sheathed filter may cause it to be caught on protruding stent struts. This is especially likely if the hoop of the filter is not sheathed or the filter is quickly and forcibly pulled back. Filter retrieval should be monitored on fluoroscopy and any resistance should trigger gentle advancement and full collapse. Larger caliber catheter can be used to fully collapse debris containing filters without extruding the particles through filter pores.

Filter Potential Pitfalls

- Undersizing to vessel diameter
  - Incomplete particle capture
- Oversizing to vessel diameter
  - Increased risk of dissection or spasm
- Filter occlusion
  - Never retrieve without first performing aspiration
- Retrieval problems
  - Make sure basket is completely collapsed
  - If basket is full, collapse to ensure the hoop is in the retrieval sheath
  - Do not forcibly pull through the stent: when resistance encountered, advance, postdilate stent, and try again

Clinical Pointers

Carotid Artery Interventions

- Consider using a 0.014-in. "buddy" wire to facilitate advancing DEP across a tortuous internal carotid artery.
- Gentle predilation with a 2.0-mm coronary balloon may be required to advance some DEP devices across the lesion.
- A "no reflow" phenomenon after stent placement is likely related to filter occlusion or filter-induced vessel dissection. Always aspirate the stagnant column before retrieving the filter.
- Difficulty advancing the retrieval catheter through the stented segment may be overcome by stent postdilation, advancing the sheath into the stent or

by using a more flexible catheter of appropriate caliber.

Renal Artery Interventions

- A rigid stent may be difficult to place over a less supportive 0.014-in. wire due to the acute angle between the aorta and renal artery. Careful deep seating of the guide or sheath over a more flexible balloon acting as an obturator can allow the stent to be advanced, "desheathed," and deployed.
- In renal arteries with proximal bifurcation, protect the branch supplying the majority of renal tissue. In special circumstances when intervening in a solitary kidney or on a thrombotic, ulcerated plaque with high embolization potential, consider protecting both branches and deploying a 0.035-in. wire-compatible stent over both DEP wires. The benefit of such advanced techniques has to be weighed against the higher risk of vessel injury.
- After stent deployment and postdilation of its ostium with partly withdrawn stent balloon, deep seat the guide over the balloon to facilitate advancement of the retrieval catheter without traversing the transition between the angled, protruding stent and the guide withdrawn into the aorta.

Lower Extremity Interventions

- The primary goal of DEP in lower extremity interventions is prevention of embolic occlusion of the tibial trifurcation or pedal vessels.
- The Spider FX and Emboshield NAV6 filters allow deployment in common and superficial femoral arteries measuring up to 7 mm in caliber. Protection of tibial or popliteal arteries allows the use of wider spectrum of 3–5 mm devices.

- A larger diameter 5 Fr coronary multipurpose guide can be used to retrieve a filter full of debris without losing its content.
- Consider using monorail designs to minimize longitudinal filter motion when advancing and withdrawing angioplasty balloons over long distances typical in lower extremity interventions.
- The Emboshield NAV6 DEP device allows filter retrieval while maintaining wire position across the treated lesion, a valuable feature in some complex interventions. Its hypotube design tolerates more wire movement and rotation without affecting filter's position in the vessel.

Bibliography

1. Dubel GJ, Murphy TP. Distal embolic protection for renal arterial interventions. Cardiovascular and Interventional Radiology 2008;31:14–22.
   → *This review article describes embolic protection devices used in renal interventions and succinctly discusses published outcomes in renovascular interventions with and without their use.*
2. Roffi M, Mukherjee D. Current role of embolic protection devices in percutaneous coronary and vascular interventions. American Heart Journal 2009;157:263–70.
   → *This article outlines the stages in development of embolic protection devices and summarizes the rationale for their use in cerebrovascular, coronary and peripheral arterial interventions.*
3. Cooper CJ, Haller ST, Colyer W, et al. Embolic protection and platelet inhibition during renal artery stenting. Circulation 2008;117:2752–2760.
   → *This is the only published randomized trial designed to evaluate the benefit of distal embolic protection and platelet inhibition in renovascular interventions.*

4. Kastrup A, Groschel K, Krapf H, et al. Early outcome of carotid angioplasty and stenting with and without cerebral protection devices: a systematic review of literature. Stroke 2003; 34:813–9.
→ *This systematic literature review compared reported CAS outcomes with and without DEP and paved the way towards widespread acceptance of DEP in carotid interventions.*
5. Clair DG, Hopkins LN, Mehta M, Kasirajan K, Schermerhorn M, Schonholz C, Kwolek CJ, Eskandari MK, Powell RJ, Ansel GM. Neuroprotection during carotid artery stenting using the GORE flow reversal system: 30-Day outcomes in the EMPiRE clinical study. Catheter Cardiovasc Interv 2011; 77:420–429.
→ *Proximal protection devices are the most recent addition to the armamentarium of carotid interventions. This trial describes procedural outcomes using the GORE flow reversal proximal protection system.*
6. Ansel GM, Hopkins LN, Jaff MR, Rubino P, Bacharach JM, Scheinert D, Myla S, Das T, Cremonesi A. Safety and effectiveness of the INVATEC MO.MA proximal cerebral protection device during carotid artery stenting: results from the ARMOUR pivotal trial. Catheter Cardiovasc Interv. 2010; 76:1–8.
→ *This article describes results from the pivotal trial investigating outcomes of carotid stenting using the second proximal protection system approved for clinical use.*
7. Lam RC, Shah S, Faries PL et al. Incidence and clinical significance of distal embolization during percutaneous interventions involving the superficial femoral artery. J. Vascular Surgery 2007;46:1155–1159.
→ *This study used ultrasound to detect distal embolization during various stages of infrainguinal interventions and correlated these events to clinical outcomes.*

Chapter 6
Principles of Diagnostic Angiography

Sujal M. Nanavati, Rajiv Sawhney, and Christopher D. Owens

Monitoring radiation exposure is a concern for the health care worker and patients. Health care workers are usually monitored and restricted to 100 mSv effective dose every 5 years and a maximum of 50 mSv in any given year. Patients on the other hand are exposed to ever increasing utilization of radiographic procedures for diagnostic or therapeutic purposes. The effects of radiation exposure are cumulative and no level of exposure can be considered to be "safe." Therefore vigilance of radiation exposure is absolutely critical in the safe performance of cardiovascular fluoroscopy.

R. Sawhney
Interventional Radiology Division, Department of Radiology and Biomedical Imaging, University of California – San Francisco and VA Medical Center, San Francisco, CA, USA
e-mail: rajiv.sawhney@va.gov

S.M. Nanavati
Interventional Radiology Division, Department of Radiology and Biomedical Imaging, University of California – San Francisco, San Francisco, CA, USA
e-mail: sujal.nanavati@ucsf.edu

C.D. Owens (✉)
Division of Vascular Surgery, Department of Surgery, University of California – San Francisco, San Francisco, CA, USA
e-mail: christopher.owens@ucsfmedctr.org

C.D. Owens and Y. Yeghiazarians (eds.),
Handbook of Endovascular Peripheral Interventions,
DOI 10.1007/978-1-4614-0839-0_6,

Growth of Computed Tomography (CT) and Nuclear Medicine Examinations in the United States

Examination	1980	2005
CT	3,000,000	60,000,000
Nuclear medicine	7,000,000	20,000,000

Safety

Tips for Safe Procedures

- Accurate History and Physical
- Thorough review of labs and prior imaging. Prior imaging is critical to determine access site planning and may minimize fluoroscopy time. For example, if you are planning a femoral artery intervention and the patient has a recent contrast-enhanced magnetic resonance angiogram demonstrating patent aorta and iliacs then the pelvic portion of the angiogram can be omitted
- Correctly performed timeout (at a minimum, confirm patient identity, procedure to be performed, side/site, allergies, and outstanding lab values)
- Universal precautions including safe handling of all sharps
- Appropriate patient monitoring
- Clearly labeled medications such as heparinized-slaine, contrast, nitroglycerine, or lidocaine to avoid medication errors
- Meticulous angiographic technique

Radiation Safety: Operators and Patients

- Know your fluoroscopy room and all of the safety measures, Fig. 6.1
- Be vigilant about limiting fluoroscopy

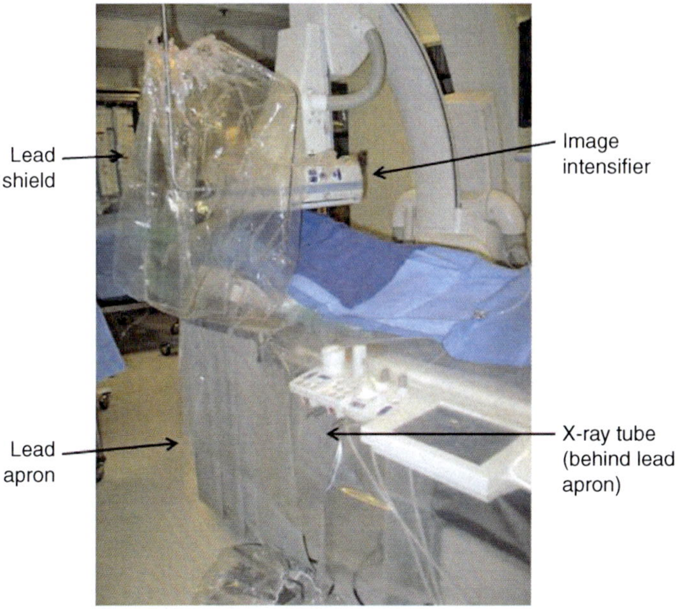

FIGURE 6.1 Anatomy of the interventional suite

- Practice proper beam collimation. Collimation at the target brings about a genuine dose reduction and also produces better image quality. Collimation is performed using cones and collimators (multi-leaf collimators or iris diaphragms) that are attached directly in front of the X-ray tube. Collimation at the target is the most effective radiation protection for the patient and personnel, because it narrows the area that the radiation can strike
- Minimize the distance between the image intensifier and the patient and maximize source to patient distance
- Use the radiation-reducing features available in the newer angiography suites (pulse fluoroscopy, last-image hold, virtual collimation; automated recording of radiation dose)
- For the operator, the cumulative exposure to radiation is important: practice judicious use of lead shielding and use

Radiation Safety Pearls

- Avoid excessive fluoroscopy times – when your eyes are not looking at the monitor, step off of the pedal. Perform non-critical wire exchanges without fluoroscopy. Document fluoroscopy times in your procedure notes
- Minimize scatter radiation: minimize the distance between the image intensifier and the patient, see Fig. 6.2 below
- Reduce radiation exposure: lead shields, use radiation-reducing safety features, leaded glasses
- Use collimation
- Position yourself in a low scatter area

radiation badges, regularly-tested lead aprons, thyroid shields, and leaded glasses should be worn at all times (the recently reported higher rate of cataracts among IR physicians underscores the importance of regular use of leaded glasses)

- Patient radiation injury: prolonged fluoroscopic times as seen with particularly complex interventions
- Appropriate changes in the tube angles during complex cases will help minimize the chances of radiation injury to the skin
- Always adhere to the ALARA principle, "As Low As Reasonably Achievable"
  - There is no known absolutely safe dose of ionizing radiation
  - The smaller the dose, the less the risk of adverse effect
  - Incremental radiation exposures have cumulative effects (Tables 6.1 and 6.2)

Table 6.1 Radiation safety terminology

Quantity	Units of measurement	What it is	What it measures	Why it is useful	Conversion between old and new units
Absorbed dose	Gray (Gy) or milligray (mGy) [rad or millirad (mrad)]	The amount of energy locally deposited in tissue per unit mass of tissue	Measures concentration of energy deposition in tissue	Assess the potential biological risk to that specific tissue	1 rad = 10 mGy
Effective dose	Sievert (Sv) or millisievert (mSv) [rem or millirem (mrem)]	An attributed whole-body dose that produces the same whole-person stochastic risk as an absorbed dose to a limited portion of the body	Converts any localized absorbed or equivalent dose to a whole-body risk factor	Permits comparison of risks among several exposed individuals, even though the doses might be delivered to different sets of organs in these individuals	1 rem = 10 mSv
Air kerma	Gray (Gy) or milligray (mGy) [rad or millirad (mrad)]	The sum of initial kinetic energies of all charged particles liberated by the X-rays per mass of air	Measures amount of radiation at a point in space	Assesses the level of hazard at the specified location	1 rad = 10 mGy

(continued)

Table 6.1 (continued)

Quantity	Units of measurement	What it is	What it measures	Why it is useful	Conversion between old and new units
Exposure	millicoulomb•kg^{-1} [roentgen (R) or milliroentgen mR]	The total charge of ions of one sign produced by the radiation per unit of mass of air	Measures amount of radiation at a point in space	Assesses the level of hazard at the specified location	1 millicoulomb•kg^{-1} = 4Roentgen (R)
Equivalent dose	Sievert (Sv) or millisievert (mSv) [rem or millirem (mrem)]	A dose quantity that factors in the relative biological damage caused by different types of radiations	Provides a relative dose that accounts for increased biological damage from some types of radiations	This is the most common unit used to measure radiation risk to specific tissues for radiation protection of personnel	1 rem = 10 mSv

Source: From A Report of the American College of Cardiology Foundation/American Heart Association American College of Physicians Task Force on Clinical Competence Training. Adopted from the Journal of the American College of Cardiology Decmeber 7th 2004:2259–82

TABLE 6.2 Patient safety thresholds

Single dose effect	**Threshold (Gy)**	**Onset**
Early transient erythema	2	Hours
Main erythema	6	≈ 10 days
Late erythema	15	≈ 6–10 weeks
Temporary epilation	3	≈ 3 weeks
Permanent epilation	7	≈ 3 weeks
Dry desquamation	14	≈ 4 weeks
Moist desquamation	18	≈ 4 weeks
Secondary ulceration	24	>6 weeks
Ischemic dermal necrosis	18	>10 weeks
Dermal atrophy 1st phase	10	>14 weeks
Dermal atrophy 2nd phase	10	>1 year
Induration (invasive fibrosis)	10	Not known
Telangiectasia	10	>1 year
Lat edermal necrosis	>12	>1 year
Skin cancer	Not known	>5 years

The importance of judicial use of table height and image intensifier (II) position is illustrated in Fig. 6.3. It is good practice to keep the X-ray tube away from the patient while having the II close to the patient. As a consequence of placing the X-ray tube in close proximity to the patient and having the II away from the patient, the patient on the left receives over 200% of the skin dose as the patient on the right. In addition, the image generated by the configuration on the left is 40–50% larger owing to geometric magnification caused by the elevated II.

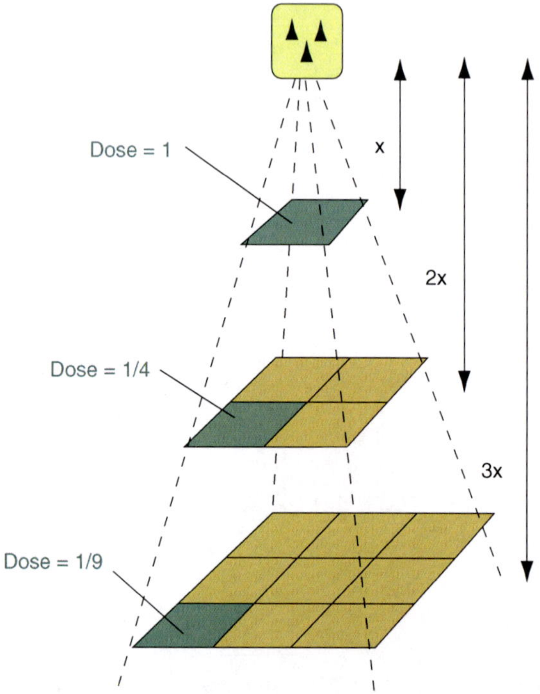

FIGURE 6.2 The principle of the inverse square law. Doubling the distance between the operator and X-ray tube decreases the radiation dose by 1/4th and tripling the distance minimizes exposure by 1/9th

Infectious Disease Safety

- The risk of transmission of pathogens from the patients to physicians is of concern, therefore universal precautions must be observed at all times.
- The obvious risk of hepatitis B or C and HIV transmission has mandated the use of universal precautions:
  - Routine use of surgical gowns
  - Masks (preferably with face shields)
  - Protective eyewear, and double gloves

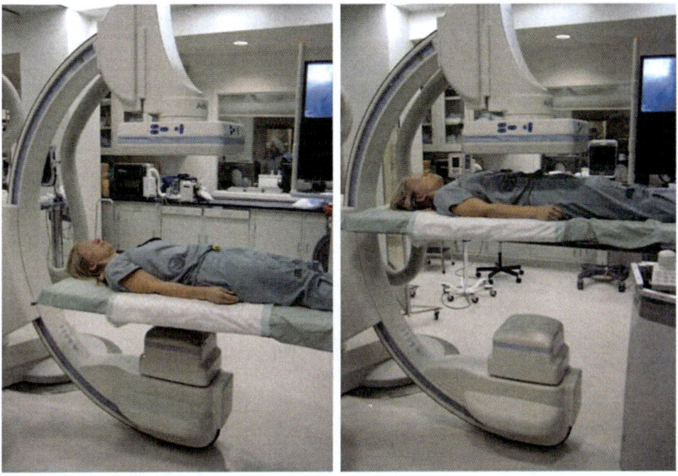

FIGURE 6.3 The importance of judicial use of table height and image intensifier (II) position is illustrated. It is good practice to keep the X-ray tube away from the patient while having the II close to the patient. As a consequence of placing the X-ray tube in close proximity to the patient and having the II away from the patient, the patient on the left receives over 200% of the skin dose as the patient on the right. In addition, the image generated by the configuration on the left is 40–50% larger owing to geometric magnification caused by the elevated II

  - Gloves should be changed during prolonged cases or whenever gloves have been damaged
  - Sharps should be safely handled: never recap needles, use safety needles, place all needles in sharp containers and all other sharp instruments should be kept in a known secure place on the angiographic table
  - If a needle stick occurs, the appropriate safety experts should be consulted immediately
- Concern about patient to patient infectious transmission and MRSA infections also mandates:
  - Use of universal precautions

Sedation Safety

- Minimal sedation (anxiolysis) is defined as a drug-induced state in which patients respond normally to verbal stimulation. Although cognitive function and coordination may be impaired, ventilator and cardiovascular functions are unaffected.
- Moderate sedation should be administered only by trained personnel. Moderate sedation is defined as the degree of sedation during which the patient can purposefully respond to verbal and light tactile stimulation. The airway remains patent and spontaneous ventilation is adequate. Cardiovascular function is usually maintained Moderate sedation is administered for reduction of anxiety and pain induced from the procedure

American Society of Anesthesiologists (ASA) Physical Status Classification

Class I: A normal healthy patient
Class II: A patient with mild systemic disease
Class III: A patient with severe systemic disease
Class IV: A patient with severe systemic disease that is a constant threat to life
Class V: A moribund patient who is not expected to survive without the operation
Class VI: A declared brain-dead patient whose organs are being removed for donor purposes

- It is required that the physician responsible for the administration of moderate sedation be trained in ACLS or pass a local standard test for moderate sedation and a nurse whose primary function during the procedure is to administer medications under the direction of the physician be present and monitor/record the patient's physiologic parameters throughout the case.
- Management during sedation include intravenous access, homeothermia should be preserved, supplemental oxygen should be available, suction should be immediately available, and a defibrillator with back-up emergency power

and emergency cart, including equipment for intubation and ventilation, should be immediately available.

- Patients who are ASA class I or II qualify for sedation/analgesia. Patients who are ASA class III or IV may require consultation with and/or presence of the anesthesiology service in order for the procedure to be performed safely.
- Patients with obstructive sleep apnea must be evaluated carefully. Consultation with the anesthesiology service is recommended.
- Most diagnostic angiogram and endovascular interventions can be performed using moderate sedation. If deeper sedation or general anesthesia is required, the anesthesiology team must be present.
- Appropriate patient monitoring including continuous cardiac monitoring, continuous pulse oximetry, and blood pressure measurement is required.
- Typical doses of medications commonly used: Versed 1 mg IV and fentanyl 50 μg IV or versed 0.5 mg IV and Fentanyl 25 μg IV given at appropriate intervals (for elderly patients or patients with poor liver function the doses are reduced to even Versed 0.25 mg IV, fentanyl 12.5 μg IV). Caution in patients with liver disease, renal failure, or preload-dependent cardiac states (such as severe aortic stenosis or advanced pulmonary hypertension).
- Anesthesia service may need to be present for a procedure to be performed safety and successfully.
- Appropriate post-procedure patient monitoring is equally important.

Clinical Pearls: Our Discharge Criteria Following Moderate Sedation

1. Vital signs are stable
2. Nausea, vomiting, and dizziness are minimal
3. Swallow, cough, and gag reflexes are present
4. Respiratory distress is absent
5. Patient's dressing is intact
6. The patient is able to ambulate
7. The patient's mental status has returned to baseline

8. The patient is able to initiate urinary stream
9. If appropriate, discharge medications or prescriptions are given
10. If the patient is to be discharged home, written instructions are given
11. If the patient meets discharge criteria, he/she must not drive; a responsible adult will escort the patient home

Diagnostic Angiography of Specific Vascular Beds

Purpose

- To obtain detailed diagnostic information, especially in smaller blood vessels (since cross-sectional imaging is very good for larger vessels)
- For planning and performing interventions

Tools

- Flush catheters (e.g., Pigtail, Omni, straight, etc.) and selective end-hole catheters (e.g., Cobra, Sos selective, RIM, Headhunter, Simmons, etc., tailor to anatomy and operator familiarity)
- Wires – floppy vs. stiff; non-hydrophilic vs. hydrophilic; 0.035″ vs. 0.018″ or 0.014″
- Sheaths

Pre-procedure Considerations

- Non-invasive alternatives (can consider CTA/MRA for Aortic arch, carotids, aorta, pelvis, femoropopliteal) to answer or simplify the particular question
- Renal function – catheter angiography, especially selective, may utilize less contrast than CTA [MRA not feasible in renal insufficiency due to risk of nephrogenic systemic fibrosis (NSF)]
- Single-procedure vs. staged (diagnostic, then later therapeutic) – determined by patient tolerance, renal function, need for consultation with referring clinician.

- Figures 6.4–6.9 give examples and practical tips for obtaining anatomical specific views.
- Table 6.3 outlines techniques for obtaining quality views in specific anatomic beds.

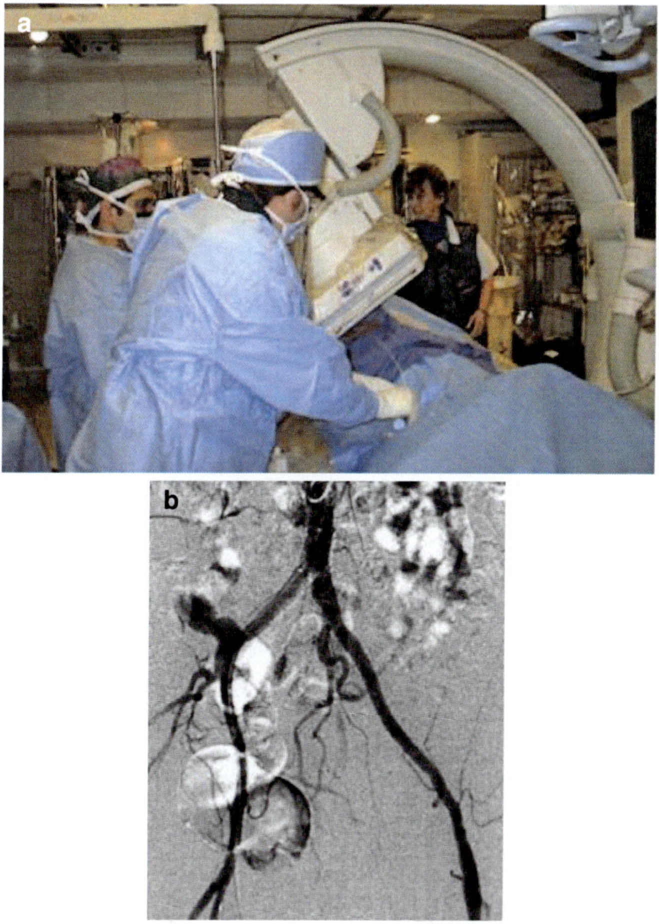

FIGURE 6.4 Right anterior oblique positioning for the pelvis. The right anterior oblique allows better visualization of the left internal and external iliac artery. A complete view of the pelvis would include an AP pelvis and right and left oblique view. (**a**) Right anterior oblique C-ARM positioning. (**b**) Pelvic arteriographic image in the right anterior oblique projection optimally demonstrating the left iliac bifurcation and the right femoral bifurcation

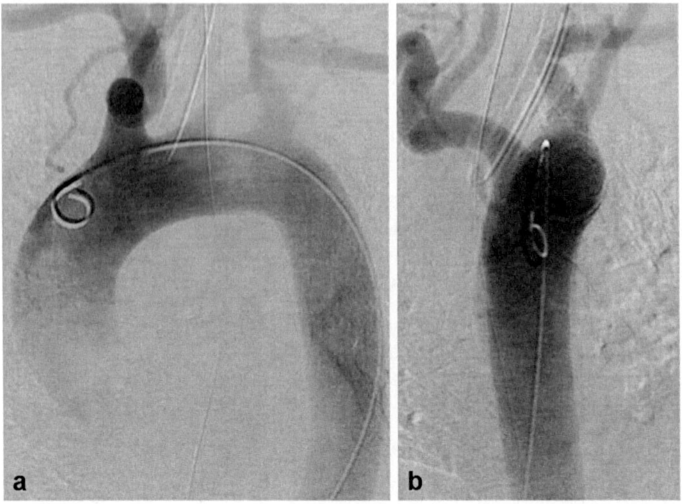

FIGURE 6.5 Aortic arch. Aortic arch angiogram with the pigtail catheter positioned above the aortic valve and the image intensifier obliqued approximately 45° LOA, contrast injection was 20 cc/s for a total of 40 cc (**a**). In the near AP view, the ascending aorta and descending aorta are superimposed as are the origins of the great vessels (**b**)

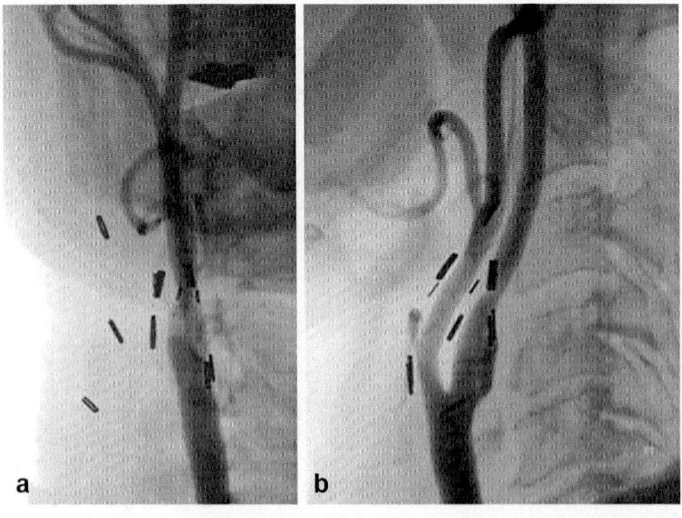

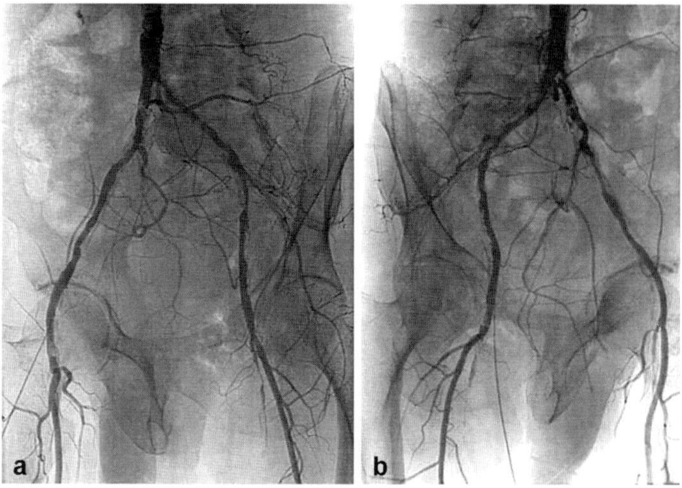

FIGURE 6.7 Iliac/common femoral arteries. Pelvic angiogram with the pigtail catheter positioned just above the aortic bifurcation. The image intensifier is positioned approximately 35° LAO. This obliquity typically lays out the contralateral iliac vessel (R internal iliac origin) and opens the ipsilateral femoral bifurcation. The contrast injection was 8 cc for a total of 16 cc (**a**). Pelvic angiogram with the pigtail catheter positioned just above the aortic bifurcation. The image intensifier is positioned approximately 35° RAO (**b**)

FIGURE 6.6 Carotid vessels. Right common carotid angiogram with the catheter positioned in the proximal common carotid artery and the image intensifier near the AP position. The external and internal carotid arteries are essentially overlapped. The contrast injection was 4 cc/s for a total of 8 cc (**a**). Right common carotid angiogram with the catheter positioned in the proximal common carotid artery and the image intensifier in the lateral position. Now the external and internal carotid arteries are separated nicely. The contrast injection was 4 cc/s for a total of 8 cc (**b**)

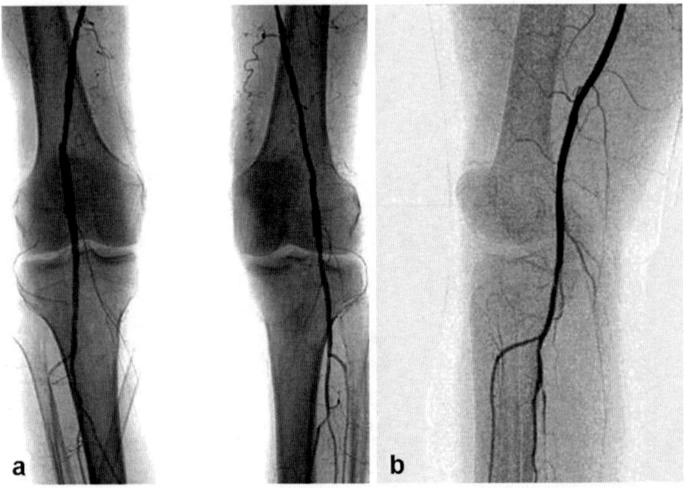

FIGURE 6.8 Trifurcation vessels. Angiogram of both trifurcations with the pigtail catheter positioned just above the Aortic bifurcation. The contrast injection was 10 cc/s for a total of 30 cc. The left foot is slightly turned in (LAO view of the calf) when compared to the right and this can open up the trifurcation and take the vessels off of the bones (**a**). Lateral angiogram of the left trifurcation with a straight catheter in the left external iliac artery and the image intensifier in the 90° lateral position. This view nicely shows the origins of the trifurcation vessels (**b**)

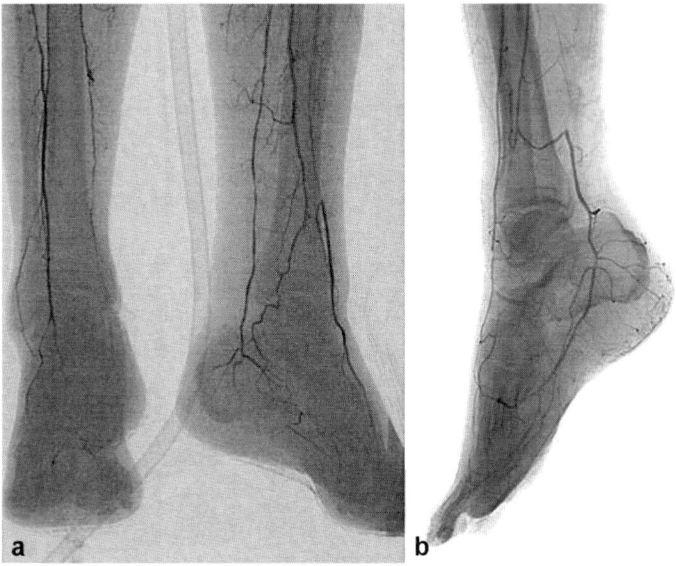

FIGURE 6.9 Foot vessels. Angiogram of both feet with the pigtail catheter in the distal aorta and a contrast injection of 10 cc/s for a total of 40 cc. The right foot is in the near AP position and the left foot has been turned out laterally. This demonstrates the value of a lateral foot view in separating the vessels as they supply the foot (**a**). Another lateral foot angiogram with the a straight catheter in the left external iliac artery and the foot turned out completely laterally showing the nice separation of the foot vessels. The contrast injection was 5 cc/s for a total of 25 cc (**b**)

TABLE 6.3 Techniques for obtaining quality views in specific anatomic beds

Vascular bed	Injection rate of mL per s/total volume in mL	II angle	Preferred selective catheter	Catheter location	Special comments	Other considerations
Aortic arch	20/40	LAO 45	5 Fr Pigtail or other flush-type catheter	Just above the aortic valve	Candycane view to open up the arch	Avoid air bubbles, avoid excessive arch manipulation
Carotids	4–6/6–12	Lateral or steep ipsilateral oblique	Headhunter Simmons Vitek	Common carotid artery	Use RAO to separate right subclavian from right common carotid	Meticulous attention to avoid even the smallest air bubbles during injections/flushes
Pelvis (See Fig. 6.4)	7–10/14–20	RAO and LAO 30–35	Pigtail or other flush-type catheter	Just above the aortic bifurcation	RAO opens left iliac and right femoral bifurcations LAO opens right iliac and left femoral bifurcations	Breath-hold with rapid filming rate

Bilateral lower extremities – bolus-chase	7/77	AP with legs in anatomic position	Pigtail or other flush-type catheter	Just above the aortic bifurcation		Initial breath-hold
Bilateral lower extremities – stages	7–10/14–15 7–10/14–20	AP	Pigtail or other flush-type catheter	Just above the aortic bifurcation	Legs in anatomic position	Diminish filming rate and consider imaging delay as moving distally
Proximal thighs	7–10/21–25					
Distal thighs						
Knees and prox legs						
Distal legs and ankles/feet	7–10/28–30					
Unilateral lower extremity – bolus chase	4/44	IAO 30 Ipsilateral to extremity being studied	4 or 5 Fr, sheath OR selective, end-hole catheter – cobra, sos selective, etc.	Tip in external iliac artery	Leg in anatomic position	

(continued)

Table 6.3 (continued)

Vascular bed	Injection rate of mL per s/total volume in mL	II angle	Preferred selective catheter	Catheter location	Special comments	Other considerations
Unilater lower extremity – stages	4–5/8–10	IAO 30 IAO 30–45	4 or 5 Fr, sheath OR selective, end-hole catheter	Tip in external iliac artery	Steeper II angle if imaging femoral bypass origin	Intermediate filming rate for thigh and knee
Femoral bifurcation and thigh	4–5/12–15					Slower filming rate for leg
Knee	4–5/16–20	IAO 30–45				
Proximal and distal calf	4–5/20–25				Angle to widen interosseous space – will separate infrapopliteal arteries proximally	
Ankle/foot		Lateral view of ankle/foot				Slow filming rate and consider imaging delay for ankle/foot

Bibliography

LaBerge JM, Gordon RL, Kerlan RK, Wilson MW. Interventional Radiology Essentials. Philadelphia: Lippincott Williams & Wilkins.

→ *Small textbook providing concise review of interventional radiology, including diagnostic and interventional vascular procedures; includes numerous images.*

Valji K. Vascular and Interventional Radiology. Philadelphia: W.B. Saunders.

→ *Medium-sized textbook that is well-organized and contains many images for vascular and non-vascular procedures.*

Reza Fazel, M.D., M.Sc., Harlan M. Krumholz, M.D., S.M., Yongfei Wang, M.S., Joseph S. Ross, M.D., Jersey Chen, M.D., M.P.H., Henry H. Ting, M.D., M.B.A., Nilay D. Shah, Ph.D., Khurram Nasir, M.D., M.P.H., Andrew J. Einstein, M.D., Ph.D., and Brahmajee K. Nallamothu, M.D., M.P.H. Exposure to Low-Dose Ionizing Radiation from Medical Imaging Procedures. N Engl J Med 2009; 361:849–857.

→ *Article describing ionizing radiation exposure resulting from medical imaging procedures.*

Comparing Strategies for Operator Eye Protection in the Interventional Radiology Suite, Raymond H. Thornton, Lawrence T. Dauer, Joaquin P. Altamirano, Keith J. Alvarado, Jean St. Germain, Stephen B. Solomon JVIR 2010; 21: 1703–1707.

→ *Article describing effects of ionizing radiation to eyes of operator and ways to diminish exposure.*

Practice Guidelines for Sedation and Analgesia by Non-Anesthesiologists: An updated report by the American Society of Anesthesiologists Task Force on sedation and analgesia by non-anesthesiologists. Anesthesiology 2002; 96:1004–17.

→ *Practical society guidelines for sedation and analgesia by non-anesthesiologists.*

American College of Radiology. ACR technical standard for management of the use of radiation in fluoroscopic procedures. Practice Guidelines and Technical Standards 2003. Reston, VA: American College of Radiology, 2003;669–673. Board guidelines summarized.

Stecker MS, Balter S, Towbin RB, et al. Guidelines for Patient Radiation Dose Management. J Vasc Interv Radiol 2009; 20: S263-S273.

→ *Society guidelines for patient radiation dose management.*

Chapter 7 Prevention of Contrast-Induced Nephropathy

Andrew Lin and Kerry C. Cho

Definition of Contrast-Induced Nephropathy

- There is no consensus definition of contrast-induced nephropathy (CIN). Commonly used definitions include an increase in serum creatinine of 0.5 mg/dL or a 25% increase above baseline within 48 h of contrast.
- Acute renal failure that develops more than 3 days after contrast exposure is not likely to be CIN. Atheroembolic disease should be considered as a diagnosis in these cases, especially in patients thought to be at lower risk for CIN who develop acute renal failure post-procedure. Other stigmata of atheroembolic disease include embolization, livedo reticularis, peripheral eosinophilia, non-recovery of kidney function, recent anticoagulation, or vascular instrumentation.

A. Lin • K.C. Cho (✉)
Division of Nephrology, Department of Medicine,
University of California – San Francisco,
San Francisco, CA, USA
e-mail: alin000@hotmail.com; kerry.cho@ucsf.edu

C.D. Owens and Y. Yeghiazarians (eds.),
Handbook of Endovascular Peripheral Interventions,
DOI 10.1007/978-1-4614-0839-0_7,

Pathophysiology

CIN is thought to be caused by a combination of vasoconstriction, direct renal tubular damage, and formation of reactive oxygen species caused by IV contrast administration.

Risk Factors

- Most commonly cited risk factors for CIN: pre-existing kidney disease (estimated GFR < 60 mL/min/1.73 m^2) and particularly diabetic nephropathy, diabetes mellitus, large contrast volume, congestive heart failure, hemodynamic instability.
- Other risk factors: Age >75 years old, intra-arterial administration > intravenous administration of contrast, concomitant use of NSAIDs/nephrotoxins, baseline anemia.

Calculating Risk of CIN

- One simple algorithm to estimate risk of CIN is shown in Table 7.1.
- Each risk factor is assigned a point score in the chart on the left. Add up the points for all the risk factors to determine a total score. Use the total score with the chart on the right to determine the risk of CIN and risk of dialysis after contrast.

Contrast and Osmolality

- There are three categories of radiocontrast media: hyperosmolar (1,400–2,100 mosm/kg), low osmolar (500–900 mosm/kg), and isoosmolar (290 mosm/kg) (Table 7.2).
- Normal serum osmolality is 285–295 mosm/kg.

TABLE 7.1 Risk score for predicting CIN

Risk factor	Points	Score	Risk of CIN (%)	Risk of dialysis (%)
Hypotension	5	≤5	7.5	0.04
IABP	5	6–10	14	0.12
CHF	5	11–16	26.1	1.09
Age > 75	4	≥16	57.3	12.6
Anemia	3			
DM	3			
Contrast volume	1 point per 100 mL			
Serum Cr > 1.5	4			
OR				
eGFR:				
40–60	2			
20–40	4			
<20	6			

Source: Mehran et al. *J Am Coll Cardiol* 2004; 44(7):1393–9
IABP intra-aortic balloon pump, *DM* diabetes mellitus, *Cr* creatinine

Table 7.2 Osmolalities of various radiocontrast media

Hyperosmolar	Osm	Low osmolar	Osm	Isoosmolar	Osm
Diatrizoate (Hypaque 50)	1,550	Ioxaglate (Hexabrix 320)	580	Iodixanol (Visipaque 320)	290
Metrizoate (Isopaque Coronar 370)	2,100	Iopamidol (Isovue 370)	796		
		Iohexol (Omnipaque 350)	884		
		Ioxilan (Oxilan 350)	695		
		Iopromide (Ultravist 370)	774		
		Iopentol (Imagopaque 350)	810		

Contrast Osmolality and Risk of CIN

- Low osmolar contrast is associated with lower rates of CIN compared with hyperosmolar contrast.
- Differences in CIN risk between various low osmolar contrast dyes (ionic vs. non-ionic, monomeric vs. dimeric) have not been established.
- Studies comparing isoosmolar and low osmolar contrast are mixed, however, a meta-analysis by McCullough et al. in 2006 showed a lower rate of CIN when using isoosmolar contrast vs. low osmolar contrast (1.4% vs. 3.5%, $p<0.001$).

Potential Agents for CIN Prophylaxis

Administration of isotonic IV fluids is the mainstay of CIN prophylaxis. Other means of preventing CIN such as IV sodium bicarbonate and *N*-acetylcysteine are not well proven.

Isotonic Saline (0.9%) vs. Half-Isotonic Saline (0.45%)

- Mueller et al. in Archives of Internal Medicine 2002 showed that administration of isotonic saline showed significantly lower rates of CIN after cardiac cath compared with half-isotonic saline with 5% dextrose (0.7% vs. 2%).
- Fluids were given at a rate of 1 mL/kg, starting at 8 a.m. on the morning of procedure and continued until 8 a.m. the next day. Emergent cases received a 500 mL bolus of Lactated Ringer's solution and then received saline at 1 mL/kg until 8 a.m. the next day.

Potential Pitfalls

- Administration of IV sodium bicarbonate can decrease serum potassium and calcium levels

- Isotonic saline is a reasonable alternative to IV sodium bicarbonate for CIN prophylaxis in patients with low potassium or calcium
- Careful with hydration of patients who are in a fluid-overload state prior to the procedure (e.g., heart failure)

Sodium Bicarbonate vs. Isotonic Saline

- One of the first studies comparing sodium bicarbonate and saline was published by Merten et al. in JAMA 2004.
- IV Sodium Bicarbonate (154 mEq/L) or IV saline (154 mEq/L) were given 3 mL/kg/h × 1 h prior to contrast, then 1 mL/kg/h × 6 h after contrast. Sodium bicarbonate reduced the risk of CIN compared to saline (1.7% vs. 13.6%).
- Several prospective studies and meta-analyses have been done since then with mixed results.

N-Acetylcysteine (NAC)

- Effectiveness of NAC in preventing CIN is uncertain. Multiple studies have been done with both positive and negative results (Kagan and Sheikh-Hamad. Clin Cardiol 2002).
- Patients who received NAC + half-normal saline had a reduced risk of CIN compared with those who received half-normal saline alone (Tepel et al. in NEJM 2000). The protocol used was 600 mg PO BID on the day prior to contrast and the day of contrast administration.
- Various NAC protocols have been used since then. Doses range from 600 to 1,200 mg, given once or twice per day, beginning 1–2 days prior to contrast and continuing 1–2 days after contrast, given both PO and IV. IV NAC may be difficult to obtain and more expensive than PO NAC and has been associated with anaphylaxis.
- A meta-analysis by Trivedi et al. in 2009 suggests high dose of NAC may be beneficial. High dose is defined as a daily

dose >1,200 mg or a single peri-procedural dose >600 mg (given within 4 h prior to contrast). The authors suggest a NAC protocol of 1,200 mg × 1 prior to contrast administration followed by 1,200 mg BID × 48 h.

- Although evidence supporting use of NAC is weak, NAC administration is generally recommended because of its low cost and relative safety.
- Given the wide variability of NAC studies in terms of methods and outcomes, the optimal protocol for NAC administration is not known. The NAC protocol suggested in the original study by Tepel et al. would be a reasonable choice, although higher dose protocols could be considered.

Renal Replacement Therapy (Hemofiltration and Hemodialysis)

- Hemodialysis immediately after contrast has been shown not to be effective in preventing CIN in many small studies.
- Continuous veno-venous hemofiltration (CVVH) for CIN prophylaxis was studied by Marenzi et al. in 2003. CVVH with NS initiated 4–8 h prior to cardiac catheterization and continued 18–24 h after contrast compared with NS alone showed decreased rate of CIN and decreased mortality. Some question the validity of the results, since CVVH itself removes creatinine from the serum, and therefore decreases serum creatinine without any true improvement in kidney function or prevention of CIN.

Diuretics

- Diuretics such as mannitol and furosemide may increase the risk of CIN due to volume contraction.

Preventing Contrast-Induced Nephropathy: How I Do It

- Determine patient's risk for CIN based on risk factors and clinical situation. The risk score proposed by Mehran et al. can provide a rough estimate of a patient's risk for developing kidney injury after contrast (see Table 7.1).

- Patients with eGFR < 60 mL/min should be considered for prophylaxis, especially in the presence of additional risk factors.
- Administer isotonic IV fluids, either 154 mEq/L sodium bicarbonate or 154 mEq/L saline (0.9% saline). A common protocol is 3 mL/kg × 1 h prior to contrast, then 1 mL/kg/h × 6 h after contrast.
- Although the effectiveness of sodium bicarbonate is not completely established, it is relatively safe and has some evidence of possible benefit, and therefore it is generally favored over saline. Bottom line: the administration of IV fluids is more important than the composition of the IV fluids.
- If patient has low serum potassium or calcium, use caution when giving IV sodium bicarbonate and strongly consider giving isotonic saline instead, since sodium bicarbonate can cause hypokalemia and hypocalcemia.
- Evidence for NAC is weak, but it is safe and inexpensive. The optimal protocol for NAC administration is not known. The protocol used in the original study by Tepel et al. would be a reasonable choice (600 mg PO BID the day before and the day of contrast), although higher dose protocols could be considered.
- In high-risk patients, use iso-osmolar contrast if possible, or if unavailable use low osmolar contrast.
- Consider performing catheterizations/interventions as staged procedures with separation of the diagnostic and interventional portions by at least several days to minimize the volume of contrast administered at one time.
- CVVH and hemodialysis are not routinely recommended for CIN prophylaxis.
- High-risk patients should be monitored for development of CIN with routine labs, BUN, and creatinine 2–3 days following contrast administration. Clinical utility of urinary markers such as NGAL, IL-18, and cystatin C have not yet been fully established and are not routinely recommended.

Bibliography

1. Kagan A and D Sheikh-Hamad. Contrast-induced Kidney Injury: Focus on Modifiable Risk Factors and Prophylactic Strategies. Clin Cardiol. 2010; 33(2): 62–66.

   → *An excellent overview of risk factors, pathophysiology, and prevention of CIN.*

2. Jawdeh B, AA Kanso, JR Schelling. Evidence-based Approach for Prevention of Radiocontrast-induced Nephropathy. J Hosp Med. 2009 Oct; 4(8): 500–506.

   → *Another review of CIN with more in-depth discussion of CIN prophylaxis.*

3. Mehran R, ED Aymong, E Nikolsky, et al. A Simple Risk Score for Prediction of Contrast-Induced Nephropathy After Percutaneous Coronary Intervention: Development and Initial Validation. J Am Coll Cardiol. 2004 Oct 6; 44(7): 1393–1399.

   → *Provides a method to calculate risk of CIN based on patient risk factors.*

4. Mueller C, G Buerkle, HJ Buettner et al. Prevention of contrast media-associated nephropathy. Arch Int Med. 2002; 162: 329–336.

   → *Prospective randomized controlled trial comparing isotonic saline vs. half-isotonic saline in prevention of contrast induced nephropathy.*

5. Merten GJ, WP Burgess, LV Gray, et al. Prevention of contrast-induced nephropathy with sodium bicarbonate. JAMA 2004; 291: 2328–2334.

   → *One of the first prospective trials showing IV sodium bicarbonate reduces the risk of CIN.*

6. Hoste E, De Waele JJ, Gevaert SA, et al. Sodium bicarbonate for prevention of contrast-induced acute kidney injury: a systematic review and meta-analysis. Nephrol Dial Transplant. 2010; 25: 747–758.

   → *A recent meta-analysis showing reduced rates of CIN when using sodium bicarbonate vs. saline.*

7. Tepel M, vander Giet M, Schwarzfeld C et al. Prevention of radiographic-contrast-agent-induced reductions in renal function by acetylcysteine. N Engl J Med. 2000; 343: 180–4.

   → *First clinical trial showing benefit of NAC in CIN prevention.*

8. Trivedi H, S Daram, A Szabo, et al. High-dose N-acetylcysteine for the prevention of contrast-induced nephropathy. Am J Med. 2009; 122: 874.e9-874.e15.

   → *A meta-analysis showing benefit of high dose N-acetylcysteine for CIN prevention.*

9. McCullough PA, Bertrand ME, Brinker JA, Stacul F. A meta-analysis of the renal safety of isoosmolar iodixanol compared with low-osmolar contrast media. J Am Coll Cardiol. 2006; 48(4): 692–699.
   → *A meta-analysis showing a lower rate of CIN with iodixanol (isoosmolar contrast) compared with low osmolar contrast media.*
10. Marenzi G, Marana I, Lauri G et al. The prevention of radiocontrast-agent-induced nephropathy by hemofiltration. N Engl J Med. 2003; 349: 1333–1340.
   → *Prospective clinical trial comparing CVVH vs. control to prevent contrast-induced nephropathy.*

Chapter 8
Anticoagulation, Thrombolysis, and Mechanical Thrombectomy for Acute Limb Ischemia

Lincoln Roland and Andres Schanzer

Acute Limb Ischemia (ALI)

A sudden decrease in arterial perfusion of an extremity resulting in a potential threat to limb viability.

> **Clinical Pointers: Embolus vs. Thrombosis**
> Differentiating embolization from thrombosis has direct implications on prognosis and treatment.
> Emboli usually lodge at arterial bifurcations (where there is a change in vessel caliber) with the most frequent locations being the bifurcation of the common femoral artery, popliteal artery, and brachial artery.
> Thrombosis of a chronically diseased artery may be accompanied by large collaterals thereby causing less severe ischemia as compared to an embolic event.

L. Roland (✉) • A. Schanzer
Department of Vascular Surgery,
University of Massachusetts Medical School, Worcester, MA, USA
e-mail: rolandl@ccf.org; andres.schanzer@umassmemorial.org

C.D. Owens and Y. Yeghiazarians (eds.), *Handbook of Endovascular Peripheral Interventions*,
DOI 10.1007/978-1-4614-0839-0_8,

Etiology

Embolization: Most common source is mural thrombus originating in the heart followed by atherosclerotic debris from a diseased proximal artery.

Thrombosis: Occurs secondary to progressive atherosclerotic obstruction, often in the setting of a low flow or hypercoagulable state.

Dissection: Disruption of flow (arterial malperfusion) due to either static or dynamic obstruction by an intimal flap.

Background

Anticoagulation: Goal is to prevent thrombus progression above and below the site of clot which has already formed.

Thrombolysis: Goal is to lyse thrombus through activation of plasminogen.

Mechanical thrombectomy: Goal is to break up and aspirate thrombus.

Prevalence

Based on the largest studies to date assessing the efficacy of anticoagulation, thrombolysis, and mechanical thrombectomy in patients with ALI, the Surgery vs. Thrombolysis for Ischemia of the Lower Extremity (STILE) trial and the Thrombolysis of Peripheral Arterial Surgery (TOPAS) trial, approximately 50% of patients with ALI present with symptoms within 14 days and may be suitable candidates.

The Rutherford classification (Table 8.1) may be helpful in stratifying patients according to their severity and thereby assist in determining who might benefit from immediate surgical revascularization as opposed to endovascular attempts at revascularization (i.e., Rutherford 2b and Rutherford III). On presentation, of affected extremities, 45% are viable, 45% are threatened, and 10% are nonviable.

TABLE 8.1 Rutherford classification and stratification of limb viability

		Findings		Doppler signals	
Category	**Description**	**Sensory loss**	**Muscle weakness**	**Arterial**	**Venous**
I. Viable	Not immediately threatened	None	None	Audible	Audible
II. Threatened					
(a) Marginal	Salvageable if properly treated	Minimal (toes) or none	None	Often inaudible	Audible
(b) Immediate	Salvageable with immediate revascularization	More than toes, associated with rest pain	Mild, moderate	Usually inaudible	Audible
III. Irreversible	Major tissue loss or permanent nerve damage inevitable	Profound, anesthetic	Profound, paralysis (rigor)	Inaudible	Inaudible

Adapted from TASC II

Clinical Presentation

Pulselessness: Absence of pulse or doppler signal signifies impaired arterial perfusion.
Pain: The majority of patients report severe pain at rest.
Pallor: Color changes can be subtle and misleading due to accompanying dependent rubor or a mottled appearance.
Parasthesia: Sensory loss implies ongoing nerve injury.
Paralysis: A late finding consistent with severe ischemia.
Poikilothermia: The classic finding of a "cold extremity" can be variable depending on the ambient environment and may be absent when external warming devices are utilized (i.e., bear hugger).

Clinical Pointers
Diagnosis can be difficult and clinical sequelae resulting from a delay in diagnosis may be severe. Although variable, irreversible nerve injury followed by muscle necrosis is observed approximately 6 h from the onset of ischemia. ALI is an emergency and an appropriate treatment plan should be instituted immediately.

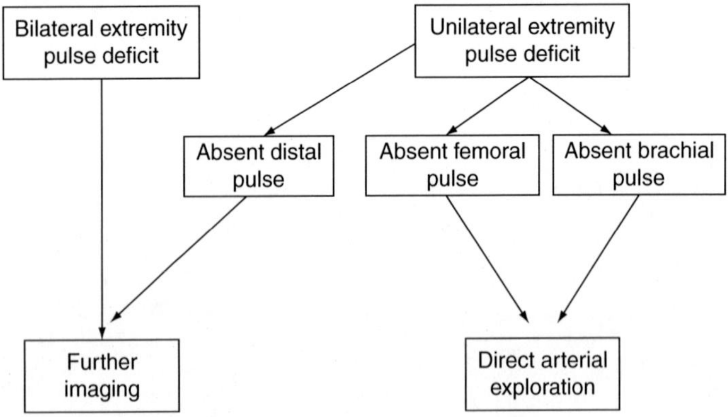

FIGURE 8.1 Pulse exam often guides management

Initial Evaluation

History: there is absolutely no substitute for a good history. Duration of symptoms, time of onset, location, and previous revascularization, all provide important clues. Past history of claudication and recent instrumentation should be explored.

A complete history and physical examination is imperative with a special emphasis on the following factors (Figs. 8.1 and 8.2):

- Vascular risk factors
- Prior vascular disease

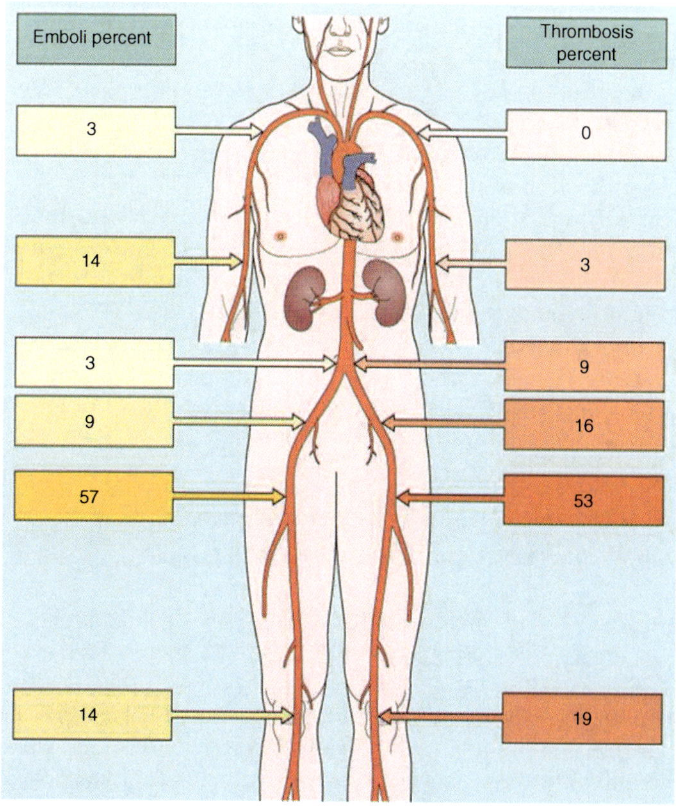

FIGURE 8.2 The relative frequency of embolic events by anatomic location

- Arrhythmias
- Coagulation disorders
- Cardiac exam (i.e., cardiac myxoma)
- Pulse exam
- Motor and sensory exam
- Careful examination of the unaffected extremity to assess for asymmetry

Attempt to Determine Etiology

Embolus: arrhythmia (past or current), cessation of anticoagulation, known thoracic/abdominal aneurysm, or atherosclerotic disease.
Native thrombosis: previous revascularization, known peripheral arterial disease.
Dissection: acute onset chest and back pain.
Quantification of the Severity of Ischemia.
Ankle-Brachial Index (ABI): objective measure of arterial perfusion. The presence of a pulse or Doppler signal does not necessarily rule out ALI. A decrease in ABI of at least 0.15 from previous documentation is significant.
Arterial Imaging: In cases where the affected limb is not immediately threatened (no motor or sensory changes); duplex and/or CTA can assist in localization of the lesion.

Randomized Trial Data Assessing the Role of Thrombolysis in Patients with ALI

Surgery vs. Thrombolysis for Ischemia of the Lower Extremity (STILE) Trial

In patients with acute (symptoms less than 14 days) lower extremity ischemia, catheter-directed thrombolysis with recombinant tissue plasminogen activator or urokinase was associated with improved amputation-free survival and shorter hospital stays in comparison to surgery.

Rochester Study

Patients with ALI randomized to thrombolysis had decreased perioperative mortality rates compared to those randomized to surgical revascularization.

Thrombolysis or Peripheral Artery Surgery Trial (TOPAS)

This study demonstrated equivalent 1-year amputation-free survival in the thrombolysis and surgical groups. However, the magnitude of open surgery required was significantly reduced in the thrombolysis group.

Treatment

- Patients with stage I or stage IIa ischemia are appropriate candidates for anticoagulation, thrombolysis, and mechanical thrombectomy.
  - Anticoagulation: In order to halt the clotting process and avoid further propagation of clot, all patients with suspected ALI should be treated with intravenous heparin. An initial bolus of 80 U/kg and an intravenous drip at 18 U/kg/h should be instituted. Heparin also plays a role in preventing pericatheter thrombosis during thrombolysis therapy.
  - In the case of heparin-induced thrombocytopenia (HIT), we use bivalirudin. This has the shortest half life among the heparin substitutes, provided the patient is not dialysis-dependent. In dialysis-dependent patients argatroban is used due to its shorter half-life. There are no data to support the use of antiplatelet agents in the acute period (i.e., aspirin, clopidogrel, Gp 2b, 3a inhibitors).
    - BIVALIRUDIN DOSING: Bolus 0.4 mg/kg over 1 min followed by an infusion of 1 mg/kg/h. An ACT is performed 5 min after the loading dose. If less than twice control a smaller bolus of 0.2 mg/kg over 30 s is administered. An ACT is checked every hour during infusion until a goal of 2–2.5 times control is maintained.

TABLE 8.2 Contraindication to thrombolysis

Absolute contraindications
1. Established cerebrovascular event (excluding TIA within previous 2 months)
2. Active bleeding diasthesis
3. Recent gastrointestinal bleeding (within previous 10 months)
4. Intracranial trauma within previous 3 months
Relative contraindications
1. Cardiopulmonary resusitation within previous 10 days
2. Major nonvascular surgery or trauma within previous 10 days
3. Uncontrolled hypertension (systolic >180 mmHg or diastolic >110 mmHg)
4. Puncture of noncompressible vessel
5. Intracranial tumor
6. Recent eye surgery
Minor contraindications
1. Hepatic failure, particularly those with coagulopathy
2. Bacterial endocarditis
3. Pregnancy
4. Active diabetic proliferative retinopathy

  - ARGATROBAN DOSING: Bolus 2 mcg/kg over 1 min followed by adjusting the dose until a steady state aPTT of two to three times normal is reached.
- Thrombolysis: Several different agents have been used and tested including prourokinase, urokinase, streptokinase, reteplase, and tissue plasminogen activator. Considering the potential grave nature of the consequences, a contraindication to thrombolysis must be ruled out prior to institution of therapy (Table 8.2).
- Mechanical Thrombectomy: The simplest form is manual aspiration through an end-hole catheter (i.e., pronto catheter or export catheter). We tend to prefer utilizing the angiojet catheter which is a hydrodynamic

Potential Pitfalls

Cerebral bleed can occur at any time (1.2% and 1.6%, respectively in STILE and TOPAS trial).

Life-threatening hematoma – as high as 12.5% in the TOPAS and 5.6% for the STILE trial.

Access-related hematomas are common.

Progression of limb ischemia can occur during thrombolytic therapy.

thrombectomy device. This device uses hydrodynamic energy to break up thrombus into fine particles which are then simultaneously aspirated and removed. An alternative device is the bacchus trellis which consists of a dual balloon system that permits isolation of the segment being treated. Drug infusion and mechanical thrombectomy takes place between the balloons followed by aspiration of debris from side-holes.

- *Strengths*: Functions synergistically with thrombolytic agents but also can be used as a stand-alone therapy if lytic agents are contraindicated. Rapid restoration of limb perfusion with decreased time required for clot extraction. Relatively easy to use.
- *Weaknesses*: The device is expensive. The hydrodynamic therapy can cause damage to the endothelial layer.
- Patients with stage IIB or stage III ischemia should go directly to the operating room for surgical revascularization in order to provide the most timely revascularization strategy possible.

Anticoagulation, Thrombolysis, and Mechanical Thrombectomy: How I Do It

- Access remotely with a 4–6 Fr sheath. Utilization of the contralateral femoral artery is preferred.
- A brachial artery approach may be necessary in select cases when an "up-and-over" approach is not possible (i.e., aortobifemoral bypass or occluded iliac system)

- Begin with a pararenal aortogram using an ultraflush catheter with 20–30 mL of contrast.
- Advance the catheter up and over the aortic bifurcation into the contralateral external iliac artery to obtain an extremity arteriogram.
- Position a 6-Fr guide sheath (Ansel, Balkin, or Arrow) up and over the aortic bifurcation into the external iliac artery in order to provide adequate support for cannulating and crossing the occluded arterial segment.
- A 0.035 Terumo Glidewire and a 4 Fr glide catheter are usually adequate for canulation and crossing of the occluded arterial segment.
- Place a side-hole infusion catheter across the occluded segment and infuse 5 mg of tissue plasminogen activator (tPA) through the catheter. Depending on the length of the clot burden, an infusion catheter with an appropriate infusion length is chosen.
- Begin an infusion of tPA at 1 mg/h through the catheter and an infusion of heparin at 500 U/h through the sheath. Admit the patient to the intensive care unit for 12–24 h of infusion with close monitoring (Fig. 8.3).
- A standardized thrombolysis protocol guides monitoring of the patient and relevant laboratory values – fibrinogen levels, CBC, PT, PTT are checked Q 4 h (Fig. 8.4).
- Neurological and vital signs are checked Q 1 h. Pulse or Doppler exam are performed Q 1 h for the first 4 h and Q 4 h thereafter. Thrombolysis therapy is stopped if fibrinogen level decreases to <100 mg/dL. Please refer to Fig. 8.4.
- Reimage at 12–24 h intervals to assess for progress of clot lysis. We generally do not extend thrombolysis infusion beyond 72 h due to an increased risk of bleeding.
- After successful lysis, flow will often be restored but some residual thrombus will often still be present. Our general practice is to extract this residual thrombus using mechanical thrombectomy.

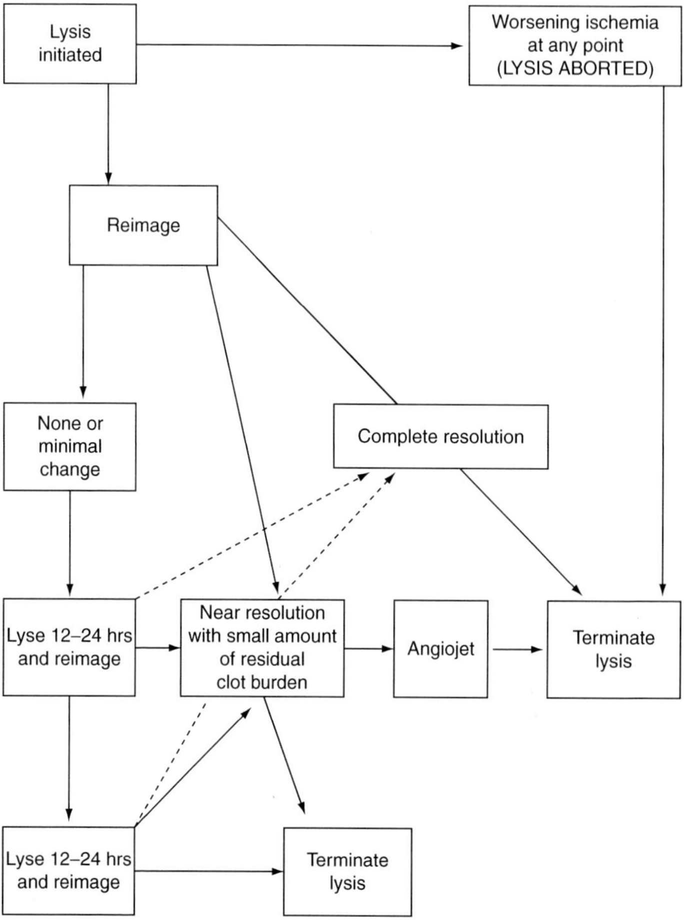

FIGURE 8.3 Treatment algorithm for thrombolysis

- Once arterial flow has been restored, careful completion imaging should be carried out with a focus on identifying any underlying lesion(s) that may have predisposed the patient to the initial thrombotic event.

ALL OTHER ORDERS	DATE	TIME	MEDICATION ORDERS ONLY
Admit to: ICU			☐ D5 1/2 NS w/ 20 mEq KCl/L @ ______ mL/hr IV
Procedure: Angiography & Thrombolysis Catheter			☐ 154 mEq Sodium Bicarbonate in 1 L D5W
placement			@ ______ mL/Hr x 3 hours
Condition:			**Scheduled Medications:**
			☐ 50mg of tPA in 500 mL NS @ ______ mL/hr intraarterial
Diagnosis:			via thrombolysis catheter. D/C if Fibrinogen <100 and
			start NS @ 10 mL/hr
Nursing:			☐ Heparin 500 units/hr via arterial sheath
			☐ NS @ 30 mL/hr if Heparin not infusing
☐ Record vital signs q 1 hour, neurologic check q1 hour			☐ Cefazolin 1 gm IV q 8 hr (patient < 60 kg) while sheath in place
☐ Document hourly intake and output with vital signs			☐ Cefazolin 2 gm IV q 8 hr (patient > 60 kg) while sheath in place
☐ Foley to gravity and record output hourly			**Choose all that apply:** ☐ Penicillin allergy ☐ High MRSA
☐ Weigh patient and record on flow chart by 0600			rate in facility ☐ Known prior colonization with MRSA
☐ ABI every morning			☐ Vancomycin 1000 mg IV q 12 hr (patient 50–70 kg)
			while sheath in place
☐ Check pulses or doppler signals - DP, PT.			☐ Vancomycin 1250 mg IV q 12 hr (patient 71–90 kg)
q1hr x 4 h then q4h			while sheath in place
☐ Incentive spirometry, ten times every hr while awake			☐ Vancomycin 1500 mg IV q 12 hr (patient 91–110 kg)
			while sheath in place
☐ Notify HO if urine output is < 30 mL/hr; MAP <60 or			☐ Vancomycin 2000 mg IV q 12 hr (patient >110 kg) while
>90mmHg; HR <60 or >100, RR <8 or > 20, Temp >38.5;			sheath in place
Any Bleeding, Mental status change, Fibrinogen <100,			☐ Aspirin ______ mg PO/PR daily. Start:
Drop in Fibrinogen >50 between consecutive			☐ Clopidogrel (Plavix) 75 mg po daily
labs, Drop in hemoglobin > 1 between consecutive			☐ Metoprolol ______ mg IV Q6H
labs, PTT > 40			Hold for SBP < 100 and/or HR < 60
☐ Check groin puncture for bleeding/hematoma Q1H			☐ Famotidine 40mg IV daily
Diet:			☐ Ketorolac ______ mg IV q 6hrs x 48 hrs
☐ NPO			☐ Docusate sodium 100 mg PO q 12 hours
☐ Medications with sip of water			**Glucose Control**
			☐ Adult ICU Glycemic Control orders (see sheet)
			☐ Adult Subcutaneous insulin orders (see sheet)
ALL OTHER ORDERS	DATE	TIME	MEDICATION ORDERS ONLY
Activity:			**PRN Medications:**
☐ Bed rest with HOB > 30 degrees;			
☐ R/L leg in knee immobilizer			☐ KCl Protocol via central line IV per standard mix
Diagnostics:			For serum K 3.8–4.0, give KCL 10 mEq over 30 min x 2
			For serum K 3.5 –3.7, give KCl 10 mEq over 30 min x 4
☐ STAT CBC, BMP, Mg, PT, PTT,			and Recheck K in the AM
Fibrinogen on arrival to ICU			For serum K < 3.5, give KCl 10 mEq over 30 min x 6 and
☐ STAT CBC, PT, PTT, Fibrinogen Q4H			Recheck K in the AM
☐ FSBS per insulin protocol			☐ Ondansetron (Zofran) 2 mg IV q 6 hrs PRN for nausea
☐ BMP, Mg QAM			**Pain Medications:**
☐ STAT CT Head for any change in neurological exam			☐ PCA (see sheet)
			☐ Morphine 2–5 mg IV Q1H PRN Pain
			☐ Lorazepam (Ativan) 0.5–2 mg IV Q6H PRN Agitation
			or Anxiety
			☐ Acetaminophen 650 mg OGT/NGT/PO q 4hrs PRN
			Temp > 38.5°
			☐ Other
			Lipid Lowering:
			☐ Simvastatin (Zocor) ______ mg NGT/PO daily
			☐ Other
			☐ See Medication Reconciliation form

Signature of MD/DO/NP/PA: ______ Printed Name: ______ Pager: ______ Date: ______

Signature of RN: ______ Printed Name: ______ Date: ______

FIGURE 8.4 Thrombolysis order set – an example

Tips of the Trade

- Avoid groin bleeding complications with precise common femoral artery puncture.
  - Fluoroscopically mark area of puncture over femoral head
  - Ultrasound guided puncture
- Access from the arm may be necessary and feasible in certain cases. Generally, current catheter lengths preclude treatment beyond the mid thigh from this approach.
- Quickly recognize worsening ischemia or when endovascular techniques will fail and move directly to surgical revascularization.

Follow-Up After Anticoagulation, Thrombolysis, and Mechanical Thrombectomy

- Patients are maintained on heparin postoperatively and then transitioned to coumadin for a treatment course of 6 months.
- Patients who are identified to have an embolic source are maintained on life-long anticoagulation.
- Patients suspected to have had an embolus with no clear source are evaluated with a transthoracic echocardiogram and a CT angiogram of the chest, abdomen, and pelvis.
- Patients are screened for a hypercoagulability disorder. This testing is associated with a higher pretest positive probability if the patient is young, has a history of prior embolic event or a family history. Of note, ethnicity may influence lab ranges for protein C, protein S and antithrombin III. Black Africans and Black Caribbeans have a lower level than Whites, and may be diagnosed inappropriately.
- Patients in whom patency has been restored to an occluded bypass graft are placed on a graft duplex surveillance protocol with a scan at 4 weeks, 3 months, 6 months, 12 months, and annually thereafter.

Hypercoagulability Workup

- CBC
- PTT, PT
- Factor V Leiden
- Protein S
- Protein C
- Antithrombin III (AT III)
- Antiphospholipid antibody
- Prothrombin 20210A
- Fibrinogen
- Homocysteine
- Anticardiolipin antibody
- Lupus anticoagulant antibody
- Homocystein

Equipment List

Sheaths

- 4–6-Fr standard short sheaths

Guiding Sheaths

- Ansel (Cook)
- Balkin (Cook)
- Arrow (Arrow International)

Guide Wires: Generally an 0.035 Platform Is Adequate for These Types of Procedures

- Benson (Boston Scientific)
- Glidewire (Terumo)
- Versacore (Abbot)

Lytic Catheters

- Fountain (Merit)
- Katzen wire (Boston Scientific)

Mechanical Thrombectomy Device

- Angiojet (Possis)
- Baccus Trellis

Balloons/Stents

As necessary depending on lesion

Drugs

- Tissue plasminogen activator
- Heparin

Bibliography

Inter-Society Consensus for the Management of Peripheral Arterial Disease (TASC11). Society of Vascular Surgery 2007.

→ *A document that details international guidelines for treatment of peripheral arterial disease.*

Results of a prospective randomized trial evaluating surgery versus thrombolysis for ischemia of the lower extremity. The STILE trial. JVS 1994;220: 251–66.

→ *A multicenter trial with patients randomized into three groups – Thrombolysis with tPA, thrombolysis with urokinase and surgery.*

Thrombolysis or peripheral arterial surgery: phase 1 results. TOPAS Investigators. JVS 1996; 23:64–73. TOPAS 1

→ *A multicenter study involving 213 patients to determine the effective dose range for urokinase.*

A comparison of recombinant urokinase with vascular surgery as initial treatment for acute arterial occlusion of the legs. Thrombolysis or Peripheral Arterial Surgery (TOPAS) Investigators. TOPAS 2. N Engl J Med 1998; 338:1105–11.

→ *A multicenter trial with patients randomized to surgery or thrombolysis. The primary endpoint evaluated was amputation free survival at 6 months.*

A comparison of thrombolytic therapy with operative revascularization in the initial treatment of acute peripheral arterial ischemia. J Vasc Surg 1994;19:1021–30.

→ *A single center study recruiting patients with symptoms of less than or equal to 7 days. Patients were randomized to thrombolysis or surgery.*

Rheolytic thrombectomy in the management of acute and subacute limb-threatening ischemia. J Vasc Interv Radiol 2001;12 (4):413–21 Kasirajan.

→ *A retrospective study analyzing the use of mechanical thrombectomy in two groups – acute (<2 weeks) and subacute (2 weeks to 4 months).*

Chapter 9
Antiplatelet Therapy in the Management of Peripheral Artery Disease

Nihar R. Desai and Joshua A. Beckman

Definition

Peripheral Artery Disease (PAD): Atherosclerotic occlusive disease of the distal abdominal aorta and lower extremity arteries sufficient to reduce perfusion pressure at the ankle below 90% of brachial artery pressure. Although approximately half of all PAD patients are without symptoms when present, the most common clinical presentation is intermittent claudication with atypical features. Critical limb ischemia develops in 1–2% of PAD patients.

Prevalence

In a study of subjects in the National Health and Nutrition Survey (NHANES), 4.3% of Americans older than 40 years had PAD. In a study of nearly 7,000 consecutive primary care patients with the entry criteria of age >70 years or between the ages of 50 and 69 years with a history of smoking or diabetes mellitus, 29% of this population had PAD. The disease is common in both men and women.

N.R. Desai • J.A. Beckman (✉)
Cardiovascular Division, Brigham and Women's Hospital, Harvard Medical School, Boston, MA, USA
e-mail: nrdesai@partners.org; jbeckman@partners.org

C.D. Owens and Y. Yeghiazarians (eds.), *Handbook of Endovascular Peripheral Interventions*, DOI 10.1007/978-1-4614-0839-0_9,

Clinical Presentation/Clues

- Lower extremity muscular pain with walking. Typically described as a burning, aching, heaviness, or fatigue of the hip, thigh, or calf muscle.
- The symptoms occur repeatedly with a similar amount of exertion and resolve with a similar amount of rest.
- The development of foot pain at rest, exacerbated by elevation; an ulcer that does not heal within 2 weeks, or gangrene
- The absence of a pulse or the presence of an abdominal or femoral artery bruit
- The presence of coronary or cerebrovascular atherosclerosis.

Clinical Pointer: Risk Factors

Conventional	Novel
Age	Chronic kidney disease
Smoking	Homocysteine
Diabetes mellitus	C-Reactive protein
Hyperlipidemia	
Hypertension	

Clinical Pointer: The Dual Threat

1. Patients with PAD have three-fold risk of mortality and a six- to seven-fold risk of cardiovascular death compared to patients without PAD. The most recent data reports a 25% 5-year death and cardiovascular event rate.
2. Patients with claudication have a lifestyle limitation equivalent to New York Heart Association Class III heart failure or severe chronic obstructive pulmonary disease.
3. More than half of all amputations in the United States occur in diabetic patients with PAD.

Diagnostic Tools

Functional Assessment

- Ankle Brachial Index (ABI)
  - Strengths: Safe, inexpensive, and diagnostic of disease. An ABI of <0.9 requires no confirmatory test.
  - Limitations: In the evaluation of patient with claudication or CLI, this test does not localize the segment of occlusive disease.
  - Vascular calcification may falsely elevate arterial pressure in the ankle.
- Segmental Pressure Examination
  - Strengths: Safe, inexpensive, and diagnostic of disease. It can localize occlusive disease to a leg segment.
  - Limitations: Thigh compression may be painful and intolerable to patients.
- Pulse Volume Recording
  - Strengths: Confirmatory plethysmographic evaluation of arterial blood flow. May provide information in the setting of arterial calcification.
  - Limitations: Less accurate than arterial pressure gradients
- Treadmill Exercise ABI
  - Strengths: In patients with borderline ABIs at rest, yet symptoms suggestive of claudication, exercising them will cause a reduction in ankle perfusion pressure with maintenance or elevation of brachial artery pressure, lowering the ABI and confirming the diagnosis of PAD
  - Limitations: Arterial calcification limits the use of this study. Older patients may be afraid of treadmill walking, limiting their participation prior to the onset of claudication.

Anatomic Assessment

The following tests are not needed to diagnose PAD, but should be reserved for surgical or endovascular therapeutic planning.

- Duplex Ultrasonography
- Magnetic Resonance Angiography

- Computed Tomographic Angiography
- Contrast Angiography

Antiplatelet Treatment

Cardiovascular Event Reduction

Aspirin

Currently, the use of aspirin in patients with PAD is recommended and receives a Class I indication with a Level of Evidence A in the ACC/AHA Guidelines for the Management of Patients With Peripheral Arterial Disease. However, recent data will likely attenuate this recommendation.

The Antithrombotic Trialists' Collaboration (ATC) examined 287 randomized trials of over 135,000 subjects and reported a highly significant 22% relative risk reduction in the rate of a major cardiovascular event (including death, MI, and stroke) with aspirin as compared with placebo. This effect was mirrored in the subgroup of patients with PAD ($n=9,214$) and was consistent in patients medically treated for claudication as well as those undergoing revascularization with bypass grafting or angioplasty.

Berger et al. systematically analyzed the efficacy of aspirin (with or without dipyridamole) in patients with peripheral arterial disease across 18 trials and 5,269 subjects. There was a non-significant 12% RRR in the primary endpoint – CV death, MI, or stroke and a significant 34% RRR in the secondary endpoint, non-fatal stroke. This analysis may have been underpowered and examined trials which had heterogeneous ABI criteria.

The Aspirin for Asymptomatic Atherosclerosis trial screened 28,980 men and women aged 50–75 years living in central Scotland who were free of clinical cardiovascular disease. Subjects with an ABI of 0.95 or lower were randomized to aspirin 100 mg daily or placebo. Over the course of 8 years of follow-up, the administration of aspirin did not significantly reduce death, myocardial infarction, or stroke.

Thienopyridines

Currently, clopidogrel is recommended as monotherapy for patients with PAD to reduce cardiovascular events.

Clopidogrel

The Clopidogrel versus Aspirin in Patients at Risk of Ischemic Events (CAPRIE) Trial randomized 19,185 patients with a recent history of MI or stroke, or with PAD to clopidogrel or aspirin. There was a marginally significant ($P=0.043$), 8.7% relative risk reduction in the primary endpoint, a composite of CV death, MI, and stroke at 3 years. Of note, the subgroup of patients with PAD ($n=6{,}452$) had the greatest benefit a 24% RRR with clopidogrel as compared with aspirin.

The Clopidogrel for High Atherothrombotic Risk and Ischemic Stabilization, Management, and Avoidance (CHARISMA) Trial found no benefit with clopidogrel added to aspirin compared with aspirin alone in high-risk patients, including those with PAD.

Currently, clopidogrel receives a Class I recommendation with level of evidence B for use in patients with PAD in the ACC/AHA Guidelines for the Management of Patients With Peripheral Arterial Disease.

Ticlopidine

The Swedish Ticlopidine Multicenter Study tested the efficacy of ticlopidine (250 mg twice daily) versus placebo in 687 patients with intermittent claudication and found a significant 34% RRR in the rate of major adverse cardio- and cerebro-vascular events.

Use of ticlopidine is limited by its side effect profile which includes thrombotic thrombocytopenia purpura and leukopenia.

Antiplatelet Therapy for Symptomatic Treatment

Cilostazol

Cilostazol is a phosphodiesterase (PDE) type 3 inhibitor, inhibiting platelet aggregation as well as inducing systemic vasodilation. A meta-analysis of eight randomized trials with 2,702 patients demonstrated that treatment with cilostazol was associated with increased pain-free walking distance and longer maximum walking distances. Importantly, it has not been shown to reduce cardiovascular events and is contraindicated in patients with congestive heart failure.

Neither aspirin nor clopidogrel has evidence of improving walking distance or wound healing in patients with PAD.

Antiplatelet Therapy in Patient with PAD Undergoing Revascularization

Percutaneous Revascularization

There are no randomized trial data which have examined the adjunctive antiplatelet therapy for patients undergoing percutaneous revascularization for PAD. Dual antiplatelet therapy is commonly used in accordance with bare-metal stenting in the coronary bed.

Surgical Revascularization

Recently, the Clopidogrel and Acetylsalicylic acid in bypass Surgery for Peripheral Arterial disease (CASPAR) trial was reported. In this trial, 851 patients undergoing unilateral, below-knee bypass graft for PAD were randomized to clopidogrel 75 mg/day plus ASA 75–100 mg/day or placebo plus ASA 75–100 mg/day. Over a median follow up of 364 days, there was no difference between the groups in the primary outcome (index-graft occlusion or revascularization, above-ankle amputation of the affected limb, or death). In a prespecified secondary analysis, outcomes varied according to graft type. Subjects whose index graft was prosthetic and were treated with aspirin and clopidogrel had a significant reduction in the primary endpoint compared to aspirin alone, resulting from reductions in graft occlusion and amputation. *Combination therapy may be reasonable after surgical revascularization in patients treated with a prosthetic graft.*

Bibliography

1. Hirsch AT, Haskal ZJ, Hertzer NR, Bakal CW, Creager MA, Halperin JL, Hiratzka LF, Murphy WR, Olin JW, Puschett JB, Rosenfield KA, Sacks D, Stanley JC, Taylor LM, Jr., White CJ, White J, White RA, Antman EM, Smith SC, Jr., Adams CD, Anderson JL, Faxon DP, Fuster V, Gibbons RJ, Hunt SA, Jacobs AK, Nishimura R, Ornato JP, Page RL, Riegel B. ACC/AHA 2005 Practice Guidelines for the management of patients with peripheral arterial disease (lower extremity, renal, mesenteric, and abdominal aortic): a collaborative report from the American Association for Vascular Surgery/Society for Vascular Surgery, Society for Cardiovascular Angiography and Interventions, Society for Vascular Medicine and Biology, Society of Interventional Radiology, and the ACC/AHA Task Force on Practice Guidelines (Writing Committee to Develop Guidelines for the Management of Patients With Peripheral Arterial Disease): endorsed by the American Association of Cardiovascular and Pulmonary Rehabilitation; National Heart, Lung, and Blood Institute; Society for Vascular Nursing; TransAtlantic Inter-Society Consensus; and Vascular Disease Foundation. *Circulation.* 2006;113(11):e463-654.
   → *This is the most comprehensive review and set of expert recommendations available on the treatment of patients with PAD.*
2. A randomised, blinded, trial of clopidogrel versus aspirin in patients at risk of ischaemic events (CAPRIE). CAPRIE Steering Committee. *Lancet.* 1996;348(9038):1329–1339.
   → *This study demonstrated the superiority of clopidogrel monotherapy compared to aspirin monotherapy in patients with coronary heart, cerebrovascular, or peripheral artery disease.*

3. Cacoub PP, Bhatt DL, Steg PG, Topol EJ, Creager MA. Patients with peripheral arterial disease in the CHARISMA trial. *Eur Heart J.* 2009;30(2):192–201.
   → *In the PAD subgroup of the CHARISMA trial, the addition of clopidogrel to aspirin did not reduce the primary endpoint of death, myocardial infarction, or stroke. A secondary analysis showed that dual antiplatelet therapy did reduce myocardial infarction.*
4. Belch JJ, Dormandy J. Results of the randomized, placebo-controlled clopidogrel and acetylsalicylic acid in bypass surgery for peripheral arterial disease (CASPAR) trial. *J Vasc Surg.* 2010.
   → *In PAD subjects who underwent lower extremity bypass grafting, the combination of dual antiplatelet therapy was not superior to aspirin alone in the endpoint of death, graft occlusion, or above-ankle amputation. A secondary analysis showed that subjects who received a prosthetic graft did have a reduction in the rate of graft occlusion and amputation suggesting a potential benefit in this subset.*
5. Anand S, Yusuf S, Xie C, Pogue J, Eikelboom J, Budaj A, Sussex B, Liu L, Guzman R, Cina C, Crowell R, Keltai M, Gosselin G. Oral anticoagulant and antiplatelet therapy and peripheral arterial disease. *N Engl J Med.* 2007;357(3):217–227.
   → *The WAVE trials shows that the addition of warfarin with a target INR of 2.0–3.0 to aspirin does not reduce cardiovascular events in patients with PAD, but does significantly increase the rate of life-threatening bleeding.*

Chapter 10
Risk Factor Management of Atherosclerotic Peripheral Vascular Disease

Reena L. Pande and Mark A. Creager

Introduction

Individuals with atherosclerotic peripheral vascular disease (APVD) are at significantly increased risk of adverse cardiovascular events such as myocardial infarction, stroke, and death.[1,2] Accordingly, the management of all patients with APVD should include comprehensive risk factor modification that is focused on the secondary prevention of cardiovascular events.

Smoking

Tobacco smoking is one of the most potent risk factors associated with development and progression of APVD. For example, the risk of peripheral artery disease (PAD) among current smokers is as high as five-fold greater than non-smokers. Smoking also increases the incidence of lower extremity symptoms, such as intermittent claudication and critical limb

---

R.L. Pande • M.A. Creager (✉)
Cardiovascular Division, Brigham and Women's Hospital, Harvard Medical School, Boston, MA, USA
e-mail: rpande@partners.org; mcreager@partners.org

C.D. Owens and Y. Yeghiazarians (eds.), *Handbook of Endovascular Peripheral Interventions*, DOI 10.1007/978-1-4614-0839-0_10,

ischemia. Cigarette smoking increases the severity of carotid artery atherosclerosis, doubles the risk of ischemic stroke, and is associated with a three- to four-fold greater risk of abdominal aortic aneurysm (AAA). The magnitude and duration of cigarette smoking correlates with the risk of AAA.

Although there are no prospective studies of smoking cessation, multiple observational studies in patients with APVD have shown better cardiovascular outcomes in individuals who stop smoking compared to those who continue to smoke. A meta-analysis of smoking cessation studies in patients with coronary heart disease showed a 36% reduction in the crude relative risk of mortality for those who quit compared to those who continued smoking (RR 0.64, 95% CI 0.58 – 0.71).[3] Smoking cessation also has beneficial effects on limb outcomes in PAD. Individuals with intermittent claudication have been shown to have improved walking times after smoking cessation compared with patients who continue smoking, and reduced risk of amputation or development of critical limb ischemia. Furthermore, lower extremity bypass graft patency rates at 1 year have been shown to be lower in patients who continue to smoke compared to those who quit smoking, and long-term survival is improved in patients undergoing peripheral vascular surgery who quit smoking. The number of cigarettes smoked appears directly related to outcomes after bypass surgery with heavy smokers (considered ≥15 cigarettes/day) having significantly reduced survival rates and greater amputation rates compared to moderate smokers (<15 cigarettes/day). Smoking cessation reduces the risk of stroke. In addition, smoking cessation is associated with a reduced risk of AAA.

How I Do It

An algorithm to assist patients with tobacco cessation is shown in Fig. 10.1. Without any intervention, the smoking cessation rates at 1 year are less than 1%.[4] Physician counseling for smoking cessation is effective, but results in only a 2.5% increase in cessation rate with higher success rates for intensive advice compared to minimal advice. Smoking cessation

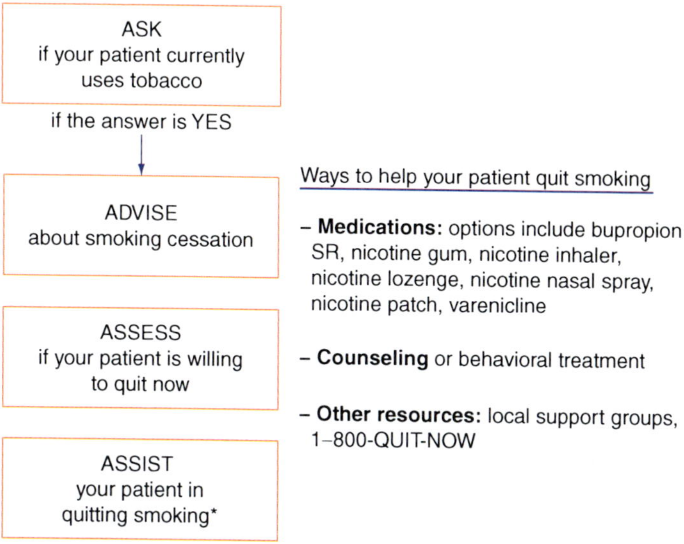

FIGURE 10.1 Algorithm to assist patients with smoking cessation (Adapted from the Surgeon General's guidelines on Treating Tobacco Use and Dependence[4])

success rates are notably higher with pharmacologic interventions, and physicians should encourage use of these agents unless specifically contraindicated. The following medical therapies have established benefits for smoking cessation in multiple populations.

- Nicotine replacement therapy
- Bupropion
- Varenicline

Various forms of nicotine replacement therapy are available (gum, inhaler, lozenges, nasal spray, or patch) with the intent to replace the nicotine otherwise obtained in cigarettes in order to reduce the severity of nicotine withdrawal symptoms. All forms of nicotine replacement have demonstrated efficacy with an estimated abstinence rate at 6 months of 19.0–26.7%.[4]

Bupropion is a non-nicotine medication that is thought to reduce the craving for cigarettes, possibly by blocking dopamine and norepinephrine neuronal reuptake and blocking nicotinic acetylcholine receptors, although the exact mechanism of action is poorly understood. Bupropion, alone or in combination with nicotine replacement therapies, has been shown to double the likelihood of long-term abstinence from tobacco, with average cessation rates of approximately 24.2%,[4] and as high as 35.5% in combination with nicotine patch.

Varenicline is a recently approved non-nicotine medication presumed to work by partial agonism/antagonism of the nicotine receptor. The overall effect is to make smoking less rewarding and to reduce the urge to smoke. Varenicline (2 mg/day) has been shown to result in mean 6-month abstinence rates of 33.2%, with effective but lower rates of smoking cessation at a lower dose (1 mg/day) of 25.4%.[4] The use of varenicline has been specifically studied in patients with cardiovascular disease, including patients with PAD, with abstinence rates as high as 47.0% after 12 weeks compared to 13.9% in the placebo group, although lower abstinence rates at 1 year (19.2%).[5]

Potential Pitfalls

- Although varenicline is generally well-tolerated, there are reports that varenicline is associated with depressed mood, behavioral changes, and suicidal ideation in some patients, particularly those with pre-existing psychiatric illness. However, it is unclear if these symptoms are due to the medication itself or to nicotine withdrawal symptoms.

- Smoking cessation is very difficult to achieve and often requires repeated intervention and multiple attempts to quit.

Summary Recommendations for Smoking Cessation

- Smoking cessation is a key component of secondary prevention of cardiovascular disease and should be attempted in all smokers with APVD
- Physician advice regarding smoking cessation is better than no advice
- Medications (nicotine replacement therapy, bupropion, and varenicline) are effective smoking cessation aids

Diabetes Mellitus

There is a strong and consistent association of diabetes with APVD. Several epidemiologic studies have shown that the risk of PAD in particular is two- to four-fold higher in patients with diabetes with increasing risk of PAD with greater severity of diabetes. Furthermore, the presence of diabetes is associated with increased frequency of lower extremity symptoms and poorer peripheral vascular outcomes in patients with recognized PAD. Patients with diabetes have greater frequency of intermittent claudication and higher rates of rest pain, ischemic ulceration, and need for amputation. Diabetes also adversely affects outcomes of peripheral revascularization with lower rates of primary and secondary patency of peripheral bypass grafts and stents, as well as increased perioperative morbidity and mortality related to cardiovascular disease. Diabetes also increases carotid atherosclerosis and the risk of ischemic stroke but is associated with lower risk of AAA.

Rigorous glycemic control prevents microvascular and cardiovascular complications in patients with type 1 diabetes.[6,7] In type 2 diabetes, although clinical trials have clearly demonstrated that tight glycemic control can reduce microvascular complications, the benefits of glycemic control for the prevention of major cariodvascular events is less clear.[8] The United Kingdom Prospective Diabetes Study (UKPDS) evaluated the benefit of an intensive diabetes treatment regimen in newly diagnosed type 2 diabetic patients over 10 years of follow-up. Average hemoglobin A1C was 7.0% in the intestive therapy group compared to 7.9% in the conventional therapy group. The study showed a significant 25% reduction in the risk of microvascular complications, but no significant difference in the rate of macrovascular complications over 10 years follow-up.[8] However, a benefit appeared to emerge after longer term follow-up (17 years) even after completion of the intervention period with significant reductions in myocardial infarction (RR 0.85, 95% CI 0.74–0.97, $p = 0.01$) and total mortality (RR 0.87, 95% CI 0.79–0.96, $p = 0.007$) in the intensive therapy group. More recent studies in patients with established diabetes, such as the Veteran's Affairs Diabetes Trial, ACCORD, and ADVANCE studies have failed to show a significant benefit of even more intensive therapy with a target hemoglobin A1C of 6.0% in reducing cardiovascular complications of diabetes.[9-11] Indeed, the ACCORD study was halted earlier than expected based on a higher number of total and cardiovascular deaths in the intensive therapy arm of the study (HR 1.22, 95% CI 1.01–1.46). Finally, the PROactive study evaluated the effect of pioglitazone, a thiazolidinedione, on cardiovascular events in patient with type 2 diabetes at risk for CVD. There was no significant difference in the primary outcome, including total mortality, MI, stroke, coronary or peripheral revascularization, or leg amputation (HR 0.90, 95% CI 0.80–1.02, $p = 0.095$). However, there was a significant 16% reduction in the secondary endpoint, a composite of all-cause mortality, non-fatal myocardial infarction, and stroke (0.84, 0.72–0.98, $p = 0.027$). A meta-analysis comprising all of these studies (including UKPDS, VADT, ACCORD, ADVANCE, and PROactive) did suggest a reduction in the overall risk of coronary heart disease (RR 0.89, 95% CI 0.81–0.96) (Fig. 10.2) and non-fatal MI (RR 0.84, 95% CI 0.75–0.94) with intensive therapy but no benefit in stroke or all-cause mortality.[12]

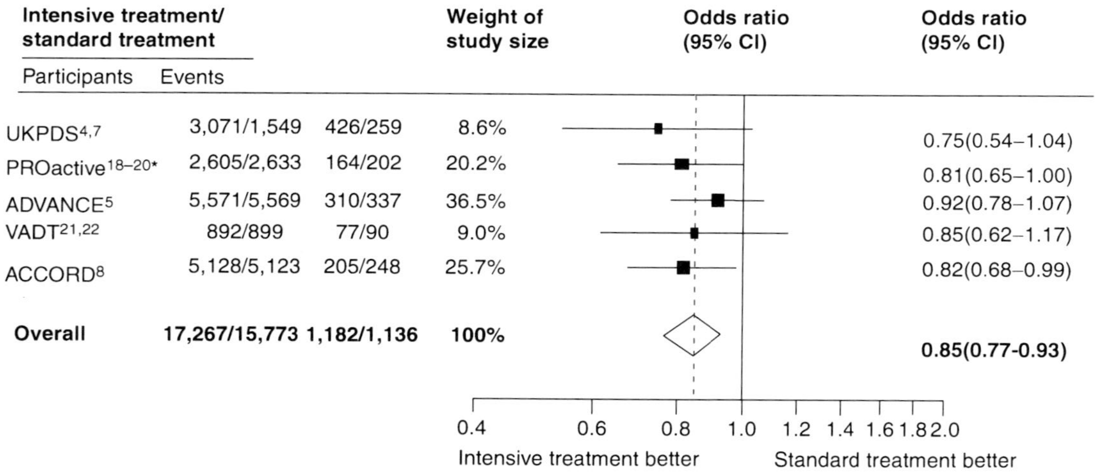

FIGURE 10.2 Meta-analysis of the effect of intensive glucose lowering on coronary heart disease events, including non-fatal myocardial infarction and cardiovascular mortality (Reprinted from Ray, KK et al. *The Lancet*. 2009; 373(9677):1765[12] With permission from Elsevier)

How I Do It

- Treatment should always include non-pharmacologic options such as diet, exercise, and weight loss.
- Several pharmacologic options exist for the management of blood glucose. Absent any contraindications, metformin is considered first-line therapy and consensus guidelines recommended that metformin be initiated along with lifestyle medication when diabetes is first diagnosed.[13] Other options for treatment include sulfonylureas (e.g., glyburide or glipizide), thiazolidenediones (e.g., pioglitazone), DDP-IV inhibitors (e.g., sitagliptin), GLP-1 agonists (e.g., exenatide), and insulin.
- Referral to a diabetes specialist may be helpful for management.

Potential Pitfalls

- Symptomatic hypoglycemia, particularly with intensive therapy

Summary Recommendations for Diabetes Management in PAD

- Diabetes increases risk of developing APVD such as PAD and increases risk of symptoms and cardiovascular complications in patients with known PAD and cerebrovascular disease
- Intensive glycemic control to reduce hemoglobin A1C level to <7% can reduce microvascular complications and possibly cardiovascular outcomes

Hypertension

Hypertension is a potent risk factor for carotid atherosclerosis and stroke, and is associated with AAA. Hypertension has a more modest effect as a risk factor for PAD. Treatment of hypertension prevents MI, stroke, and congestive heart failure.[14] It is not known whether antihypertensive therapy prevents AAA rupture.

Few trials have specifically evaluated the benefit of blood pressure control in the PAD population. The ABCD (Appropriate Blood Pressure Control in Diabetes) trial compared intensive versus modest blood pressure control in patients with diabetes. In a substudy of patients with PAD, intensive antihypertensive therapy significantly decreased the risk of cardiovascular events in patients with lower ankle-brachial index (ABI).[15] The Heart Outcomes Prevention Evaluation (HOPE) study evaluated the role of the angiotensin-converting enzyme (ACE) inhibitor, ramipril, in primary and secondary prevention of cardiovascular events in high-risk patients.[16] Patients with PAD were included based on symptoms of intermittent claudication, prior peripheral revascularization, amputation, or based on an ABI less than 0.9. Over a mean follow-up period of 5 years, there was a significant 22% reduction in the composite endpoint of MI, stroke, and cardiovascular death with a specific benefit in the PAD population and with benefits evident irrespective of baseline blood pressure. These findings were true even among patients with subclinical PAD identified only by ABI.

Despite initial concerns about the safety of certain classes of anti-hypertensive agents (particularly beta-blockers) in patients with symptoms of intermittent claudication, a meta-analysis of small randomized controlled trials of beta-blockers in patient with PAD and claudication showed no significant adverse effects on pain-free or maximal walking distance. Studies of ACE inhibitors also showed no significant adverse effects on claudication walking times.

How I Do It

- Optimal treatment of hypertension should achieve a target blood pressure of <140/90 mmHg in most patients, and <130/80 mmHg in patients with diabetes or chronic renal insufficiency according to guidelines (ref 1).

- Several classes of medications have proven efficacy in the management of hypertension, although studies in patients specifically with APVD are uncommon. Given the data regarding reduction in cardiovascular outcomes with ramipril, ACE inhibitors may be considered first-line for the treatment of hypertension in patients with vascular disease. However, any class of medication can be safely utilized in this population. Other classes of medications for treatment of hypertension include diuretics, calcium channel blockers, angiotensin receptor blockers (ARBs), beta-blockers, and vasodilators. Lifestyle modification with diet and exercise should be recommended for all hypertensive patients.

Potential Pitfalls

- Substantial reductions in blood pressure (>20 mmHg) may worsen intermittent claudication or exacerbate critical limb ischemia in some patients. Nonetheless, blood pressure should still be treated to achieve guideline targets and if limb symptoms worsen, consider specific therapies to improve these symptoms.
- Antihypertensive agents can have side effects, including lightheadedness, hypotension, bradycardia, and electrolyte disturbances depending on the mechanism of action. Patients should be closely monitored with measurement of blood pressure, heart rate, and blood tests as appropriate.

Recommendations for Blood Pressure Control in APVD

- Antihypertensive therapy should be administered to hypertensive patients with PAD to achieve a goal blood pressure <140/80 mmHg in patients without diabetes or <130/80 mmHg in patients with diabetics or chronic renal

disease to reduce the risk of MI, stroke, congestive heart failure, and cardiovascular death
- ACE inhibitors have been shown to have specific benefit in reducing cardiovascular events in patients with PAD
- Any class of anti-hypertensive agent can be safely used (including beta-blockers and ACE inhibitors)

Hyperlipidemia

Hyperlipidemia is recognized as a major risk factor for the development of cardiovascular disease and epidemiologic studies have established that elevated total cholesterol increases the risk of APVD. Elevated cholesterol is associated with the incidence and progression of PAD, and the prevalence of carotid artery stenosis and AAA.

Several studies have evaluated the benefits of lipid-lowering therapy on cardiovascular outcomes in patients with APVD. The Scandinavian Simvastatin Survival Study (4S) was the first major trial to demonstrate significant benefit in reduction of cardiovascular events and total mortality with aggressive treatment with an HMG CoA reductase inhibitor ("statin") to reduce event in patients with CAD and hyperlipidemia.[17] The more recent Heart Protection Study (HPS) studied the use of statin for primary and secondary prevention and specifically included patients with PAD based on a history of intermittent claudication or prior lower extremity bypass surgery. Overall, there was a significant 24% relative risk reduction in the occurrence of any major vascular event among those randomized to simvastatin.[18] Among the 6,748 patients with PAD, there was a 25% risk reduction over 5 years of follow-up.

Based on a limited data, it appears that cholesterol-lowering therapy with statins may also have a beneficial impact on peripheral vascular symptoms. The 4S study showed a significant 38% reduction in new or worsening claudication symptoms. A prospective trial of statin therapy in patients with claudication showed a reduction in pain-free, but not maximal, walking distance. Statin therapy also limits progression of carotid atherosclerosis and reduces the risk of stroke in patients with atherosclerosis (Fig. 10.3).[19]

The National Cholesterol Education Program (NCEP) has recommended that secondary prevention of vascular events in patients with atherosclerotic vascular disease be targeted to a goal low density lipoprotein (LDL) of <100 mg/dL or a more aggressive target of <70 mg/dL in individuals at particularly high risk of recurrent vascular events.[20]

Although non-LDL cholesterol (such as high-density lipoprotein, or HDL) is known to be an independent risk factor for vascular disease, the efficacy of other lipid-lowering therapies, such as niacin, bile acid sequestrants, or ezetimibe in reducing cardiovascular events in patients with APVD is not established. Moreover, there is controversy regarding the efficacy of fibric acid derivatives which increase HDL cholesterol. In patients with CAD, treatment of low HDL cholesterol levels with gemfibrozil in the Veterans Affairs High-Density Lipoprotein Intervention Trial (VA-HIT) reduced cardiovascular events by 11% for every 5 mg/dL increase in HDL ($p=0.02$).[21] In a placebo-controlled randomized study, bezafibrate did not reduce the incidence of coronary artery disease events or strokes in patients with PAD. In a randomized trial involving patients with type 2 diabetes and atherosclerosis, fenobibrate did not decrease the incidence of coronary events, which was the primary outcome, but did decrease total cardiovascular events, a prespecified secondary outcome, which included the composite of cardiovascular death, myocardial infarction, stroke, and coronary and carotid revascularization.[22]

How I Do It

- Based on NCEP ATP III guidelines, all patients with APVD are considered to be coronary heart disease risk equivalents and merit aggressive management of hyperlipidemia. Goal LDL cholesterol level should be <100 mg/dL for patients with APVD and <70 mg/dL in individuals considered to be at particularly high risk. Lifestyle modification with diet and exercise should be

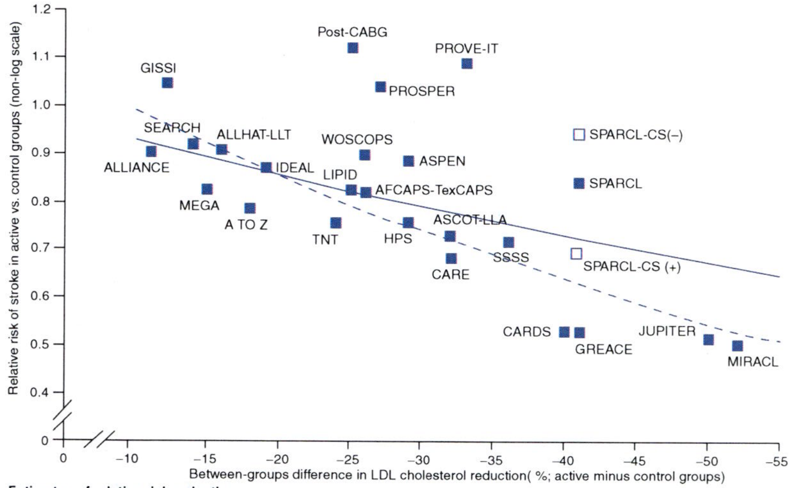

Estimates of relative risk reduction

- 10% LDL reduction: relative risk reduction 7.5% (2.3,12.5) overall)
  relative risk reduction 13.5% (7.7,18.8) for primary prevention of stroke
- 1mmol/L (39 mg/dL) LDL reduction: relative risk reducation 21.1% (6.3,33.5) overall
  relative risk reducation 35.9% (21.7,47.6) for primary prevention of stroke

FIGURE 10.3 Association of greater LDL cholesterol lowering with greater reduction in the relative risk of stroke (Reprinted from Amarenco, P and Labreuche, BS. *Lancet Neurology.* 2009; 8(5):453[19] With permission from Elsevier) recommended for all patients. Given the available clinical trial data showing clear benefit of statins in reduction of overall mortality and cardiovascular events, statins are the first choice for treatment of hyperlipidemia in patients with APVD. Additional treatment options for lowering LDL cholesterol include ezetimibe and bile acid sequestrants (e.g., cholestyramine and colestipol), but the efficacy of these agents for reducing cardiovascular events is not established. For the specific management of low HDL cholesterol or elevated triglycerides, further treatment with fibrates, nicotinic acid, and/or fish oil supplements may be considered.

Potential Pitfalls

- Potential side effects of statin medications include myalgias with rare cases of rhabdomyolysis and elevated liver function tests.

Summary Recommendations for Treatment of Hyperlipidemia in AVPD

- Lipid-lowering therapy with a statin is indicated for all patients with PAD to achieve a goal LDL cholesterol level of <100 mg/dL
- More aggressive lipid-lowering therapy (goal LDL < 70 mg/dL) may be indicated for individuals at high-risk of recurrent vascular events

Bibliography

1. Hirsch AT, Haskal ZJ, Hertzer NR, Bakal CW, Creager MA, Halperin JL, Hiratzka LF, Murphy WR, Olin JW, Puschett JB, Rosenfield KA, Sacks D, Stanley JC, Taylor LM, Jr., White CJ, White J, White RA, Antman EM, Smith SC, Jr., Adams CD, Anderson JL, Faxon DP, Fuster V, Gibbons RJ, Hunt SA, Jacobs

AK, Nishimura R, Ornato JP, Page RL, Riegel B. ACC/AHA 2005 Practice Guidelines for the management of patients with peripheral arterial disease (lower extremity, renal, mesenteric, and abdominal aortic): a collaborative report from the American Association for Vascular Surgery/Society for Vascular Surgery, Society for Cardiovascular Angiography and Interventions, Society for Vascular Medicine and Biology, Society of Interventional Radiology, and the ACC/AHA Task Force on Practice Guidelines (Writing Committee to Develop Guidelines for the Management of Patients With Peripheral Arterial Disease): endorsed by the American Association of Cardiovascular and Pulmonary Rehabilitation; National Heart, Lung, and Blood Institute; Society for Vascular Nursing; TransAtlantic Inter-Society Consensus; and Vascular Disease Foundation. *Circulation.* 2006;113:e463-654.

2. Norgren L, Hiatt WR, Dormandy JA, Nehler MR, Harris KA, Fowkes FG. Inter-Society Consensus for the Management of Peripheral Arterial Disease (TASC II). *J Vasc Surg.* 2007;45 Suppl S:S5-67.

   → *The preceding two references provide a comprehensive review of the management of patients with atherosclerotic peripheral vascular disease, including detailed review of the existing literature and inter-societal guidelines for specific management of atherosclerotic risk factors.*

3. Critchley JA, Capewell S. Mortality risk reduction associated with smoking cessation in patients with coronary heart disease: a systematic review. *Jama.* 2003;290:86–97.

4. Fiore MC JC, Baker TB, et al. Treating Tobacco Use and Dependence: 2008 Update. Quick Reference Guide for Clinicians. *Rockville, MD: U.S. Department of Health and Human Services. Public Health Service.* April 2009.

   → *A clinical practice guideline for smoking cessation compiled by the United States Public Health Service.*

5. Rigotti NA, Pipe AL, Benowitz NL, Arteaga C, Garza D, Tonstad S. Efficacy and safety of varenicline for smoking cessation in patients with cardiovascular disease: a randomized trial. *Circulation. 2010;*121:221–229.

6. The effect of intensive treatment of diabetes on the development and progression of long-term complications in insulin-dependent diabetes mellitus. The Diabetes Control and Complications Trial Research Group. *New England Journal of Medicine.* 1993;329:977–986.

7. Nathan DM, Cleary PA, Backlund JY, Genuth SM, Lachin JM, Orchard TJ, Raskin P, Zinman B. Intensive diabetes treatment and cardiovascular disease in patients with type 1 diabetes. *N Engl J Med.* 2005;353:2643–2653.
8. Intensive blood-glucose control with sulphonylureas or insulin compared with conventional treatment and risk of complications in patients with type 2 diabetes (UKPDS 33). UK Prospective Diabetes Study (UKPDS) Group. *Lancet.* 1998;352:837–853.
   → *The preceding three references represent landmark clinical trials examining the effect of intensive glucose lowering on macrovascular and microvascular complication in patients with diabetes.*
9. Duckworth W, Abraira C, Moritz T, Reda D, Emanuele N, Reaven PD, Zieve FJ, Marks J, Davis SN, Hayward R, Warren SR, Goldman S, McCarren M, Vitek ME, Henderson WG, Huang GD. Glucose control and vascular complications in veterans with type 2 diabetes. *N Engl J Med.* 2009;360:129–139.
10. Gerstein HC, Miller ME, Byington RP, Goff DC, Jr., Bigger JT, Buse JB, Cushman WC, Genuth S, Ismail-Beigi F, Grimm RH, Jr., Probstfield JL, Simons-Morton DG, Friedewald WT. Effects of intensive glucose lowering in type 2 diabetes. *N Engl J Med.* 2008;358:2545–2559.
11. Patel A, MacMahon S, Chalmers J, Neal B, Billot L, Woodward M, Marre M, Cooper M, Glasziou P, Grobbee D, Hamet P, Harrap S, Heller S, Liu L, Mancia G, Mogensen CE, Pan C, Poulter N, Rodgers A, Williams B, Bompoint S, de Galan BE, Joshi R, Travert F. Intensive blood glucose control and vascular outcomes in patients with type 2 diabetes. *N Engl J Med.* 2008; 358:2560–2572.
12. Ray KK, Seshasai SR, Wijesuriya S, Sivakumaran R, Nethercott S, Preiss D, Erqou S, Sattar N. Effect of intensive control of glucose on cardiovascular outcomes and death in patients with diabetes mellitus: a meta-analysis of randomised controlled trials. *Lancet.* 2009;373:1765–1772.
    → *Meta-analysis of existing randomized clinical trials, including the three preceding references, on the impact of glucose lowering for reduction of cardiovascular outcomes in patients with diabetes.*
13. Nathan DM, Buse JB, Davidson MB, Ferrannini E, Holman RR, Sherwin R, Zinman B. Medical management of hyperglycemia in type 2 diabetes: a consensus algorithm for the initiation and

adjustment of therapy: a consensus statement of the American Diabetes Association and the European Association for the Study of Diabetes. *Diabetes Care.* 2009;32:193–203.

→ *Consensus statement from the American Diabetes Association and the European Association for the study of diabetes on guidelines for the medical management of diabetes.*

14. Major cardiovascular events in hypertensive patients randomized to doxazosin vs chlorthalidone: the antihypertensive and lipid-lowering treatment to prevent heart attack trial (ALLHAT) ALLHAT Collaborative Research Group. *JAMA.* 2000; 283:1967–1975.

    → *The ALLHAT study was a landmark clinical trial demonstrating the benefit of anti-hypertensive medications on reducing major caridovascular events.*

15. Estacio RO, Jeffers BW, Hiatt WR, Biggerstaff SL, Gifford N, Schrier RW. The effect of nisoldipine as compared with enalapril on cardiovascular outcomes in patients with non-insulin-dependent diabetes and hypertension. *N Engl J Med.* 1998; 338:645–652.

16. Yusuf S, Sleight P, Pogue J, Bosch J, Davies R, Dagenais G. Effects of an angiotensin-converting-enzyme inhibitor, ramipril, on cardiovascular events in high-risk patients. The Heart Outcomes Prevention Evaluation Study Investigators. *N Engl J Med.* 2000;342:145–153.

17. Randomised trial of cholesterol lowering in 4444 patients with coronary heart disease: the Scandinavian Simvastatin Survival Study (4S). *Lancet.* 1994;344:1383–1389.

18. Heart Protection Study Collaborative Group. MRC/BHF Heart Protection Study of cholesterol lowering with simvastatin in 20,536 high-risk individuals: a randomised placebo-controlled trial. *Lancet.* 2002;360:7–22.

    → *The preceding two references highlight two large clinical trials in greater than 20,000 patients establishing the role of cholesterol lowering and statin medications in particular in cardiovascular risk reduction in patients with vascular disease.*

19. Amarenco P, Labreuche J. Lipid management in the prevention of stroke: review and updated meta-analysis of statins for stroke prevention. *Lancet Neurology.* 2009;8:453–463.

    → *Meta-analysis of the impact of statin therapy on prevention of stroke.*

20. Expert Panel on Detection, Evaluation, And Treatment of High Blood Cholesterol In Adults. Executive Summary of The Third Report of The National Cholesterol Education Program (NCEP) Expert Panel on Detection, Evaluation, And Treatment of High Blood Cholesterol In Adults (Adult Treatment Panel III). *JAMA*. 2001;285:2486–2497.
→ *Summary of the recommendations from the NCEP ATP III on the management of patients with hyperlipidemia.*
21. Robins SJ, Collins D, Wittes JT, Papademetriou V, Deedwania PC, Schaefer EJ, McNamara JR, Kashyap ML, Hershman JM, Wexler LF, Rubins HB. Relation of gemfibrozil treatment and lipid levels with major coronary events: VA-HIT: a randomized controlled trial. *JAMA*. 2001;285:1585–1591.
22. Keech A, Simes RJ, Barter P, Best J, Scott R, Taskinen MR, Forder P, Pillai A, Davis T, Glasziou P, Drury P, Kesaniemi YA, Sullivan D, Hunt D, Colman P, D'Emden M, Whiting M, Ehnholm C, Laakso M. Effects of long-term fenofibrate therapy on cardiovascular events in 9795 people with type 2 diabetes mellitus (the FIELD study): randomised controlled trial. *Lancet*. 2005;366:1849–1861.

Chapter 11
Intracerebral Interventions for Acute Ischemic Stroke

Muneer Eesa, Randall T. Higashida, and Philip M. Meyers

Etiology

- Two main etiologies of stroke: ischemic vs. hemorrhagic
- About 85% of strokes are ischemic in nature
- Ischemic Etiologies include:
  - Arterial thrombotic (i.e., in-situ clot)
  - Embolic
  - Hypoperfusion
  - Venous Thrombotic
- Hemorrhagic stroke can be classified as:
  - Intra-axial (i.e., intra-ventricular or intra-parenchymal bleed)
  - Extra-axial (i.e., epidural, subdural, or sub-arachnoid bleed)

M. Eesa • P.M. Meyers (✉)
Interventional Neuroradiology, Columbia University, College of Physicians and Surgeons, New York Presbyterian Hospitals, New York, NY, USA
e-mail: pmm2002@columbia.edu

R.T. Higashida
Interventional Neuroradiology, University of California – San Francisco, San Francisco, CA, USA
e-mail: randall.higashida@ucsf.edu

C.D. Owens and Y. Yeghiazarians (eds.), *Handbook of Endovascular Peripheral Interventions*, DOI 10.1007/978-1-4614-0839-0_11,

Historical Background of Interventional Neuroradiology

- Interventional neuroradiology has evolved rapidly from its beginnings in the early twentieth century to a highly specialized field that involves the treatment of patients with a variety of neurovascular diseases.
- The first reports of attempted endovascular methods to treat problems in the cerebrovascular territories date back to the early twentieth century.
- In 1904, James Dawbarn described embolization of malignant tumors in the external carotid circulation using a mixture of vaseline and paraffin.
- In 1930, Barney Brooks described treatment of a carotid-cavernous fistula using muscle tissue.
- During the middle part of the twentieth century, flow-directed treatment for highly vascular lesions such as cerebral arteriovenous malformations (AVMs) evolved.
- In 1960, Alfred J. Luessenhop and colleagues described embolization of AVMs using silastic pellets injected into the carotid artery.
- In 1980s, with the introduction of over-the-wire microcatheter systems, the field of neurointervention advanced from a less-targeted flow guidance to highly specific transcatheter therapy, with the ability to address a wider spectrum of cerebrovascular diseases. This includes patients with cerebral vascular aneurysms, malformations, tumors, symptomatic intracranial atherosclerotic stenosis, and thromboembolic occlusions causing acute ischemic stroke.
- In some cases, endovascular management complements open surgical techniques; in others, endovascular interventions have become the method of first choice.

Prevalence

- ~750,000 strokes/year in the USA
- Higher incidence in African Americans

Clinical Pointers

- Three-fourths of strokes occur in patients older than 75 years of age
- Fourth leading cause of death
- Significant morbidity and cost associated with stroke

Clinical Presentation and Evaluation (Table 11.1)

- Symptoms typically start suddenly without prodrome and depend on the area of the brain affected.
- History and neurological examination not only serve to localize the patient's neurological problem and define the etiology and duration of the problem, but also serve as a baseline to assess procedural success and possible iatrogenic complications from the intervention.
- Patients with acute injury require immediate neurological imaging to guide further treatment.
- Assays of coagulation and platelet function have particular importance in neurointerventions both to prevent iatrogenic thromboembolic stroke during procedures and to reduce the likelihood of hemorrhage, a common response to neurological injury.
- For elective procedures, assays of renal function are important as iodinated contrast dosages are often significant during complex interventions. Knowledge of a patient's medications and allergies are important to maintain hemodynamic stability and reduce the risk of seizures.

Tips on Which Imaging Study to Perform As an Initial Evaluation?

- Cross-sectional imaging recommended prior to intervention.
- Unenhanced CT brain scan remains critical to exclude intracranial hemorrhage, and has a high negative predictive value.

- Further imaging should be tailored to the clinical scenario and the acuity of presentation as well as institutional preferences to better plan the intervention.
- MR or CT angiography, including 3D reconstructed views, is helpful in planning intervention.
- Perfusion, functional, diffusion-weighted and tensor imaging, computational flow dynamics and nuclear medicine techniques to evaluate cerebral blood flow and oxygen extraction fraction are finding their way into routine evaluation and treatment.
- Diffusion imaging depicts cytotoxic edema related to the ischemic insult as early as minutes. Perfusion imaging reveals areas of mismatch and potentially salvageable ischemic penumbra.

TABLE 11.1 Evaluation of patients undergoing intra-arterial stroke treatment

Clinical evaluation
Brief but relevant history and examination to ascertain
Rule out stroke mimics such as seizures, hypoglycaemia, neoplasm
Cardiovascular and cerebrovascular medical history
Medications
Blood pressure, pulse rate, respiratory rate
12 lead ECG
Determine contraindications such as recent surgery/trauma
Time of onset
Neurological impairment scales – e.g., NIH stroke scale
Disability scales – e.g., modified Rankin scale
Laboratory evaluation
Hematology – hematocrit, hemoglobin, platelets
Coagulation parameters – PT (INR), aPTT
Kidney function – BUN, creatinine

TABLE 11.1 (continued)

Imaging
Unenhanced CT of the head to rule out hemorrhage and completed infarction >1/3 of the vascular territory
Vascular and perfusion imaging, depending on institutional protocols to characterize level of occlusion and tissue at risk

Therapeutic Options for Acute Ischemic Stroke: Lytic vs. Endovascular Interventions

- Treatment of acute ischemic stroke requires a well-coordinated multidisciplinary approach which includes all aspects of care from emergency medical services to post-stroke rehabilitative care.
- A number of trials have evaluated the safety and efficacy of intravenous (IV) and intra-arterial (IA) fibrinolysis for the treatment of acute ischemic stroke [1–3].
- Most recently, mechanical devices for clot retrieval, alone or in combination with fibrinolytic therapy, are under evaluation in registry and NIH-funded randomized trials [4, 5].

Contraindications to Lysis

- Minor stroke symptoms
- Rapidly resolving symptoms
- Active GI Bleeding
- Seizure at presentation
- Uncontrollable Hypertension
- Anticoagulant use with INR >1.7
- Recent brain surgery

- *At this time, the only acute ischemic stroke therapy scientifically shown to improve clinical outcomes as defined by the various stroke scales, is IV fibrinolysis using rt-PA administered within 3 h of stroke onset, at a dose of 0.9 mg/kg, to a maximum of 90 mg. Ten percent of the dose is administered as an initial bolus and the remainder infused over a period of 60 min.*

- Based on the recent publication of ECASS-III many investigators now extend the window for intravenous fibrinolysis to 4.5 h of stroke onset [2].
- Endovascular treatment, in conjunction with intravenous treatment forms a small but important part in the whole process of stroke care.

Clinical Pointers on Intra-arterial (IA) Thrombolysis

- Although IA fibrinolysis has become community standard, it has not been proven effective in two independent trials and thus is not FDA-approved with a stroke indication.
- Technical advances in the field of neurointervention, with the development of soft microcatheters and microwires, high-resolution fluoroscopy and digital subtraction angiography, and non-ionic contrast agents, have made it feasible and safe to access the major intracranial blood vessels from a transfemoral approach.
- Rapid, local delivery of fibrinolytic agents or immediate access of thrombolytic devices is now feasible with these techniques.
- Currently IV therapy is the treatment of choice in patients presenting within 3 h of onset. IA thrombolysis is performed in patients who are ineligible for IV thrombolysis.
- IA dose is tailored based on each individual case at the discretion of the interventionalist

Percutaneous Endovascular Treatment

Pre-procedural Issues

Various peri-procedural technical aspects relevant to performing safe interventions on the cerebral vasculature are outlined below:

Consent

- A detailed discussion must be undertaken with the patient and family members about the proposed procedure whenever possible.
- In many cases, both the disease requiring treatment and the procedure itself carry substantial risk.
- These issues should be described in simple language accessible to those involved. It is imperative to address all of the patient's questions and concerns about the procedure including the risks and benefits.
- During the interview process, both the treating team and the patient should together establish realistic goals. Certain treatments may require a staged approach, or neurological recovery may be prolonged.
- For many neurovascular procedures, the scientific evidence remains limited and technological developments outstrip the time required to accumulate high-level evidence.
- A frank discussion of any off-label or experimental application of drugs or technology is important in the interest of full disclosure. For this reason, a facile knowledge of the relevant medical literature is very important.

Anesthesia

- The cerebral vasculature is delicate and complex. For these reasons, many neurovascular interventions are performed using some form of general anesthesia.
- Experts disagree, but most will acknowledge that motion reduction is needed for high-level spatial and temporal resolution. The use of roadmap imaging is essential for safe navigation of the cerebral and spinal vasculature.
- Most centers specializing in the treatment of neurovascular diseases have a good working relationship with anesthesiologists specialized in neurological disease.
- Specific needs for patient paralysis requiring endotracheal intubation for mechanical ventilation or strict blood pressure control can be communicated.

- Diagnostic cerebral arteriography is generally performed with moderate sedation with the assistance of nursing staff. In acute situations where availability of the anesthesia team may be delayed due to resource issues, such as intra-arterial thrombolytic therapy for acute ischemic strokes, the type of anesthesia may be tailored to the situation based on institutional practices pending development of additional scientific evidence, societal guidelines, or recommendations for practice.

Scrub Team

- Many procedures are facilitated by good assistants.
- Consequently, communication among the members of the scrub team is important for performance of safe intracranial interventions. All members of the team must know institutional protocols for designation of syringes, flush lines, and sharp disposal practices.
- The team should ideally include the attending (lead) interventionalist, trainees or partners, and sometimes a scrub nurse or technologist.
- Surgical sterility should be observed in all cases, particularly those in which prosthetic implants will be used.

Angiography Equipment

- Biplane digital subtraction angiography on machines now designed and configured for neurovascular imaging and intervention is ideal. These units use x-ray tubes with micro-focal spots for high resolution imaging and high heat capacity for prolonged magnification fluoroscopy and high frame-rate angiography.
- Most units include the capability for rotational angiography, three dimensional reconstruction, and neurovascular analysis packages to facilitate treatment. These suites are modified operating rooms with laminar flow ventilation for infection control, gases, suction, and data links to accommodate anesthesia machines and life-support equipment.
- With a profusion of modern technology, storage for various catheter systems and implants must allow rapid access.

Despite optimization of equipment for neurological procedures, the interventionist should at all times be cognizant of radiation safety practices to minimize exposure both to patients and to hospital staff.

Potential Pitfalls

- Imaging is essential to rule out hemorrhage and stroke mimics
- Delays may occur in obtaining anesthesia support
- "Time is brain" – Efficient teamwork is essential; get things moving as quickly as possible

Endovascular Therapy for Acute Ischemic Stroke: How I Do It

The basic principles of intracerebral interventions as outlined above are illustrated in the following scenario including the endovascular treatment of acute ischemic stroke. Tables 11.2 and 11.3 outline some of the common intraprocedural equipments/devices used in the interventional neuroradiology suite.

Procedural Technique

After obtaining femoral vascular access, a short vascular sheath is placed. Larger diameter sheaths such as 8–9 Fr sheaths may be necessary if using large balloon guiding catheters required for mechanical clot retrieval (MERCI device).

Diagnostic Angiography

The gold standard for demonstrating occlusion is angiography. A three- or four-vessel pre-intervention diagnostic cerebral angiogram, including both internal carotid arteries and the dominant vertebral artery with delayed imaging into the

TABLE 11.2 Common equipment used in interventional neuroradiology suite-access, catheters, wires, and closure devices

Arterial access

Needles

Micropuncture set

18-gauge single wall access needle

Vascular sheaths

5–9 Fr short and long vascular sheaths

Flush lines

Pressure bags with heparinized saline (1–5 IU heparin per cc normal saline) for all indwelling intravascular catheters

Air-removal devices are becoming standard equipment for neurovascular procedures

Angiography catheters/guidewires

Catheters

Diagnostic catheters 3–5 Fr

Guidewires

0.035–0.038″ guidewires with and without hydrophilic coating

Exchange length (300 cm) guidewires for catheter exchanges without loss of access

Guiding catheter assembly

Catheters

5–8 Fr catheters with large internal diameter (ID)

Various tip configurations depending on location and individual anatomy

Rotational hemostatic valve connectors

To enable bloodless exchange of catheters and wires and simultaneous flushing

Microcatheters

Varying inner diameter microcatheters (multiple manufacturers)

Tip – shape-able vs. pre-shaped tip configurations

TABLE 11.2 (continued)

Microwire
0.008–0.018″ configurations
Operator shapeable
Exchange length microwires for exchanging microcatheters without losing access
Steerable microwires for precision control
Arterial closure devices
Starclose, angioseal, perclose, etc.

TABLE 11.3 Common equipment used in interventional neuroradiology suite-embolics, stents, balloons, and other devices

Embolic agents
Detachable coils
Varying thickness 0.010–0.018″ from 2 to 20 mm diameter sizes
Coated vs. bare platinum coils
Variable detachment mechanisms
Mechanically deployed coils
Passed through microcatheter and delivered using a pusher wire (bleeding/tumor)
Liquid embolic agents
n-butyl cyanoacrylate
Ethylene vinyl alcohol copolymer
Particulate embolic agent
PVA particles for tumor embolization
Detachable balloons
Intracranial stents
Stent-assisted aneurysm coiling
Enterprise, leo stent, neuroform, solitaire, etc.

(continued)

TABLE 11.3 (continued)

Intracranial atherosclerotic disease
Wingspan stent
Stent-assisted endoluminal flow disruption
Pipeline embolization device, silk stent, etc.
Intracranial angioplasty balloons
Compliant balloons
Balloon-assisted aneurysm coiling (hyperglide, hyperform, ascent, etc.)
Non-compliant balloons
Intracranial angioplasty prior to stenting (gateway balloon, myriad coronary balloon catheters)
Clot retrieval systems
Mechanical retrieval
MERCI retrieval device
Vacuum-assisted clot retrieval
Penumbra stroke system

late venous phase is recommended before fibrinolysis to evaluate collateral circulation, concomitant pathology, and anatomic variations. Standard AP and lateral views and oblique projections as necessary may be required. Nearly 8–10 cc of non-ionic contrast is injected at a rate of 3–5 cc/s. The angiogram should assess the following angiographic findings among other features:

- Location of occlusion(s)
- Extent of occlusion
- Vascular territories involved
- Perfusion assessment (TIMI or TICI grading system; Table 11.4)
- Collateral blood flow sources and pattern (Table 11.5)
- Presence of shunting ("luxury perfusion")/vascular blush
- Arterial dissection, aneurysm, anomaly
- High-grade stenosis
- Non-atherosclerotic arteriopathy (e.g., vasculitis).

TABLE 11.4 Thrombolysis in cerebral infarction (TICI) perfusion categories

Grade 0	*No perfusion.* No antegrade flow beyond the point of occlusion.
Grade 1	*Penetration with minimal perfusion.* The contrast material passes beyond the area of obstruction but fails to opacify the entire cerebral bed distal to the obstruction for the duration of the angiographic run.
Grade 2	*Partial perfusion.* The contrast material passes beyond the obstruction and opacifies the arterial bed distal to the obstruction. However, the rate of entry of contrast into the vessel distal to the obstruction and/or its rate of clearance from the distal bed are perceptibly slower than its entry into and/or clearance from comparable areas not perfused by the previously occluded vessel, e.g., the opposite cerebral artery or the arterial bed proximal to the obstruction.
Grade 2a	Only partial filling (<2/3) of the entire vascular territory is visualized.
Grade 2b	Complete filling of all of the expected vascular territory is visualized, but the filling is slower than normal.
Grade 3	*Complete perfusion.* Antegrade flow into the bed distal to the obstruction occurs as promptly as into the obstruction *and* clearance of contrast material from the involved bed is as rapid as from an uninvolved other bed of the same vessel or the opposite cerebral artery.

TABLE 11.5 Collateral flow grading system: angiographic

Grade 0	No collaterals visible to the ischemic site.
Grade 1	Slow collaterals to the periphery of the ischemic site with persistence of some of the defect.
Grade 2	Rapid collaterals to the periphery of ischemic site with persistence of some of the defect and to only a portion of the ischemic territory.
Grade 3	Collaterals with slow but complete angiographic blood flow of the ischemic bed by the late venous phase.
Grade 4	Complete and rapid collateral blood flow to the vascular bed in the entire ischemic territory by retrograde perfusion.

IA Fibrinolysis Technique

- Once a site of vascular occlusion that corresponds to the patient's neurologic deficit is angiographically confirmed, IV heparin is administered by most neurointerventionalists based on the methods and results of PROACT-II [3]. A 2,000-U bolus is administered followed by 500 U/h infusion for 4 h beginning at the time of angiography.
- Systemic anticoagulation with heparin reduces the risk of catheter-related thrombo-embolism.
- Antithrombotic (anti-platelet) therapy may be useful to prevent acute reocclusion, which is more common with atheromatous plaque thrombosis than with cerebral embolism. Abciximab may be administered intravenously or intra-arterially although proper dosage is uncertain.
- These indications are counterbalanced by the potentially increased risk of cerebral hemorrhage when heparin is combined with a fibrinolytic agent.
- After the diagnostic angiogram, a guiding catheter is placed in the artery leading to the target lesion.
- Using roadmap imaging, the microcatheter is guided to the site of vessel occlusion over a micro-guidewire. Variations in treatment techniques include traversing the occlusion and lacing the clot with drug, embedding the microcatheter in the occlusion, or simple proximal drug infusion.
- Intra-arterial lytic treatment may be instituted with or without prior intravenous fibrinolysis. Single end-hole microcatheters are used most often for local cerebral fibrinolysis, depending on the extent of clot formation.
- Control angiography through the guiding catheter is performed at intervals of approximately 15–30 min to assess the degree of clot lysis.
- If there is partial clot dissolution, the microcatheter may be advanced into the remaining thrombus, where additional fibrinolysis may be performed.
- As the thrombus is dissolved, the microcatheter is advanced into more distal branches of the intracranial circulation, so

that the majority of the thrombolytic agent enters the occluded vessel and does not pass preferentially into patient blood vessels.

- Most neurointerventionalists will not perform intra-arterial fibrinolysis in the anterior cerebral circulation beyond 6 h of stroke onset although there are reports of successful therapy beyond this time point.
- The goal is to achieve rapid recanalization with as little fibrinolytic agent as possible to restore cerebral blood flow and to limit the risk of hemorrhagic transformation.

Mechanical Embolectomy Technique

- Alternatively, mechanical embolectomy is under investigation as a means to restore cerebral blood flow in acute ischemic stroke.
- Theoretical advantages include more rapid restoration of cerebral blood flow, longer time horizon to treatment, up to 8 h, and a lower risk of hemorrhage when fibrinolytic agents are avoided.
- While Concentric Merci retriever and Penumbra suction thrombectomy systems are FDA-approved foreign body retrievers with an acute ischemic stroke indication, neither device has been scientifically demonstrated to improve patient outcomes although evidence to that effect is mounting.
- Moreover, cerebrovascular stent devices are being deployed on an experimental basis to treat symptomatic acute occlusions refractory to convention revascularization methods (Fig. 11.1).

Angiographic Success

- The effect of recanalization on angiographic reperfusion should be reported with the TIMI or TICI grading system (Table 11.4) and clinical status before and after treatment using the NIH Stroke Scale.

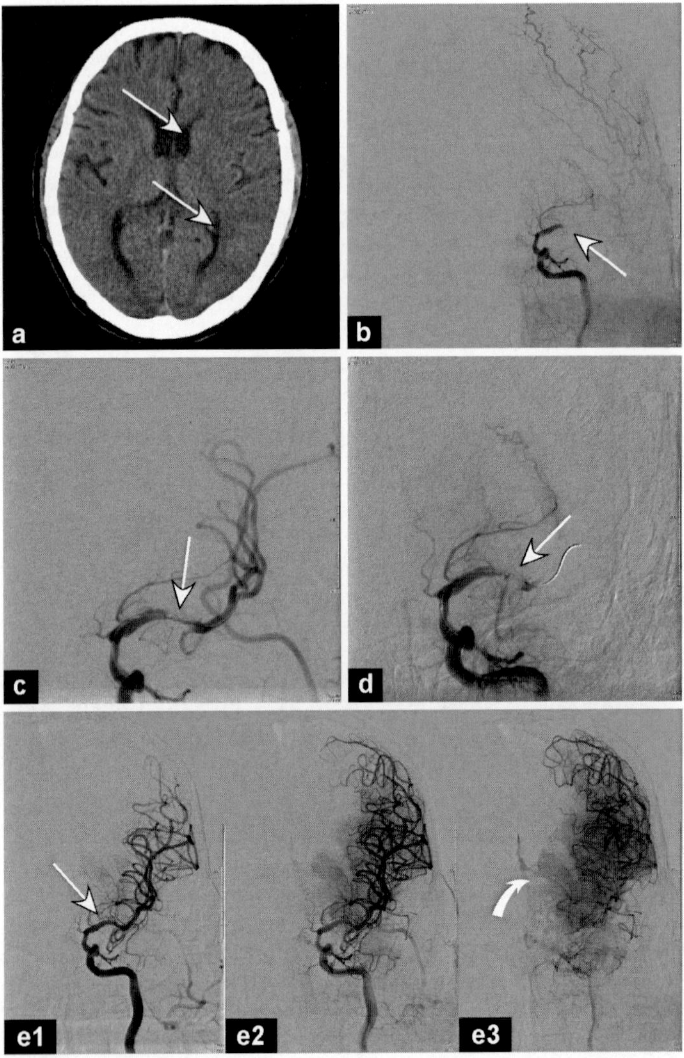
a
b
c
d
e1
e2
e3

FIGURE 11.1 A 71-year-old man with hypertension, hyperlipidemia, tobacco abuse, and peripheral vascular disease was admitted through the Emergency Department with progressive right hemiplegia and global aphasia of 2-h duration. The NIH Stroke Score was 23. (**a**) a non-enhanced CT brain scan showed early edema in basal ganglia structures and less than one third of the left middle cerebral artery distribution (*arrows*). The patient received full-dose intravenous rt-PA (0.9 mg/kg) in the ED. (**b**) When the patient showed no signs of initial improvement, he was triaged for emergency catheter arteriography. Left internal carotid arteriography in the frontal projection during the arterial phase showed proximal occlusion of the left middle cerebral artery (*arrow*). (**c**) Initial attempts to perform mechanical thrombectomy were not successful. Balloon angioplasty was then performed restoring a thin channel for antegrade blood flow in the M1 segment of the left middle cerebral artery (*arrow*). (**d**) Repeat arteriography shows re-occlusion of the left middle cerebral artery despite systemic anticoagulation with rt-PA (*arrow*). (**e**) Stent angioplasty was then performed using a 4.5×14 mm^2 self-expanding nitinol stent on a compassionate basis (*arrow*). Successive angiographic images show dramatic reperfusion of the left middle cerebral artery with luxury perfusion (*curved arrow*) in the basal ganglia indicative of tissue injury and loss of autoregulation. At the time of discharge to rehabilitation, the patient had moderate hemiparesis (strength 4+/5) and resolving expressive aphasia

- Subjects can be categorized as complete responders (TICI 3), partial responders (TICI < 3 but ≥ 1 category improvement from baseline), and nonresponders (no improvement in TICI category).

Post-procedural Care and Evaluation

- Patients undergoing stroke therapy must be closely monitored for symptomatic intracranial hemorrhage.
- Many patients require rehabilitative therapy after hospitalization. Coordination with physical medicine, rehabilitative therapies, and social services is necessary for a smooth transition to subacute or acute rehabilitative centers.

- Ongoing evaluation of treated patients is an important part of the neurointerventionalist's job. Outpatient facilities are necessary to monitor these patients longitudinally.

Potential Pitfalls

- Control of serum glucose and electrolytes correlates with patient outcome
- Neurological deterioration may be difficult to evaluate in a sedated patient

- Patients are transferred to intensive care immediately following therapy.
- Many neurointerventionalists will use a vascular closure device to obtain hemostasis at the femoral puncture site.
- Alternatively, the sheath may be left in place for invasive arterialpressure monitoring until the fibrinolytic effect abates and the sheath can be removed with manual compression alone.

Neurological Evaluation

- Unanticipated changes in level of consciousness or focal neurological signs should prompt immediate evaluation, including cross-sectional imaging.
- Repeated neurological evaluations including NIHSS (Table 11.6) determinations should be performed throughout treatment, after the final angiogram, and at defined time points after treatment per institutional protocols.
- Any signs of neurologic deterioration must be recorded and should prompt evaluation for ICH, edema with mass effect, or hydrocephalus that may require urgent intervention.

TABLE 11.6 Stroke assessment scales

Scale	Description	Range	What the score means
National Institutes of Health Stroke Scale (NIHSS)	42 point scale measuring neurological deficit across 11 subcategories	0–42	A score of 0 indicates normal neurological function; Scores of ≥22 indicate severe deficit
Modified Rankin Scale (mRS)	A simplified assessment of neurological function and dependency	0–6	0 means no symptoms; A score of 5 indicates severe disability. A score of 6 indicates death.
Barthel index	Measures the ability to perform activities of daily living	0–100	A score of 100 indicates ability to perform all activities independently.

- Functional outcomes are usually assessed by indices such as the modified Rankin Scale (mRS) and Barthel index (Table 11.6).

Imaging

- Noncontrast cerebral CT or MRI is performed following interventional procedures and within 24 h,
- Repeat imaging may be performed as needed for 7–10 days to guide therapy.
- As noted previously, abrupt neurologic deterioration requires clinical and imaging evaluation usually using cerebral CT.
- An evaluation of the presence/absence of hemorrhage, edema, and/or infarction as contributors to the clinical deterioration should be made.

Grading of Intracranial Hemorrhage Following Thrombolysis
Hemorrhagic Infarction type 1 – Small petechiae along the margins of the infarct

Hemorrhagic Infarction type 2 – More confluent petechiae within infarct, without space occupying effect
Parenchymal hematoma type 1 – hematoma <30% of area; some space-occupying effect
Parenchymal hematoma type 2 – Dense hematoma >30% with substantial space occupying effect

- Cerebral hemorrhage is categorized as either hemorrhagic infarct or parenchymal hematoma.
- Commonly used grading scales for hemorrhage as used in NINDS and IMS-III trials may be used (See box).

Bibliography

1. Tissue plasminogen activator for acute ischemic stroke. The National Institute of Neurological Disorders and Stroke rt-PA Stroke Study Group. N Engl J Med 333:1581–1587, 1995.
   → *Landmark NINDS trial demonstrating the efficacy of intravenous tPA for acute ischemic stroke when treated within 3 h of onset.*
2. Hacke W, Kaste M, Bluhmki E, Brozman M, Dávalos A, Guidetti D, Larrue V, Lees KR, Medeghri Z, Machnig T, Schneider D, von Kummer R, Wahlgren N, Toni D; ECASS Investigators. Thrombolysis with alteplase 3 to 4.5 hours after acute ischemic stroke. N Engl J Med. 2008 Sep 25;359(13):1317–29.
   → *Results of ECASS investigators demonstrating benefit of IV tPA extended to window of 4.5 h.*
3. Furlan A, Higashida R, Wechsler L, Gent M, Rowley H, Kase C, Pessin M, Ahuja A, Callahan F, Clark WM, Silver F, Rivera F: Intra-arterial prourokinase for acute ischemic stroke. The PROACT II study: a randomized controlled trial. Prolyse in acute cerebral thromboembolism. JAMA 282:2003–2011, 1999.
   → *The Original PROACT II paper, a randomized, controlled, multicenter, open-label clinical trial with blinded follow-up demonstrating improved clinical outcomes in patients with MCA occlusion treated with intra-arterial pro-urokinase within 6 h of onset.*

4. Smith WS, Sung G, Starkman S, Saver JL, Kidwell CS, Gobin P, Lutsep HL, Nesbit GM, Grobelny T, Rymer MM, Silverman E, Higashida RT, Budzik RF, Marks MP: Safety and efficacy of mechanical embolectomy in acute ischemic stroke: results of the MERCI trial. Stroke 36:1432–1438, 2005.
   → *MERCI trial which led to the FDA approval of a mechanical device for clot retrieval of acute clots in patients ineligible for IV tPA.*
5. Bose A, Henkes H, Alfke K, Reith W, Mayer TE, Berlis A, Branca V, Sit SP; Penumbra Phase 1 Stroke Trial Investigators. The Penumbra System: a mechanical device for the treatment of acute stroke due to thromboembolism. AJNR Am J Neuroradiol. 2008 Aug;29(7):1409–13.
   → *Results of Penumbra system for reducing clot burden in acute stroke due to large vessel occlusive disease.*

Chapter 12
The Carotid Artery

Warren J. Gasper, Christopher D. Owens, and Joseph Rapp

Etiology

Atherosclerosis (>95%), Fibromuscular dysplasia, Arterial redundancy and kinking, Arteritis, Radiation Therapy.

Background

Atherosclerotic plaque primarily involves the carotid bifurcation. Moderate plaque buildup frequently occurs in the common carotid but it rarely extends more than 3–4 cm into the internal carotid. Symptoms are rare due to flow reduction. *This is the only vascular lesion where embolization is the primary pathologic entity.*

W.J. Gasper • C.D. Owens (✉) • J. Rapp
Division of Endovascular and Vascular Surgery, Department of Surgery, University of California – San Francisco, San Francisco, CA, USA
e-mail: warren.gasper@ucsf.edu; christopher.owens@ucsfmedctr.org

C.D. Owens and Y. Yeghiazarians (eds.), *Handbook of Endovascular Peripheral Interventions*, DOI 10.1007/978-1-4614-0839-0_12,

Clinical Pointers
- Age of presentation is usually greater than 60-years old.
- Risk factors include: age, hypertension, dyslipidemia, smoking, diabetes, low HDL (<40 mg/dL).
- The sensitivity and positive predictive value of carotid bruit to diagnose hemodynamically significant carotid stenosis are low (50–60% and 20–30%, respectively).

Clinical Presentation

- Asymptomatic: carotid bruit or ultrasound screening
- Symptomatic: Transient Ischemic Attack (TIA) or stroke referable to a single hemisphere (Tables 12.1 and 12.2)

TABLE 12.1 Common symptoms of carotid territory transient ischemic attack

Embolic symptoms
Transient monocular blindness
Transient monocular field cuts
Dysarthria
Dysphagia
Aphasia
Monoparesis
Hemipareis
Hemisensory deficit
Hypoperfusion symptoms
Bright light amaurosis
Shaking (limb) body TIA

TABLE 12.2 Signs and symptoms unlikely to be related to carotid disease (in absence of embolism)

Unconsciousness (including syncope)
Tonic/clonic activity
Dizziness alone
Vertigo alone
Dysphagia alone
Dysarthria alone
Confusion alone
Visual loss with alteration of consciousness

TABLE 12.3 Results of a meta-analysis of the accuracy of noninvasive imaging for all stenosis groups and imaging modalities

Stenosis group (%)	Imaging	Sensitivity (95% CI)	Specificity (95% CI)
70–99%	US	0.89 (0.85–0.92)	0.84 (0.77–0.89)
	CTA	0.77 (0.68–0.84)	0.95 (0.91–0.97)
	CEMRA	0.94 (0.88–0.97)	0.93 (0.89–0.96)
50–69%	US	0.36 (0.25–0.49)	0.91 (0.87–0.94)
	CTA	0.67 (0.30–0.90)	0.79 (0.63–0.89)
	CEMRA	0.77 (0.59–0.89)	0.97 (0.93–0.99)
0–49, 100%	US	0.83 (0.73–0.90)	0.84 (0.62–0.95)
	CTA	0.81 (0.70–0.88)	0.91 (0.74–0.98)
	CEMRA	0.96 (0.90–0.99)	0.96 (0.90–0.99)

Screening

Choices based on local expertise and preferences. The results of a recent meta-analysis on the sensitivity and specificity of CTA, contrast-enhanced MRA, and duplex ultrasound are presented in Table 12.3. The anatomic and morphologic features associated with adverse outcomes after carotid artery

TABLE 12.4 Anatomic and morphologic features associated with adverse outcomes after carotid artery stenting, or that might influence the choice of protection device or stent, and relationship with imaging modalities

		Modality			
Vessel affected	Feature	US	MRA	CTA	Angiography
Aortic arch	Ulceration	X	+	++	++
	Excessive calcification	X	X	++	+
	Bovine arch variants	X	++	++	++
	Type III arch	X	++	++	++
Great vessels	Ulceration	X	+	++	+
	Tortuosity/ kinking	X	++	++	++
	Excessive calcification	X	X	++	+
	Anatomic anomalies	X	+	++	+
	Severe inflow stenosis	X	+	++	++
Common carotid	Diffuse disease	+	++	++	++
	Coiling/kinking	+	++	++	++
	Excessive calcification	+	X	++	+
Carotid bifurcation	Excessive calcification	X	X	++	+
	Angulation	++	++	++	++
Ipsilateral external carotid artery	Occlusion/ severe stenosis	++	++	++	++

TABLE 12.4 (continued)

		Modality			
Vessel affected	**Feature**	**US**	**MRA**	**CTA**	**Angiography**
Ipsilateral internal carotid artery	Excessive calcification	X	X	++	+
	Distal tortuosity/ coiling	X	++	++	++
	Plaque characterization	++	++	+	X
	Fresh thrombus	+	+	+	X
	Preocclusive stenosis	++	++	++	++
	Long lesion (>3 cm)	+	+	++	++
Contralateral internal carotid artery	Stenosis >50%	++	++	++	++
Incomplete circle of Willis		X	++	++	+

Adapted from Rutherfords Vascular Surgery, 7th edition
X not really suited for imaging, + basic information provided, ++ highly suitable for imaging, *MRA* magnetic resonance angiography, *CTA* computed tomographic angiography, *US* ultrasound

stenting and the relationship with imaging modalities are presented in Table 12.4.

Ultrasonography

Strengths

- Preferred first-line modality for identifying patients with 70–99% stenosis.
- Low cost.

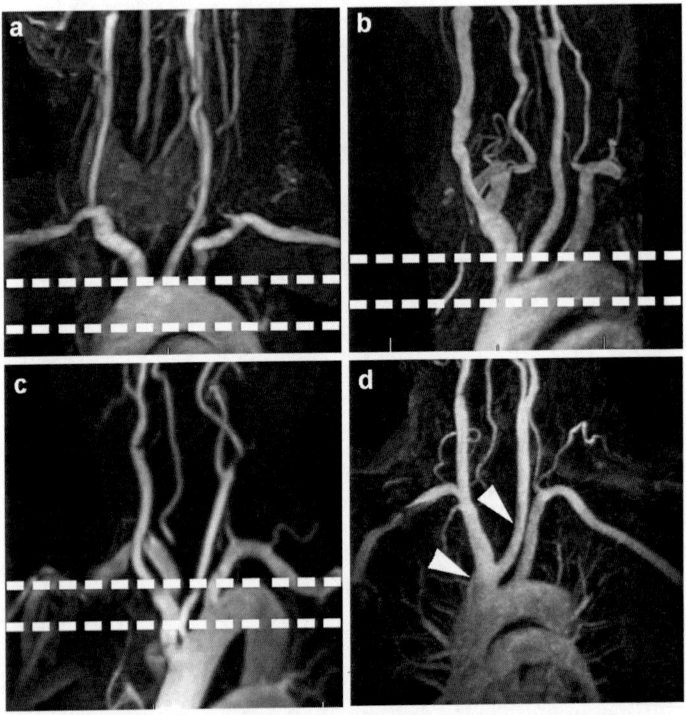

FIGURE 12.1 Types of aortic arches as seen on MRA. The location of the inominate artery takeoff in relation to the outer and inner curves of the aortic arch determines the type of aortic arch. (**a**) Type I – the inominate and left carotid origins are above the outer curve of the arch (*dotted white lines*). (**b**) Type II – the origin of the inominate and left carotid are between the outer and inner curves (*dotted white lines*). (**c**) Type III – the origin of the inominate and left carotid are below the level of the inner curve. The inferior location of the common carotid arteries make cannulating and exchanges very difficult. This often requires increased manipulation which consequently increases the risk of aortic plaque embolization. (**d**) Bovine aortic arch. The inominate and left carotid artery share a common origin on the aortic arch (*white arrows*)

- Non-invasive, highly reproducible if done by the same operator with the same machine.
- Robustness of sensitivity analysis (Table 12.3).

Limitations

- Flow rate acts as a surrogate marker for degree of stenosis.
- Echo shadowing in heavily calcified vessels.
- Proximal common carotid and arch cannot be visualized. This limitation is particularly significant when planning carotid artery stenting as may influence choice of selective catheters, stent type, or protection devices used (see Fig. 12.1).

Clinical Pointers: The UCSF ultrasound criteria and flow characteristics for all grades of stenosis

Class	**Peak systole**	**End diastole**	**ICA/CCA ratios sys dias**	**Flow character**	
Normal	<125 cm/s	–	<1.8	<2.5	Minimal or no spectral broadening during the deceleration phase of systole. Boundary layer separation within the carotid bulb present.
<50%	<125 cm/s	–	<1.8	<2.5	Plaque/intimal thickening is present
50–69%	125–230 cm/s	<100	1.8–3.7	2.6–5.5	Plaque present
≥70% to near occlusion	>230 cm/s	–	>3.7	>5.5	Visible plaque and lumen narrowing present

Class	Peak systole	End diastole	ICA/CCA ratios sys dias	Flow character	
Near occlusion	Varies	–	–	–	Markedly narrowed lumen at color Doppler
Occlusion	No flow	–	–	–	No detectable lumen
Criteria for ICA stenosis based on NASCET measurement method					
>70%	= ICA/CCA>4.0				
>60%	= ICA/CCA>3.2				

ICA internal carotid artery, *CCA* common carotid artery

Magnetic Resonance Angiography (MRA)

Strengths

- No radiation
- Excellent view of the entire arch, extracranial carotid and major intracranial vessels
- Can get highly sensitive images of brain ischemia with diffusion-weighted imaging

Limitations

- More dependent upon technical expertise to get excellent images
- Susceptible to artifacts from motion (arch vessels at arch) and tortuosity (origin vertebral arteries)
- Gadolinium toxicity may create NSF (nephrogenic systemic fibrosis) in patients with renal insufficiency
- Contraindicated in patients with pacemakers, defibrillators, cochlear implants, and spinal cord stimulators and may not be tolerated by claustrophobic patients

Computed Tomography Angiography (CTA)

Strengths

- Excellent images obtained with three-dimensional anatomy.
- Allows visualization of the vascular supply from the arch through the brain.
- Widely available, (rapid) fast study.

Limitations

- Image interpretation may be difficult due to "blooming" of overlying calcification – i.e., calcification appears larger than actual size.
- Clarity of image depends on timing of the bolus and type of CT scanner (newer multi-detector scanners are superior to older spiral CT).
- Radiation exposure; requires iodinated contrast.

Conventional Angiography/Digital Subtraction Angiography

Strengths

- Can be coupled with stenting in the same procedure.

Limitations

- Generally underestimates the true degree of stenosis because of its two-dimensional display.
- Invasive, requires groin puncture, catheterization.
- Requires contrast exposure with potential renal damage.
- Radiation exposure.
- There is a small risk of neurologic deficit from procedure.

Treatment

- General
  - Medical treatment of risk factors and smoking cessation.
  - Anti-platelet therapy:
    - Aspirin is recommended for all patients.
    - Clopidogrel (Plavix) may be added if there is symptom developed while on aspirin. However, there is no direct evidence for the efficacy of clopidogrel in this situation and aspirin + clopidogrel may be associated with more bleeding complications.
    - In symptomatic patients (prior TIA or ischemic stroke), aspirin with extended-release dipyridamole (Aggrenox) has been shown to reduce the risk of recurrent ischemic events compared to aspirin alone.
  - Statins have been shown to reduce the risk of ischemic stroke in patients with cerebrovascular disease, cardiovascular disease or diabetes regardless of cholesterol level.
- Asymptomatic stenosis.
  - Major trials of carotid endarterectomy demonstrate clinical effectiveness in preventing stroke for patients with carotid stenoses of 60–99%. To maximize the risk-benefit ratio of a preventative procedure, we favor limiting treatment of asymptomatic carotid stenosis to a lesion of ≥80%.
- Symptomatic stenosis.
  - Early treatment of symptomatic patients (small CVA or TIA) with a stenosis ≥70% is highly recommended.
  - Early treatment of symptomatic patients with an ipsilateral 50–70% stenosis is generally recommended based on the NASCET results.
  - Treatment delayed for healing of the blood/brain barrier in patients with CVA and large infarct for fear of hemorrhagic conversion.

Endarterectomy vs. Stenting for Carotid Stenosis

- A recent meta-analysis of randomized controlled trials of carotid artery stenting (CAS) vs. carotid artery endarterectomy (CEA) found that carotid stenting was associated with a higher risk of periprocedural and mid to long-term stroke or death but a lower risk of periprocedural MI and cranial nerve injury compared to carotid endarterectomy (Bangalore et al., Archives of Neurology, 2010, see references). This meta-analysis includes results from SPACE, EVA-3 S, ICSS, and CREST and the results of these four RCTs are summarized below (Table 12.5).

Clinical Pointers

- Endarterectomy preferred (see Fig. 12.2)
  - Symptomatic patients
  - Patients age ≥70 years old – asymptomatic or symptomatic (based on CREST and other randomized trials)
  - Type III aortic arch
- Stenting preferred (see Fig. 12.3)
  - Patients with hostile necks, i.e., post-radiation therapy or tracheostomy
  - Recurrent stenosis
  - Plaques extending above C-2
- Either endarterectomy or stenting
  - Asymptomatic patients <60-years old with high-grade lesions

TABLE 12.5 Summary of major trials comparing CEA and CAS

	Study population	Results
SPACE, 2008	1,196 patients	*Outcome*: ipsilateral stroke or death
	Symptomatic with ≥50% stenosis	*Results*: higher rate of ipsilateral stroke or death in CAS group at 30 days (6.84% CAS vs. 6.34% CEA, $p=0.09$)
EVA-3 S, 2008	527 patients	*Outcome*: stroke or death
	Symptomatic with ≥60% stenosis	*Results*: significantly higher rate of ipsilateral stroke or death in CAS group at 30 days (9.6% CAS vs. 3.9% CEA, $p=0.01$) and 6 months (11.7% CAS vs. 6.1% CEA, $p=0.02$)
ICSS, 2010	1,710 patients	*Outcome:* stroke, MI, or death
	Symptomatic with >50% stenosis	*Results*: significantly higher rate of ipsilateral stroke or death in CAS group at 120 days (8.5% CAS vs. 5.2% CEA, $p=0.006$)
CREST, 2010	2,502 patients	*Outcome*: stroke, MI, or death
	Symptomatic (1,321) and asymptomatic (1,181)	*Results*: no significant difference in rate of outcome at median 2.5-year follow-up (7.2% CAS vs. 6.8% CEA). However, the rate of stroke was significantly higher for stenting (4.1% CAS vs. 2.3% CEA, $p=0.01$) while the rate of MI was significantly lower (1.1% CAS vs. 2.3% CEA, $p=0.03$)

CAS carotid artery stent, *CEA* carotid endarterectomy, *SPACE* Stent-Supported Percutaneous Angioplasty of the Carotid Artery versus Endarterectomy, *EVA-3 S* Endarterectomy versus Angioplasty in Patients with Symptomatic Severe Carotid Stenosis, *ICSS* International Carotid Stenting Study, *CREST* Carotid Revascularization Endarterectomy vs. Stenting Trial

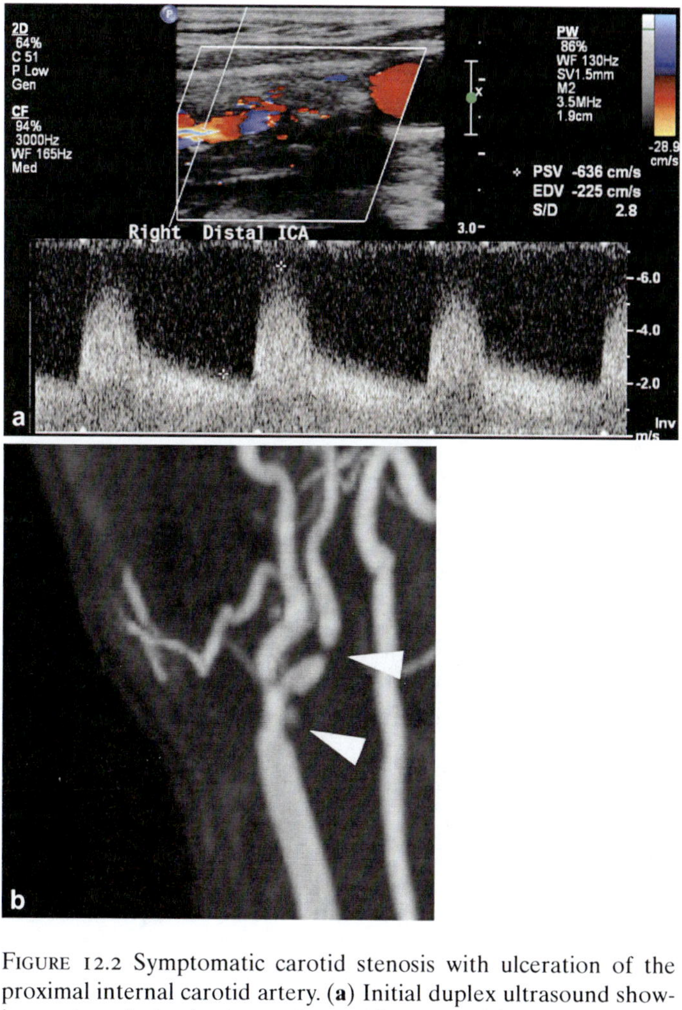

FIGURE 12.2 Symptomatic carotid stenosis with ulceration of the proximal internal carotid artery. (**a**) Initial duplex ultrasound showing a stenosis in the internal carotid artery with a peak systolic velocity (PSV) of 636 cm/s and end diastolic velocity (EDV) of 225 cm/s. (**b**) MRA of the neck showing an ulceration of the proximal internal carotid (*lower arrow*) and a critical stenosis just distal to the ulceration (*upper arrow*). (**c**) Intraoperative photograph of the ulcerated plaque in the proximal carotid artery (*arrow*) during carotid endarterectomy. (**d**) Follow-up duplex ultrasound demonstrating markedly lower velocities after endarterectomy and patch angioplasty (PSV 16.4 cm/s, EDV 2.8 cm/s)

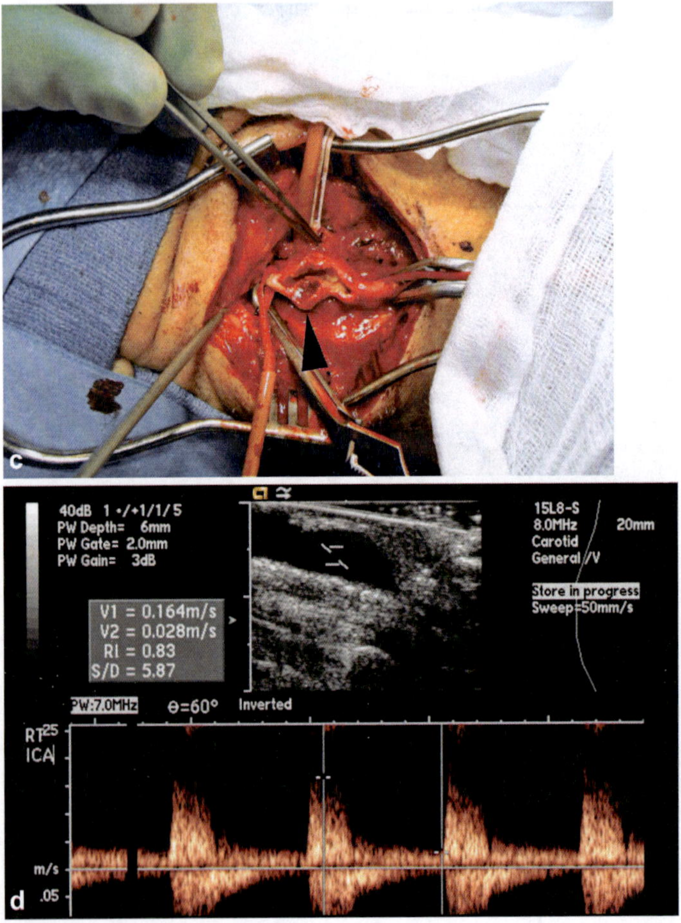

FIGURE 12.2 (continued)

Carotid Artery Angioplasty and Stenting: How I Do It

- Access
  - All patients are started on aspirin and clopidogrel (Plavix) before the procedure and are kept on dual therapy up to the time of the procedure.

- Retrograde femoral artery puncture with 6 F sheath. If ilio-femoral segment is adequate, upgrade to 9 Fr.
- Heparin is given to keep ACT >300 s and glycopyrolate 0.4 μg is given to prevent bradycardia with angioplasty.
- The patient's neurological status is monitored during the procedure by asking the patient to repeat the phrase "No ifs, ands, or buts" and squeeze a squeak toy in the contralateral hand. Failure of one of these tests should prompt an evaluation for intracranial emboli (see Potential Pitfalls).
- Berenstein 2 or JB-1 catheter and a 180-cm Bentson wire are used to negotiate the iliacs up to the arch and cannulate the carotid arteries in 90% of cases without arch

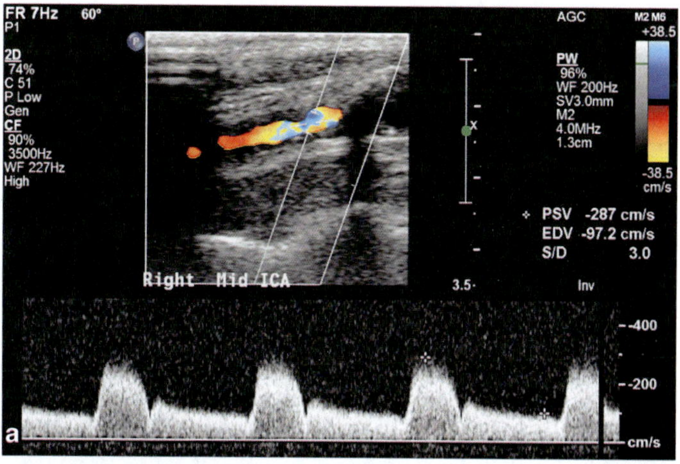

FIGURE 12.3 Stenting of a lesion in the proximal internal carotid. (**a**) Initial duplex ultrasound showing a stenosis in the internal carotid artery with a peak systolic velocity (PSV) of 287 cm/s and end diastolic velocity (EDV) of 97 cm/s. (**b**) Digital subtraction angiogram of the carotid artery demonstrating the stenosis in the proximal internal carotid artery with an ulceration just distal to the carotid bulb (*black arrow*). (**c**) Digital subtraction angiogram after placement of a stent from the common carotid artery to the internal carotid artery (*white arrows*). (**d**) Follow-up duplex ultrasound demonstrating markedly lower velocities after stenting (PSV 64.7 cm/s, EDV 21.2 cm/s)

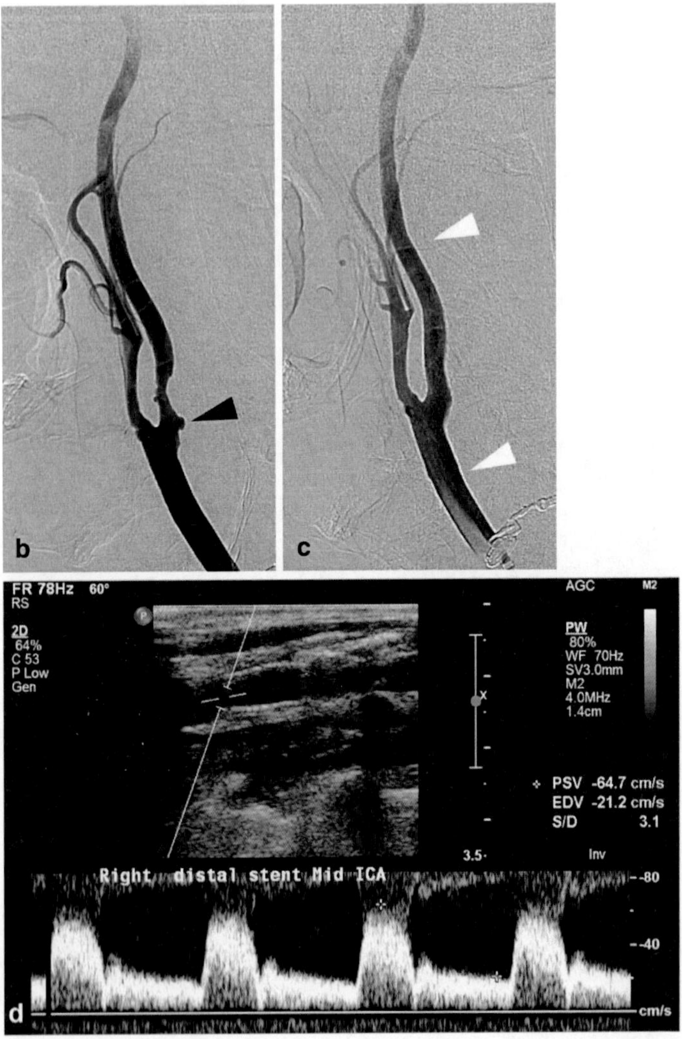

FIGURE 12.3 (continued)

TABLE 12.6 Features of embolic protection devices

	Distal filter	Flow reversal (preferred)
Advantages	– Maintain ICA blood flow	– Cerebral protection prior to crossing the lesion
	– Angiographic control throughout case	– Protection even with tortuous or friable lesions
Disadvantages	– Must cross lesion to deploy – Complete vessel wall apposition is required	– May not be tolerated by all patients, especially if contralateral carotid occluded or circle of Willis not patent
	– Filter can become clogged and require emptying during the case	– Requires 9 Fr sheath

angiography. Difficult anatomy requires a Simmon's 2 catheter, generally reformed in the left subclavian artery.

– Supracore wire (260 cm) advanced into the external carotid artery and a Gore flow-reversal device (sheath) positioned in the common carotid artery. *If you choose to use a filter-type embolic protection device, then place a long 6 F sheath into the Common Carotid Artery at this time and gently pass the protection device through the lesion into a straight segment of the ICA distal to the lesion, see* Table 12.6.
– Angiograms of the lesion are done. Obtain multiple views of the lesion in lateral and oblique projections to obtain the best vantage point for the intervention. Intracranial views are recommended but not required.
– Flow reversal is created by the balloon occlusion of the external and common carotid artery with retrograde flow being returned to the patient through a 6 F sheath in the contralateral common femoral vein. This is confirmed with slow injection of 2–4 mL of dye (see Fig. 12.4).
– Transend 0.014-in. wire is used to cross the stenosis.

- Closed-cell stents are used simply due to their improved visibility over the Nitinol self-expanding stents (see Fig. 12.5). Predilation to 3–4 mm is done if the lesion has calcification suggesting rigidity. Post-dilate the stent with an appropriate-sized balloon, generally 5 or 6 mm.
- Once post-dilation is done, aspirate 100 mL slowly through the flow-reversal device prior to re-establishing

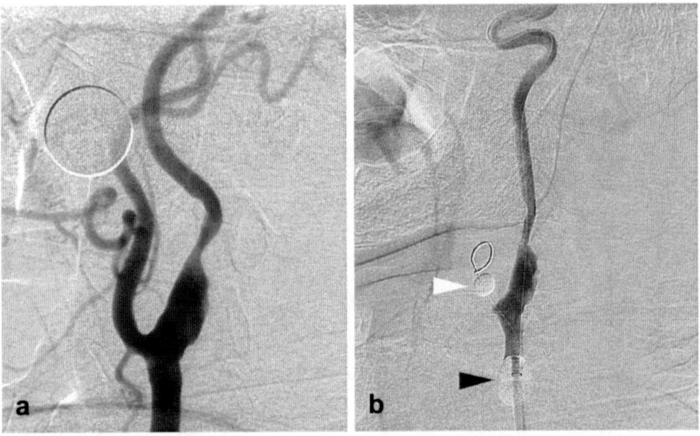

FIGURE 12.4 Flow-reversal device seen on digital subtraction angiography. (**a**) Initial angiogram showing a stenosis in the internal carotid artery. (**b**) Placement of the flow-reversal device with occluding balloons in the external carotid (*white arrow*) and common carotid (*black arrow*). Injection of contrast confirms occlusion of the external and common carotid arteries by the balloons before the device is activated and flow from the internal carotid drained into the left femoral vein. (**c**) Completion angiogram after stenting and removal of the flowreversal device. (**d**) Photographs of the GORE® Flow Reversal System (W.L. Gore and Associates, Inc. Flagstaff, AZ) demonstrating the position of the balloons and the equipment at the end of the device. Notice in the left panel that the balloon in the external carotid is positioned to exclude the superior thyroid artery. Before device activation, a sheath is placed in the contralateral femoral vein (*not shown*) and connected to the flow reversal line (*right panel*)

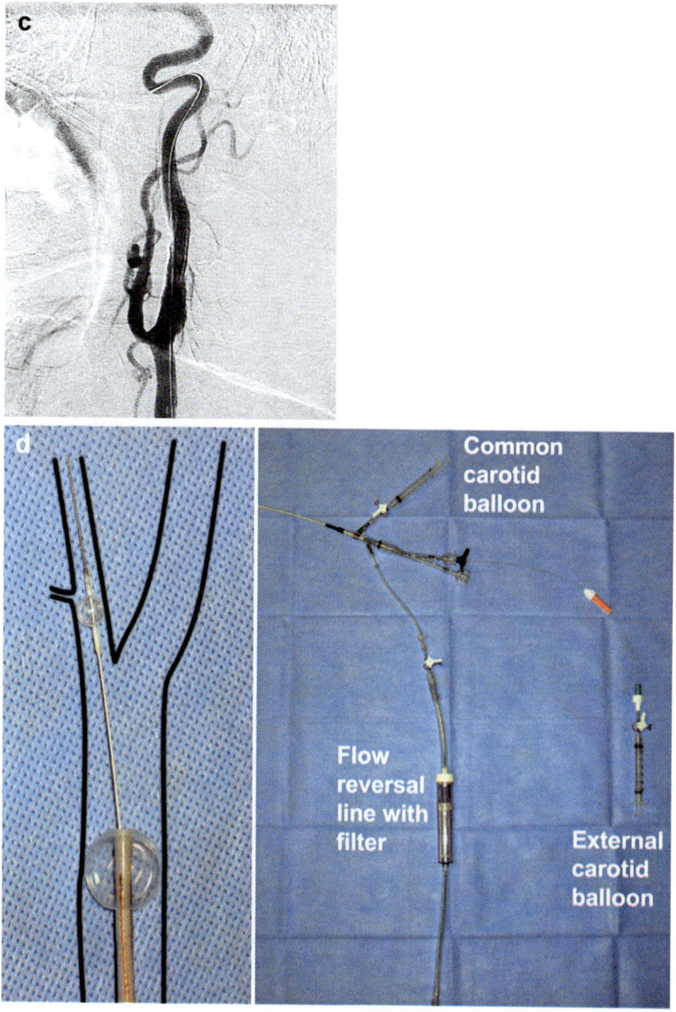

FIGURE 12.4 (continued)

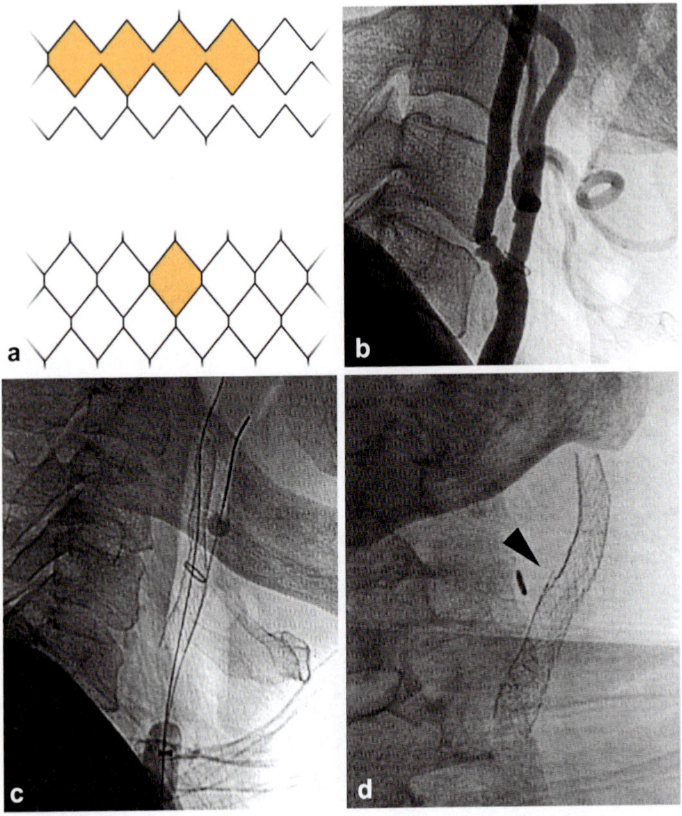

FIGURE 12.5 Open-cell stent "fish scaling" after carotid stenting. (**a**) Diagram of the difference between an open-cell (*upper panel*) and closed-cell (*lower panel*) stent construction. (**b**) Initial lateral angiogram demonstrating an irregular, calcified plaque in the internal carotid artery. (**c**) Lateral image after stent deployment with flow-reversal (notice the balloons in the external carotid and common carotid arteries). (**d**) AP image shows "fish scaling" of the stent with projection of the stent struts into the vessel intima (*arrow*). Of note, the fish scaling stent made removal of the flow-reversal balloon from the external carotid balloon difficult

antegrade flow by deflating first the external carotid and then the common carotid occluding balloons.

- Completion angiography done with the Transend wire in place. Once satisfied with the result, the Transend wire is removed.
- The external carotid balloon is intentionally "jailed" by the stent and must be completely deflated and gently pulled under the stent.
- A StarClose device is used on the arterial puncture. The venous puncture is handheld. The authors acknowledge that StarClose is not indicated for 9 Fr devices but the senior author (JR) has deployed the device in over 50 cases with 9 Fr sheaths without incident!

Tips of the Trade

- In cannulating an early-branching bovine left common carotid, it may be of value to turn the Simmon's 2 catheter slightly horizontal to reduce its angle of entry.
- If the catheter will not track over the wire, slight changes in the angle of the carotid arteries can be achieved with a deep breath by the patient or turning the head to the left or right.
- When passing a sheath from the arch into the common carotid artery, the "push–pull" technique is sometimes helpful. A gentle, steady, forward, pressure is applied to the sheath while the stiff guide wire is kept on traction and even withdrawn very slightly.
- Cannulating the external carotid with the Supracore wire may be difficult and a Glidewire may be required with advancement of the Berenstein or Simmon's 2 catheter up into the proximal external carotid artery and the Supracore wire placed through the catheter.
- If the patient does not tolerate the full flow-reversal, the sheath can simply be used for placement of the distal protection device.

Potential Pitfalls

- Avoiding emboli is paramount and requires full heparinization with ACT monitoring as well as strict avoidance of air bubbles in lines and tubing. No champagne injections!
- Calcifications of the aortic arch can be dislodged during the initial catheterization of the carotid or by "snow plowing" the sheath into the plaque and showering emboli. Excellent catheter control and a delicate touch are necessary throughout the procedure.
- When using a flow-reversal device, the external carotid balloon must be carefully withdrawn from beneath the stent. If the balloon is not completely deflated or there is "fish scaling" of the stent, the balloon may become trapped and further manipulation may risk showering emboli or dislodging the stent. If the balloon is stuck, try advancing a catheter along the wire, pulling in the balloon and then withdrawing the balloon and catheter together (see Figs. 12.4 and 12.5).
- A change in neurological status (inability to repeat the phrase "no ifs, ands, or buts" or failure to squeeze a squeak toy in the contralateral hand) should prompt an evaluation for intracranial emboli. This requires an immediate cerebral angiogram to look for filling defects and a neurointerventionalist consult.

Follow-Up and Screening After Carotid Artery Stenting

- Close post-procedure monitoring with frequent neurologic exams and early follow-up are critical as most strokes (78%) occur after stenting (20% occur after discharge from the hospital).
- The patient continues on daily clopidogrel 75 mg daily and aspirin 81 mg daily for 6 weeks after the procedure.

- After 6 weeks, single therapy with aspirin 81 mg daily is recommended.
- Ultrasound is done prior to the patient leaving the hospital, then at 6 weeks, 3 months post-procedure, and then 6 months, and then every 6 months, looking for re-stenosis. Stents tend to increase velocities measured on duplex ultrasound, so we pursue additional imaging when velocities reach what are otherwise considered critical levels, i.e., PSV > 250–300 cm/s or EDV > 80–100 cm/s.
- Evaluation for suspected re-stenosis is typically with CTA or angiogram.
- Routine monitoring and treatment of risk factors is essential.

Equipment List

Sheaths

6- to 9-Fr long sheath (90 cm) depending on ilio-femoral segment diameter
Shuttle Select (Cook)
Pinnacle Destination (Terumo)
Flow Reversal (9-Fr sheath) (W.L. Gore & Associates)

Catheters

Berenstein 2
JB-1
Simmon's 2

Guidewires

To get access to the carotid:
0.035-in. Bentson 180 cm (Boston Scientific)
0.035-in. Supracore 260 cm (Abbott)
0.035-in. Glidewire (Terumo)

For crossing the carotid stenosis:
- 0.014-in. Transend wire (Boston Scientific) – this is a neuroangiographic wire with a shapeable, radio-opaque, hydrophobic tip that is particularly suited for crossing tight, tortuous cerebrovascular lesions

Balloons

Pre-dilation of rigid, calcified lesions
- 3 or 4 mm coronary balloon

Post-dilation of stent
- Short (2 cm) 5 or 6 mm balloon

Stents

Open cell
- Acculink Carotid Stent (Abbott)
- Protégé RX Carotid Stent (ev3)

Closed cell
- Carotid Wallstent (Boston Scientific)
- Xact Carotid Stent (Abbott)

Embolic Protection Devices

Distal filters
- SpiderFX (ev3)
- FilterWire EZ (Boston Scientific)

Flow Reversal
- GORE FlowReversal System (W.L. Gore & Associates)

Bibliography

Barnett H J, Taylor D W, Eliasziw M, Fox A J, Ferguson G G, et al. Benefit of carotid endarterectomy in patients with symptomatic moderate or severe stenosis. North American Symptomatic

Carotid Endarterectomy Trial Collaborators. The New England Journal of Medicine. 1998;339(20):1415–25.

→ *The NASCET trial randomized patients with symptomatic carotid stenosis to medical therapy or carotid endarterectomy and demonstrated a reduced risk of stroke with carotid endarterectomy for symptomatic stenosis ≥70%. This follow-up report showed a modest benefit for patients with 50–69% stenosis as well.*

Endarterectomy for asymptomatic carotid artery stenosis. Executive Committee for the Asymptomatic Carotid Atherosclerosis Study. JAMA (Chicago, Ill.). 1995;273(18):1421–8.

→ *The ACAS trial randomized 1,662 patients with asymptomatic carotid stenosis to medical therapy or carotid endarterectomy. The results demonstrated a reduced stroke rate with carotid endarterectomy and asymptomatic stenosis ≥60% if the surgery was done with <3% mortality rate.*

Ederle Jrg, Dobson J, Featherstone R L, Bonati L H, van der Worp H B, et al. Carotid artery stenting compared with endarterectomy in patients with symptomatic carotid stenosis (International Carotid Stenting Study): an interim analysis of a randomised controlled trial. Lancet. 2010;375(9719):985–97.

→ *The ICSS trial randomized 1,713 patients with symptomatic carotid stenosis ≥50% to carotid endarterectomy or carotid stent. In this interim safety analysis, the data were analyzed at 120 days by intention to treat and showed that the incidence of stroke, death, or procedural MI was 8.5% in the stent group vs. 5.2% in the endarterectomy group (HR 1.69, 1.16–2.45, p = 0.006). Rates of stroke were higher in the stent group as was the mortality rate.*

Brott T G, Hobson R W, Howard G, Roubin G S, Clark W M, et al. Stenting versus endarterectomy for treatment of carotid-artery stenosis. The New England Journal of Medicine. 2010; 363(1):11–23.

→ *The CREST trial randomized 2,502 patients with symptomatic and asymptomatic carotid stenosis to carotid endarterectomy (CEA) or carotid stent (CAS). At a median 2.5 years of follow-up, there was no difference between the groups for the primary composite end point of periprocedural stroke, MI or death or ipsilateral stroke within 4 years (5.2% CAS vs. 4.5% CEA). However, the stroke rate was significantly higher for stented patients (4.1% CAS vs. 2.3% CEA) while the MI rate was significantly lower in stented patients (1.1% CAS vs. 2.3% CEA).*

Fairman R, Gray W A, Scicli A P, Wilburn O, Verta P, et al. The CAPTURE registry: analysis of strokes resulting from carotid artery stenting in the post approval setting: timing, location, severity, and type. Annals of surgery. 2007;246(4):551–6; discussion 556.

→ *An analysis of the 170 strokes after carotid stenting in the CAPTURE trial. Observations include a significantly higher rate of major strokes among patients with symptomatic disease, 19% of strokes occurred on the contralateral side and 80% of strokes were diagnosed prior to discharge (22.3% during the procedure and 57.7% after the procedure but before discharge).*

Bangalore S, Kumar S, Wetterslev Jrn, Bavry A, Gluud C, et al. Carotid Artery Stenting vs Carotid Endarterectomy: Meta-analysis and Diversity-Adjusted Trial Sequential Analysis of Randomized Trials. Archives of neurology. 2010; e-pub October 11, 2010. PMID 20937941.

→ *The most comprehensive and up-to-date meta-analysis of randomized trials for carotid stenting vs. carotid endarterectomy. This analysis found that carotid stenting was associated with an increased risk of periprocedural and mid to long-term stroke and death but decreased risk of periprocedural MI and cranial nerve injury.*

Chapter 13
Subclavian Artery Stenosis

Victor M. Ochoa and Yerem Yeghiazarians

Etiology

- Most common is atherosclerosis (~90%).
- Other causes to consider include: fibromuscular dysplasia, arteritis, neurofibromatosis, inflammation secondary to radiation, and extrinsic compression (thoracic outlet syndrome).

Prevalence

- The incidence of subclavian stenosis in the general population ranges from 3% to 4%, and can be as high as 11–18% in patients with documented peripheral arterial disease.
- Of those patients found to have subclavian or innominate lesions, 50% have concomitant coronary artery disease, 27% lower extremity artery involvement, and 29% carotid obstructive disease.

V.M. Ochoa
Division of Cardiology, Department of Medicine,
University of California – San Francisco, San Francisco, CA, USA

Y. Yeghiazarians (✉)
Division of Interventional Cardiology, Department of Medicine,
University of California – San Francisco,
San Francisco, CA, USA
e-mail: yeghiaza@medicine.ucsf.edu

C.D. Owens and Y. Yeghiazarians (eds.),
Handbook of Endovascular Peripheral Interventions,
DOI 10.1007/978-1-4614-0839-0_13,

Clinical Pointers

- Left subclavian artery is four times more likely to be affected than the right or innominate arteries.
- If there is an isolated stenosis, due to the degree of potential collateralization, the likelihood of symptoms is less than in other vascular beds.
- However, once obstructive disease affects other aortic arch vessels, namely the carotids or vertebrals, the likelihood of steal or ischemic symptoms drastically increases.

Clinical Presentations/Clues

- Upper extremity symptoms:
  1. Arm claudication
  2. Rest pain
  3. Muscle fatigue
  4. Finger necrosis from embolization
- Neurologic symptoms (characterized by vertebrobasilar hypoperfusion):
  1. Visual disturbances
  2. Syncope
  3. Ataxia
  4. Vertigo
  5. Dysphasia
  6. Dysarthria
  7. Facial sensory deficits
- Post-Coronary Artery Bypass Graft (CABG) patients with internal mammary arterial (IMA) graft may present with angina pectoris due to coronary steal

Clinical Pointers

- Bilateral arm pressures should be checked at the initial clinic visit for all patients, but especially in patients with known coronary or peripheral arterial disease.

- A systolic blood pressure difference between the two arms of greater than 20 mmHg should raise clinical suspicion for subclavian Stenosis.
- Subclavian stenosis can be more difficult to diagnose in certain patients who have a dialysis fistula in one arm or have other clinical reasons when bilateral blood pressures cannot be obtained. In these patients, a high clinical suspicion should be followed by appropriate imaging studies.

Screening

Appropriate clinical and exam findings, such as unequal arm blood pressures, absent or drastically diminished pulses in comparison to the contralateral arm, and cervical or supraclavicular bruits should prompt further imaging studies.

Ultrasound Findings of Subclavian Steal

- The identification of a 15–20 mmHg brachial artery pressure gradient should prompt investigation for vertebral to subclavian steal syndrome
- Retrograde or undulating flow in the ipsilateral vertebral artery makes vertebral to subclavian steal likely.
- The combination of reversal of flow and a 20 mmHg pressure gradient makes the diagnosis.
- Less severe subclavian stenosis may result in early systolic deceleration or bidirectional flow in the vertebral artery

Ultrasonography (US)

- *Strengths*: safe, inexpensive and widely available, images of the subclavian artery as well as blood flow velocity and pressure waveforms, can also visualize flow reversal in the event of vertebral or IMA steal.

- *Limitations*: dependent on operator expertise, limited by technical challenges related to patient habitus or subclavian course. Is more effective in detecting distal lesions rather than proximal or ostial disease.

Computed Tomography Angiography

- *Strengths*: Excellent images can be obtained (Sensitivity >91%; Specificity 85–99% with newer scans). Is useful in planning endovascular interventions as it delineates the takeoff of important vessels such as the carotid and vertebral arteries, and their proximity/involvement with the index lesion.
- *Limitations*: image interpretation may be difficult in heavily calcified arteries; involves the use of ionizing radiation and iodinated contrast medium; may not be tolerated by claustrophobic patients.

Magnetic Resonance Angiography

- *Strengths*: No iodinated contrast or radiation (Sensitivity 90–100%; Specificity 76–94%).
- *Limitations*: gadolinium-based contrast associated with nephrogenic systemic fibrosis in patients with moderate-to-end-stage renal failure; contraindications to MRI (pacemakers, defibrillators, cochlear implants, and spinal cord stimulators); may not be tolerated by claustrophobic patients. Limited utility in suspected total occlusions.

Angiography

- *Strengths*: remains the "gold standard"; evaluates the extent of vascular disease; can measure a direct gradient across the stenosis; therapeutic procedures such as percutaneous transluminal angioplasty or stenting can be carried out at the same time.

- *Limitations*: invasive technique; radiation and contrast exposure.

Treatment

- Medical treatment of risk factors (e.g., lipids, blood pressure, smoking cessation).
- Indications for invasive therapy of subclavian stenosis are not clearly known; options are balloon angioplasty alone vs. stenting vs. surgical bypass (the latter is rarely performed and usually associated with other open surgical thoracic procedures).
- Clinical reasons to consider an invasive approach: disabling upper limb ischemia (including claudication, rest pain, and digital embolization); vertebrobasilar insufficiency from steal syndrome; anginal symptoms from coronary steal via IMA graft; and to increase flow before surgical procedures such as CABG with use of IMA grafts or dialysis graft placement.
- Decision to revascularize atherosclerotic subclavian stenosis is individualized as there are no guidelines available at this time.

Subclavian and Innominate Artery Angioplasty and Stenting: How I Do It (Fig. 13.1)

- Access: This can be obtained either retrograde through the femoral artery or through the brachial artery approach, or in some cases, both may be needed. Transradial approach is less commonly used for this purpose, but can be done. Location and lesion characteristics are important in determining the access site. Majority of cases are performed from the femoral artery approach. A brachial approach can be considered in the setting of ostial total occlusions
- Initially, a standard 5 Fr short sheath can be placed in the common femoral artery. Using a 5 Fr pigtail catheter, ascending aortography can be performed to delineate the arch anatomy. If the anatomy is already known by CT scan, this step can be skipped to minimize contrast use.
- The aortic arch can be "opened up" and the origin of the great vessels better delineated by using a left anterior

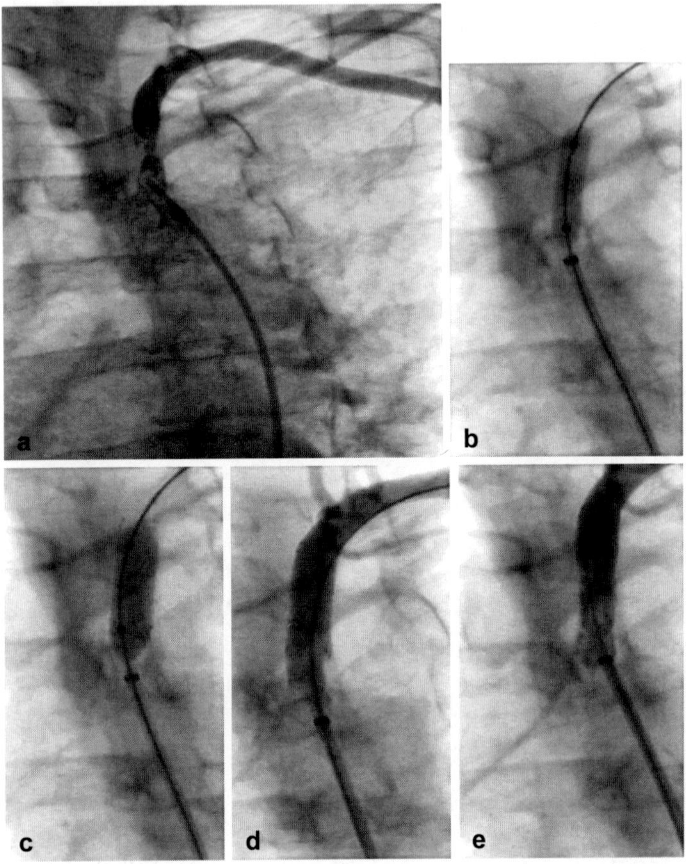

FIGURE 13.1 (**a**) Access was obtained with a 6.5 Fr standard sheath in the right femoral artery. A 6 Fr JR 4.0 catheter was used to cannulate the left subclavian and then a glidewire was used to advance the JR 4.0 catheter distal to the lesion. The glidewire was then exchanged for a Storq wire and the JR 4.0 catheter was exchanged for a long 55 cm 6 Fr sheath. (**b**) The lesion was then dilated with a PTA-PRO 5 mm × 20 mm balloon inflated to 6 ATM (**c**) The lesion was then stented with a 7 mm × 20 mm Smart Control Self-Expanding stent. (**d**) Due to residual stenosis following stent implantation, the lesion was then post-dilated with a 8 mm × 20 mm PTA-PRO balloon inflated at low pressure (2–2.5 ATM). (**e**) Post-PCI angiography revealed no residual stenosis and no residual gradient

oblique (LAO) 30–45° projection. For selective subclavian imaging, various catheters including JR-4, JB-1, or 2, IMA, multipurpose or vertebral catheter can be used. Selective angiography can be performed using a total of 10–15 cc injection over 2–3 s.

- Subclavian interventions are performed with unfractionated heparin (50–60 U/kg) to achieve an ACT ~250–300. Angiomax can also be used.
- Once the subclavian or innominate is engaged, a 0.035″ steerable hydrophilic wire (Terumo in my case) can be advanced to the axillary artery. Either the diagnostic catheter or a straight catheter can then be advanced distally in order to exchange the hydrophilic wire for a more supportive and safer 0.035″ wire such as an Amplatz, Rosen, Strorq, or Bentsen wire.
- The sheath can then be exchanged for a 6–7 Fr system (if 5 Fr was used initially). For better support, we recommend a long sheath to be used (80–100 cm for femoral access) and placed at the subclavian or innominate origin. For brachial access, a 35-cm sheath can be placed just distal to the lesion.
- Pre-dilation with an undersized balloon can be done for both vessel caliber and lesion length sizing. It should be noted that for ostial or peri-vertebral lesions, the incidence of dissection is higher with angioplasty and some operators will forgo this pre-dilatation step in these cases. Occasionally, pre-dilation is needed for stent passage and this should be done gently with an undersized compliant balloon.
- Balloon-expandable or self-expandable stents can be used depending on the lesion location. Some operators also prefer to use cover stents, making sure that main side branches will not be covered with these covered stents. For short ostial disease, including total occlusions or lesions between the right carotid and vertebral arteries (or near the left vertebral origin), a balloon-expandable stent (covered or non-covered) is recommended for better delivery precision. In the case of ostial lesions, balloon-expandable

stents are used for their enhanced radial strength in this typically heavily calcified territory. Self-expanding stents are typically better suited for post-vertebral (distal to the vertebral artery origin) lesions.

- Self-expanding stents should be oversized by 1–2 mm, and if need be, post-dilation and optimal expansion can be achieved with non-compliant balloons. When stenting ostial lesions, the balloon expandable stent should be overhung by 1–2 mm into the aorta to ensure definitive ostial coverage.
- If the retrograde brachial approach is used for total occlusions, especially at the ostium, care should be given to avoid entering dissection planes when crossing the lesion. Intra-luminal wire placement confirmation should be done by advancing a straight catheter into the ascending or descending aorta, with contrast injection distally for a conclusive assessment.

Lesion Classification by Standard of Practice Committee and Society of Interventional Radiology (by Category)

1: Stenotic lesion 3 cm or less in length not involving the right carotid artery or vertebral artery.
2: Stenotic lesion greater than 3 cm in length not involving the right carotid artery or vertebral artery.
3: Short total occlusions (less than 5 cm in length) that often involve the subclavian or innominate artery origin.
4: Stenotic lesion involving the origin of the right carotid and/or the vertebral artery or total occlusions greater than 5 cm in length.

Clinical Pointer

- In the setting of a subclavian ostial occlusion, or very proximal high-grade stenosis, it is advisable to perform an aortic angiogram. A pigtail can be placed in the proximal arch and a power contrast injection

(30 cc for 10–15 cc/s should suffice) is done to better understand the lesion characteristics and location as it relates to other great vessels and branches (i.e., the vertebral arteries or right carotid artery).

- It is important to know if the ostium of the right common carotid or the left vertebral artery is involved for safer planning of the interventional procedure.
- Knowledge of contralateral carotid and vertebral and Circle of Willis patency can also help with safer procedural planning.

Potential Pitfalls and Things to Remember

- Average diameter of the proximal subclavian artery is ~8 mm (range 7–12 mm).
- Depending on patient's body habitus, the size of the subclavian artery can be variable. To decrease the risk of complications such as perforation or dissection, the diameter should be measured prior to intervention.
- Use of a marked pigtail catheter, or quantitative angiography are commonly used methods of measuring the subclavian diameter.
- Since unfractionated heparin (UFH) can be reversed with Protamine, whereas Angiomax cannot, we find it safer to perform subclavian interventions on UFH.
- Post-dilation non-compliant balloons should be 1–2 mm smaller than the stent used to minimize the risk of perforation in cases of non-covered stent implantation.
- To accurately position the stent at the ostium of the subclavian artery, some operators prefer to advance the sheath or guide catheter past the lesion, position the stent, and then "unsheath."

- Another technique not to miss the ostium of the subclavian is to advance a second 0.014″ wire through the sheath and let this wire "straddle" the aortic arch, thus delineating the ostium of the subclavian.

Cerebral Protection

- Generally, cerebral protection is not necessary during subclavian artery interventions as it is believed that the reversal of vertebral flow that typically occurs with proximal subclavian lesions is protective. Antegrade vertebral flow is not restored for several minutes post-procedure.
- When vertebral protection is needed, this can be accomplished by inflating an appropriately sized balloon at the vertebral artery origin or with a filter device.
- There are two possible ways of doing this:
  1. The vertebral access can be obtained using transbrachial or transradial approach while the subclavian stenting procedure is performed through the femoral approach.
  2. Alternatively, two 0.014″ wires can be used through the femoral approach. One wire is positioned in the axillary artery and the other in the vertebral artery. The filter is then positioned in the vertebral artery and over *both* 0.014″ wires, appropriately sized 0.035″ balloons and stents can be advanced for the subclavian procedure. At the end of the procedure, the filter is withdrawn and the wires removed.

Follow-Up and Screening After Subclavian or Innominate Artery Stenting

- Guidelines do not exist but in our practice dual antiplatelet therapy with aspirin (325 or 162 mg daily) and clopidogrel (75 mg daily) for at least 30 days is given. Monotherapy with aspirin (81 mg daily) chronically thereafter.

- Surveillance is not standardized. We recommend a subclavian duplex ultrasound to be performed within 1–2 weeks after stenting to establish a new baseline. Depending on symptoms and/or physical exam findings during yearly clinic visits, repeat duplex ultrasounds can be considered at 6–12 month intervals. Of course, bilateral arm blood pressures should be checked at every clinic visit.
- CT and MRI are less useful given the artifact seen in the presence of the stent, but given the large size of these stents, adequate information can often be obtained.

Equipment List

This is a partial list as a variety of equipment can be successfully utilized.

Sheaths

5–6F standard short sheath.
6 Fr 80–100 cm long sheath for a trans-femoral approach.
- Terumo Pinnacle
- Cordis

6 Fr 35 mm sheath for retrograde brachial approach.
Larger sheaths (7–8F) can be considered, depending on the support needs and size of guide catheters (if used).

Diagnostic and Guide Catheters

5–8 Fr catheters with varying shapes. We find the following catheters to be useful in the majority of cases:

- JR-4
- JB-1
- JB-2
- Vertebral
- H-1

- IMA
- Multipurpose

Guidewires

We recommend 0.035″ wires given the large caliber arterial size and support needs. There are many wires that can be utilized. Commonly, we use one of the following:

- Hydrophilic: Terumo glidewire (angled for steering). Typically exchanged for the following once the lesion is crossed:
- Amplatz
- Rosen
- Storq
- Wholey

Note: in cases where 0.035″ wires cannot cross a complete subclavian occlusion, 0.014″ stiffer wires that are commonly used for coronary chronic total occlusions can be considered with caution due to risk of dissection or perforation with these wires. There are many wire choices, but some to consider include:

- Asahi series CTO coronary wires
- Cross-IT series wires
- Confianza
- Fielder XT
- Pilot
- Spartacore

Balloons

There are many balloon choices. Some include:

- OPTA-Pro (Cordis)
- AGIL-Trac (Guidant)
- Sterling (Boston Scientific)
- Maverick/Apex (Boston Scientific)
- Voyager (Abbott)
- Dura Star (Cordis)

Stents

There are various options for balloon-expandable stents. The possible options include:

- Express non-covered stent (Boston Scientific)
- Atrium ICAST covered stent (Atrium) → this is the covered stent of choice in our practice
- Cordis Genesis
- EV3 Visi-Pro
- Guidant Rx Herculink

There are various options for self-expanding stents. The options may include:

- SMART non-covered stent (Cordis)
- Viabahn covered stents (Gore)

Distal Protection

Embolic protection devices include:

- FilterWire EZ (Boston)
- GuardWire (Medtronic)

Bibliography

Prevalence of Subclavian Artery Stenosis in Patients with Peripheral Vascular Disease. *Angiology*. 2001;52:189–194.

→ *A prospective, single center, observational study assessing the incidence and prevalence of subclavian stenosis. The authors performed arch angiography in patients with manifestations of peripheral vascular disease undergoing diagnostic coronary angiography.*

Screening for Subclavian Artery Stenosis in Patients who are Candidates for Coronary Bypass Surgery. Catheterization and Cardiovascular Interventions. 2002;56:162–165.

→ *Patients referred for coronary artery bypass were prospectively screened for subclavian stenosis as guided by symptoms and physical exam findings with non-invasive imaging and in appropriate cases, angiography.*

Durability of Percutaneous Transluminal Angioplasty for Obstructive Lesions of Proximal Subclavian Artery: Long-term Results. *Journal of Vascular Surgery.* January 2005; 41(1): 19–23.

→ *An observational, single center study by de Vries et al. describing the results of 110 patients who underwent successful PTA/stenting of clinically significant subclavian stenoses.*

Endovascular Treatment of Occlusive Lesions of the Subclavian and Innominate Arteries. *Cardiovascular and Interventional Radiology*. 2006; 29: 503–510.

→ *A limited review of subclavian and innominate artery disease, it includes etiology, historical data, diagnostic classification of lesions, definitions, and treatment options including endovascular techniques.*

Catheter-Based Treatment of the Subclavian and Innominate Arteries. *Catheterization and Cardiovascular Interventions*. 2008; 71:963–968.

→ *Authors Patel, White et al. provide subclavian artery interventional outcomes from a single center. It is the largest and most recently published case series using the latest endovascular technology and techniques, as evidenced by the highest reported success for total occlusion interventions.*

Endovascular Treatment Strategies for Supra-Aortic Arterial Occlusive Disease. *Journal of Cardiovascular Surgery*. 2005; 46: 193–200.

→ *This article is a comprehensive and detailed review of procedural techniques. It systematically describes the procedure from access, guide and wire selection, balloon and stent choices as well as embolic protection.*

Endovascular Techniques for Supra-Aortic Trunk Intervention. *Perspectives in Vascular Surgery and Endovascular Therapy.* September 2007; 19(3): 231–237.

→ *A single operator review of aortic trunk intervention techniques (including carotid artery) by Dr. Frank Criado.*

Ochoa V and Yeghiazarians Y. Subclavian artery stenosis: a review for the vascular medicine practitioner. Vascular Medicine 2010 Nov 15.

→ *This article is a comprehensive review for the practitioner of the causes, diagnostic modalities, and treatment options for patients with subclavian artery stenosis.*

Chapter 14
Renal Artery Stenosis

David Lao, Christopher D. Owens, and Yerem Yeghiazarians

Etiology

Atherosclerosis (~90%), fibromuscular dysplasia, vasculitis, neurofibromatosis, congenital bands, radiation, extrinsic compression.

Background

Atherosclerotic renal artery stenosis (RAS) typically involves the ostium and/or proximal one-third of the renal artery; 70–80% unilateral.

D. Lao
Department of Medicine, University of California – San Francisco, San Francisco, CA, USA

C.D. Owens
Division of Vascular Surgery, Department of Surgery, University of California – San Francisco, San Francisco, CA, USA
e-mail: christopher.owens@ucsfmedctr.org

Y. Yeghiazarians (✉)
Division of Interventional Cardiology, Department of Medicine, University of California – San Francisco, San Francisco, CA, USA
e-mail: yeghiaza@medicine.ucsf.edu

C.D. Owens and Y. Yeghiazarians (eds.), *Handbook of Endovascular Peripheral Interventions*, DOI 10.1007/978-1-4614-0839-0_14,

Prevalence

Depends on patient subgroup (1–6% in patients with hypertension; up to 40–50% in patient with known coronary or peripheral atherosclerosis).

Clinical Presentations/Clues

- Onset of hypertension <age 30 years
- Malignant or refractory hypertension
- Unexplained renal atrophy or size discrepancy of >1.5 cm between kidneys
- Progressive renal insufficiency
- Presence of multivessel coronary artery disease or peripheral arterial disease
- Worsening renal function upon initiation of ACE-I/ARB therapy
- Abdominal bruit
- Recurrent heart failure

Clinical Pointers: Fibromuscular Dysplasia

- Younger (<50 years old), more common in women, "beads on a string" angiogram
- Progression to complete occlusion of renal artery rare
- 80% Medial fibroplasia >>intimal (~10%) or adventitial
- 60% bilateral
- In 25%, disease extends into segmental arteries
- Other arteries can also be involved (carotid, vertebral, iliac, and mesenteric). All patients need head imaging to r/o cerebral aneurysms

Clinical Pointers: Progression of Atherosclerotic RAS

- 48% of patients with <60% stenosis progress to >60% over 3 years

- 39% patients with >75% stenosis progress to complete occlusion over 1–5 years
- Average progression ~7% per year
- Note that progression of RAS and loss of renal function occur *independently* of blood pressure control

Screening

Based upon institutional expertise and patient factors.

Ultrasonography (US)

- *Strengths*: safe, inexpensive and widely available, images of the renal arteries as well as blood flow velocity and pressure waveforms, information regarding renal functional reserve as well as regarding kidney size and renal resistive index
- *Limitations*: highly dependent on operator expertise, limited by technical challenges related to obesity, kidney

Tips on Ultrasound

- Renal artery/aortic velocity ratio >3.5–60% stenosis (Sn 84%, Sp 92%)
- Renal artery Peak Systolic Velocity (PSV) >180–200 cm/s (Sn and Sp ~98%)
- End Diastolic Velocity (EDV) >150 cm/s (RAS >80%)
- Significant discrepancy in kidney size
- If renal size <9 cm and systolic velocities <10 cm/s likely consistent with renal artery occlusion
- Acceleration time (time period between the onset of systolic upstroke and the initial peak velocity (compliance peak)). Normal <100 ms (usually 40–50 ms) → if >100 ms associated with RAS ≥60%
- Renal resistive index (RRI = 1 – EDV/PSV): (Normal <0.7, nephrosclerosis >0.7)

position, and bowel gas, accessory renal arteries may be missed, mild stenosis is difficult to detect

Computed Tomography Angiography

- *Strengths*: Excellent images can be obtained (Sensitivity >91%; Specificity 85–99% with newer scans)
- *Limitations*: image interpretation may be difficult in heavily calcified arteries; involves the use of ionizing radiation and iodinated contrast medium; may not be tolerated by claustrophobic patients

Magnetic Resonance Angiography

- *Strengths*: No iodinated contrast or radiation (Sensitivity 90–100%; Specificity 76–94%)
- *Limitations*: gadolinium-based contrast associated with nephrogenic systemic fibrosis in patients with moderate-to-end-stage renal failure; contraindications to MRI (pacemakers, defibrillators, cochlear implants, and spinal cord stimulators); may not be tolerated by claustrophobic patients

Angiography

- *Strengths*: remains the "gold standard" for the diagnosis of RAS; evaluate the extent of intrarenal vascular disease; measure direct gradient across the stenosis; therapeutic procedures such as percutaneous transluminal angioplasty or stenting can be carried out at the same time.
- *Limitations*: invasive technique; contrast exposure.

Treatment

- Medical treatment of risk factors (e.g., lipids, blood pressure, smoking cessation)
- Indications for invasive therapy of RAS are controversial and not clearly known; options are balloon angioplasty alone vs. stenting vs. surgical bypass (the latter is rarely

Classification and Levels of Evidence (American Heart Association)[1]

Classification

Class I: Intervention is useful and effective
Class IIa: Weight of evidence/opinion is in favor of usefulness/efficacy
Class IIb: Usefulness/efficacy less well-established by evidence/opinion
Class III: Intervention is not useful/effective and may be harmful

Levels of Evidence

A. Sufficient evidence from randomized trials
B. Limited evidence from single, randomized, or other nonrandomized studies
C. Based on expert opinion, case studies, or standard of care

performed and usually associated with other open surgical procedures such as aorto-bifemoral bypass with concomitant renal artery stenosis)

- Young women with refractory or difficult to control HTN respond well to balloon angioplasty of the renal artery; no stenting is necessary in majority of cases if adequate angioplasty result is achieved
- Decision to revascularize atherosclerotic RAS is individualized but the following AHA recommendations can be useful:

American Heart Association Guidelines for Revascularization/Screening (adapted from *Circulation* 2006;114;1892–1895)

Asymptomatic stenosis

- Asymptomatic bilateral or solitary viable kidney with hemodynamically significant RAS (class IIb, LOE C)
- Asymptomatic unilateral hemodynamically significant RAS in a viable kidney not well-established and presently clinically unproved (class IIb, LOE C)

Hypertension

- Hemodynamically significant RAS and accelerated hypertension, resistant hypertension, malignant hypertension, hypertension with unexplained unilateral small kidney, and hypertension with intolerance to drug treatment (class IIa, LOE B)

Preservation of renal function

- Progressive chronic kidney disease with bilateral RAS or a RAS to a solitary functioning kidney (class IIb, LOE B)
- Chronic renal insufficiency with unilateral RAS (class IIb, LOE C)

Impact of RAS on congestive heart failure and unstable angina

- Hemodynamically significant RAS and recurrent, unexplained CHF or sudden, unexplained pulmonary edema (class I, LOE B)
- Hemodynamically significant RAS and unstable angina (class IIa, LOE B)

Clinical Pointer : Does the RRI Matter in Deciding Whether to Treat the RAS in a Patient?

- Despite initial studies suggesting lack of benefit of RAS therapy with RRI >0.8, more recent studies suggest that a significant response in renal function may be obtained despite an abnormal resistive index, but this response is more blunted.
- Therefore, we do not recommend using RRI as the sole decision maker to revascularize or not.

Renal Artery Angioplasty and Stenting: How I do it

- Access: Retrograde femoral artery, brachial or even radial access can be considered (Fig. 14.1).
- Renal arteries are located in L1-L2 disc space. Start with a pararenal aortogram using an Omniflush or Pigtail catheter with 10–15 ml of contrast (location of renal ostia, high-grade ostial disease, accessory artery, degree of calcification, aneurysm can be assessed without traumatizing the aorta and this initial imaging technique decreases the risk of potential distal embolization).

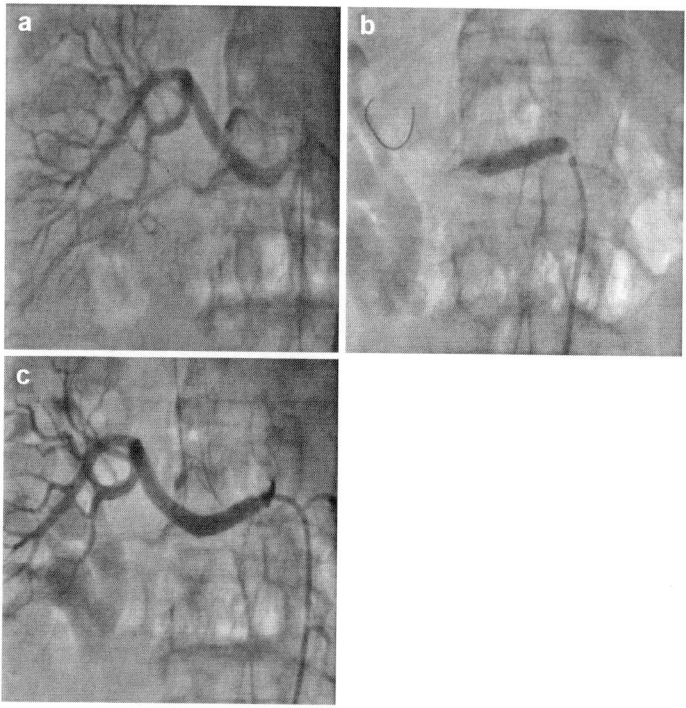

FIGURE 14.1 Percutaneous intervention of a high-grade *right* renal artery stenosis. (**a**) A 6 Fr IM guide catheter is advanced via a *right* femoral arterial sheath to the ostium of the *right* renal artery in an AP view. Selective *right* renal angiography is performed in an LAO 15° view with a hand injection of contrast. (**b**) A 0.014″ BMW wire is advanced across the target lesion to the superior ramus of the *right* renal artery. A Maverick 4.0×15 mm^2 compliant balloon is used to serially dilate the lesion at 6–9 atm, followed by placement of a Genesis 6.0×24 mm^2 Transhepatic biliary stent deployed at 8 atm. (**c**) Repeat angiography following stent implication shows no residual stenosis

- For selective renal angiography, a number of catheters can be utilized pending the take-off of the renal arteries (see Equipment list). The origins of renal arteries are posterolateral. Perform selective renal angiography ~10° ipsilateral

Tips of the Trade: Our Experiences

- For severe caudal renal artery angulations, radial/brachial access may be preferable.
- Renal arteries arise at the top of L1 vertebral body, and the right renal is typically above the left renal.
- IMA catheter is best for inferiorly directed renal arteries.
- Avoid diving catheters into the artery and wedging into the lesion. A gentle rotation with slight cranial or caudal translation to avoid storing torque in the catheter is helpful.
- Hydrophilic wires may be useful for crossing tight lesions, but these should preferably be switched to a stiffer, non-hydrophilic wire to reduce perforation risk.
- Pre-dilatation is recommended and the balloon size depends on the size of the renal artery and is usually 3–5 mm in diameter. Undersize balloon choice by at least 1 mm to minimize the risk of dissection.
- For ostial lesions, it is important to deploy the stent with the proximal segment protruding 1–2 mm inside the aorta and to flare the extending portion with a compliant balloon. There is a tendency for the stent to move slightly forward. Avoid too much stent overhang in the aorta!

oblique view; cranial or caudal views may be helpful to better estimate the severity in eccentric lesions or tortuous aorta or iliacs.

- Three to six cc of contrast over 2–3 s is usually enough with a gentle hand injection so as not to dislodge the catheter. Cine long enough to visualize the renal cortex (nephrogram) for size (normal size is anywhere between 9 and 12 mm, pending size of patient).
- Generally a 6 Fr guiding catheter is adequate to deliver the balloon-mounted stent into the renal orifice.

Potential Pitfalls

*most renal ostial lesions originate from the aortic atherosclerosis.

- It is critically important to avoid over dilation as aorta or renal artery dissection is a dreaded consequence
- As always, careful wire management to avoid renal parenchymal perforation is critical

- To cross the stenosis, we recommend either a 0.014 or 0.018 wire (see Equipment list).
- Pre-dilation over a 0.014 platform is usually recommended for all lesions, especially those that are calcified to ensure smooth passage of the stent and good apposition.
- Anticoagulation is recommended with a target ACT of 250 s.
- Use of a glycoprotein IIb/IIIa inhibitor is not recommended.
- The size of the balloon-mounted stent should be sized according to the normal renal caliber not the adjacent post stenotic dilatation that is often present distal to a hemodynamically significant stenosis. Avoid oversizing the balloon (see pitfalls).
- Efficacy of drug-eluting stents (DES) is unknown and we do not recommend the use of DES in the initial treatment of RAS at this time. For in-stent restenosis, DES can be considered pending the size of the renal artery to make sure good apposition is achieved with the DES.
- There is no general consensus on the use of be embolic protection devices.
- We do not recommend routine use of intravascular ultrasound.
- Stent boost technology (to assess adequacy of stent deployment) can be useful.

Follow up and Screening After RAS Stenting

- Dual antiplatelet therapy with aspirin (325 or 162 mg daily) and clopidogrel (75 mg daily) for at least 30 days; then monotherapy with aspirin (81 mg daily) chronically.
- Surveillance is not standardized. We recommend renal ultrasound to be performed within 1–2 weeks after RAS stenting to establish a new baseline, followed by US in 6- and 12-months. CT and MRI are less useful given the artifact seen in the presence of the stent.
- Regular monitoring of blood pressure and renal function.

Equipment List

This is a partial list as a variety of equipment can be successfully utilized.

Sheaths

5–6 Fr standard short sheath

- Terumo Pinnacle
- Cordis

6 Fr long sheath for tortuous iliac anatomy

- Cordis Brite Tip

If larger sized catheters or guides are to be used, then larger sheaths (7–8 Fr) can be considered.

Guiding Catheters

5–8 Fr guiding catheters with varying shapes. We find the following catheters to be useful in majority of cases:

- Renal Standard Curve
- Renal Double Curve
- Hockey stick
- JR4
- IMA

- Multipurpose
- Softvue Sos Omni Selective catheter for "no touch" approach

Guidewires

We recommend 0.014″ or 0.018″ wires and not 0.035″ wires. There are many wires that can be utilized. Commonly, we use one of the following:

- BMW (Abbott)
- Stabilizer (Cordis)
- Spartacore (Abbott)

Balloons

There are many balloon choices (either over-the-wire or monorail). We prefer monorail balloons and typically use one of the following:

- Maverick/Apex (Boston Scientific)
- Voyager (Abbott)
- Dura Star (Cordis)

It is preferable to avoid peripheral balloons with their large shafts and necessitating 0.035″ guidewires.

Stents

Balloon-expandable stents are recommended. We typically use one of the following:

- Genesis (Cordis)
- Express SD (Boston Scientific)

Distal Protection

Embolic protection devices:

- FilterWire EZ (Boston)
- GuardWire (Medtronic)

Bibilography

1. ACC/AHA Guidelines for the Management of Patients With Peripheral Arterial Disease. J Am Coll Cardiol. 2006 Mar 21;47(6):1239–312.
   → *This is a comprehensive review and recommends on the treatment of Peripheral Arterial Disease and it includes a detailed review of the renal artery stenosis literature.*
2. Indications for Renal Arteriography at the Time of Coronary Arteriography. *Circulation*. 2006;114:1892–1895.
   → *This is a multispecialty consensus manuscript describing the rationale for screening renal angiography at the time of cardiac catheterization.*
3. Revascularization versus Medical Therapy for Renal-Artery Stenosis. The ASTRAL investigators. N Engl J Med 2009; 361: 1953–62.
   → *The ASTRAL Trial is a randomized unblinded study of over 800 patients with RAS treated with either medical therapy alone vs. medical therapy + renal artery stenting. Patient selection for this trial is questionable but nevertheless, this is the largest study of its kind in the literature addressing percutaneous intervention of RAS.*
4. Stent revascularization for the prevention of cardiovascular and renal events among patients with renal artery stenosis and systolic hypertension: Rationale and design of the CORAL trial. Am Heart J 2006; 152:59–66.
   → *The CORAL Trial is an on-going randomized trial of stenting of renal artery stenosis and this paper discusses the rational and design of this important trial.*
5. Catheter-Based Therapy for Atherosclerotic Renal Artery Stenosis. Progress in Cardiovascular Diseases, Vol. 50, No. 2 (September/October), 2007: pp 136–150.
   → *This is an excellent review article by Dr. Christopher White on the topic of RAS.*
6. Lao D, Parasher PS, Cho KC, Yeghiazarians Y. Atherosclerotic renal artery stenosis - diagnosis and treatment. Mayo Clin Proc. 2011 Jul;86(7):649–57.
   → *This is an up-to-date comprehensive review of renal artery stenosis, it's the diagnosis and treatment.*

Chapter 15
The Superior Mesenteric and Celiac Arteries

Warren J. Gasper and Christopher D. Owens

Mesenteric Ischemia

Etiology

Atherosclerosis (most common), fibromuscular dysplasia, vasculitis, aortic dissection, isolated SMA dissection, neurofibromatosis.

Background

There is extensive collateral circulation between the celiac, superior mesenteric (SMA), inferior mesenteric (IMA), and internal iliac arteries. Atherosclerosis leading to occlusive disease of the mesenteric vessels is common and two-thirds of symptomatic patients will have symptomatic coronary,

W.J. Gasper • C.D. Owens (✉)
Division of Endovascular and Vascular Surgery,
Department of Surgery, University of California – San Francisco,
San Francisco, CA, USA
e-mail: warren.gasper@ucsf.edu; christopher.owens@ucsfmedctr.org

C.D. Owens and Y. Yeghiazarians (eds.),
Handbook of Endovascular Peripheral Interventions,
DOI 10.1007/978-1-4614-0839-0_15,

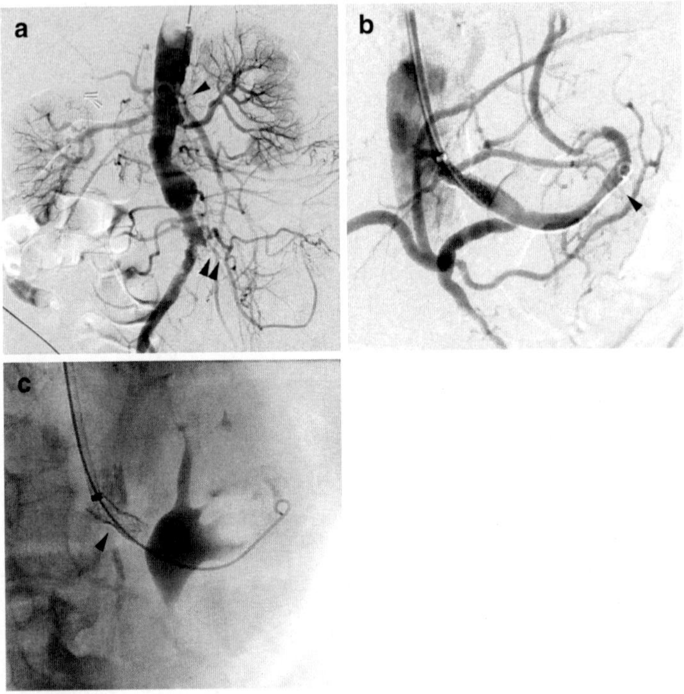

FIGURE 15.1 An 81-year-old woman with 2 years of abdominal pain after eating and a 20-lb weight loss over the past month. (**a**) Aortogram demonstrating severe aortoiliac atherosclerosis with occlusion of the celiac artery, stenosis of the proximal SMA (*arrow*), and occlusion of the left common iliac artery (*double arrow*). (**b**) Filling of the celiac axis after successful selective catheterization, balloon angioplasty, and stenting with a bare metal stent (guidewire in the splenic artery, *arrow*). (**c**) Residual waist in the celiac artery stent (*arrow*). A covered stent was placed in the initial bare-metal stent and several attempts to dilate the vessel were made with balloon angioplasty. Given the extensive aortic atherosclerosis in this patient, this result was accepted rather than risk an aortic or celiac artery dissection

cerebrovascular, renal, or peripheral arterial disease (see Fig. 15.1). Typically, symptoms are associated with a significant stenosis of two of the three vessels, although a significant isolated SMA stenosis can cause symptoms as well (see Fig. 15.2).

Prevalence

The incidence of chronic mesenteric ischemia is low. In a study reviewing aortograms, the prevalence of significant mesenteric occlusive disease was 6% and only 1.5% had

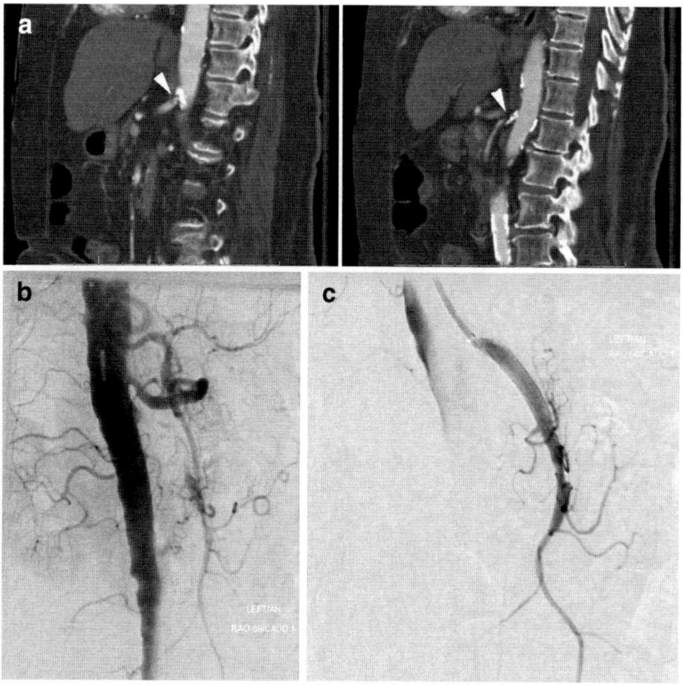

FIGURE 15.2 An 85-year-old woman with abdominal pain after eating, nausea, and vomiting. (**a**) CT angiogram demonstrating extensive calcification and stenosis at the origins of the celiac (*arrow*, *left panel*) and superior mesenteric arteries (*arrow*, *right panel*). (**b**) Aortogram demonstrating stenosis of both the celiac and superior mesenteric arteries. (**c**) Filling of the SMA after selective catheterization, balloon angioplasty, and stenting. (**d**) Stents in the celiac and superior mesenteric arteries (guidewire in the celiac artery)

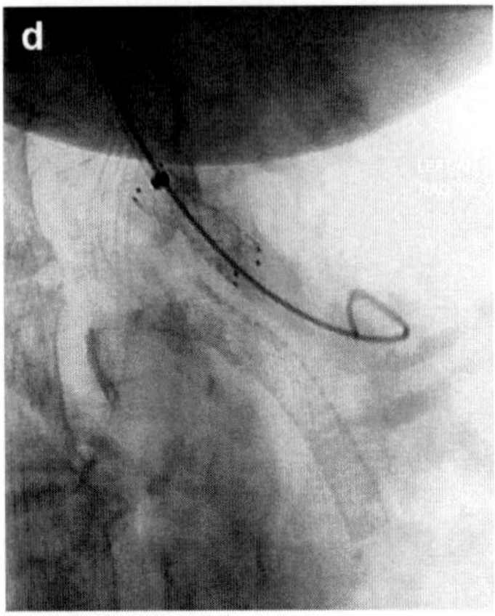

FIGURE 15.2 (continued)

three-vessel disease. However, of the patients with three-vessel disease 27% developed symptoms over a mean follow-up of 2.6 years.

Clinical Presentation

- Predominantly women, 40–70 years old with a long smoking history and hypertension.
- Abdominal pain that occurs 15–30 min after eating and lasts 1–3 h. The pain is typically in the mid-abdomen around the umbilicus and can vary from dull to crampy. Other symptoms might include weight loss and fear of food. Less common symptoms can be vague abdominal pain, nausea/vomiting, or change in bowel habits.

Clinical Pointers: Diagnosing Chronic Mesenteric Ischemia

- Frequently, the abdominal pain is long-standing and alternative explanations of the abdominal pain are sought before mesenteric ischemia is diagnosed.

- Foregut and hepatobiliary malignancies can have similar symptoms, so additional tests including CT, endoscopy, or ultrasound are often necessary.
- The mean duration of symptoms is 15 months (range 1 month to 5 years) and the mean number of diagnostic tests performed is 2.8.
- Most lesions are short and in the proximal visceral artery.

Clinical Pointers: Role of Endovascular Therapy in Acute Mesenteric Ischemia

- Endovascular therapy is limited in acute mesenteric ischemia as patients often will require a laparotomy to assess bowel viability, at which time an open thrombectomy and/or bypass can be performed.
- Hybrid procedures involving either antegrade or retrograde stenting of the SMA in combination with operative exploration have been described in small case series (see Fig. 15.3).
- Approximately 10–20% of cases of acute mesenteric ischemia will be due to non-occlusive disease, which can be treated with vasodilator medications (e.g., nitroglycerin) during an angiogram. However, intestinal necrosis is common and the prognosis is poor.

Visceral Artery Aneurysms

Etiology

- True aneurysms – degenerative/atherosclerotic, fibromuscular dysplasia, collagen vascular disease, inflammatory conditions, Ehlers-Danlos syndrome
- False aneurysms (pseudoaneurysms) – trauma, iatrogenic injury, local inflammatory processes (e.g., pancreatitis), infection

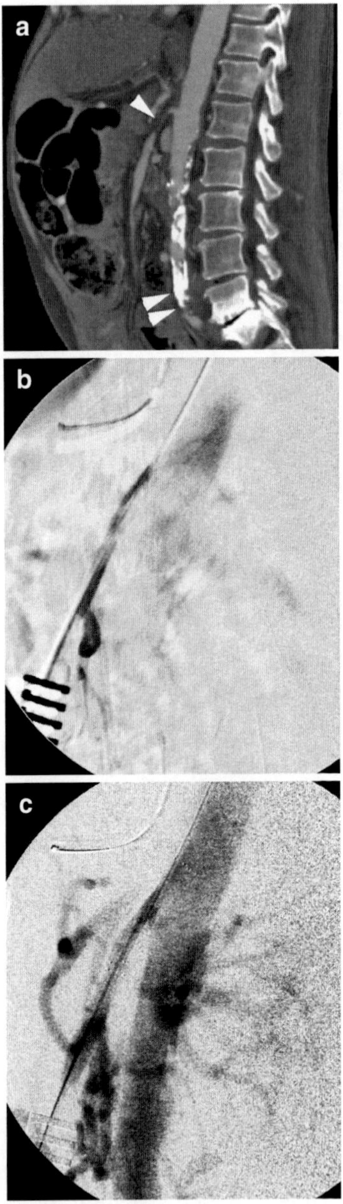

FIGURE 15.3 A 56-year-old man with 12 h of acute epigastric abdominal pain, nausea, and vomiting. (**a**) CT angiogram showing an occlusion of the SMA (*arrow*) and bowel wall thickening, concerning for acute mesenteric ischemia. Notice the extensive calcification of the distal aorta (*double arrow*). (**b**) Intraoperative retrograde angiogram of the SMA showing a near occlusion of the artery. Notice that the aorta does not fill with contrast injection. This angiogram was performed in the operating room after resection of 100 cm of gangrenous small bowel and an unsuccessful surgical embolectomy of the SMA. (**c**) Successful angioplasty and retrograde stenting of the SMA with contrast filling of the aorta

Background

A true aneurysm is a localized dilation of all three layers of the blood vessel wall, with an increase in diameter of 50% compared to the normal expected diameter. In contrast, a false aneurysm (or pseudoaneurysm) is a localized disruption of an artery that has been contained by the surrounding tissues. This can occur because of a direct injury to the vessel (trauma, iatrogenic injury), disruption of a vascular anastomosis, infection (i.e., a mycotic aneurysm), or local inflammation (e.g., pancreatitis).

Prevalence

The incidence is low – visceral artery aneurysms represent only 5% of intra-abdominal aneurysms. The most common sites are: splenic artery (60%), hepatic artery (20%), SMA (6%), celiac (4%), all other visceral arteries (10%). Some series have reported a higher incidence of hepatic artery aneurysms, possibly due to trauma or iatrogenic injuries from biliary procedures. Although up to 1/3 of true aneurysms are associated with other non-visceral artery aneurysms, there is no known pattern of particular aneurysms occurring with visceral artery aneurysms.

Clinical Presentation

- Can be symptomatic with vague abdominal pain (see Fig. 15.4).
- Typically, however, most are asymptomatic and found on intra-abdominal imaging (ultrasound, CT, MRI) for other reasons.
- Up to 25% of visceral aneurysms are diagnosed emergently after rupture with symptoms of abdominal pain, hypotension, gastrointestinal bleeding, or hemobilia. Some

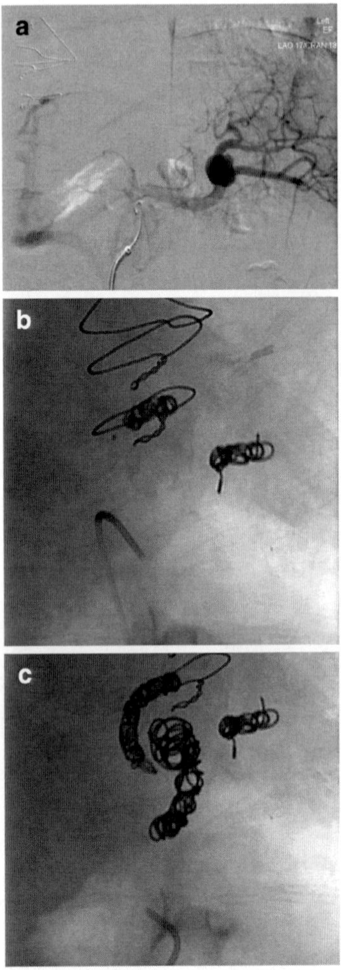

FIGURE 15.4 A 43-year-old man with a 2-cm distal splenic artery aneurysm found during a work-up for abdominal pain. (**a**) Angiogram of the splenic artery demonstrating a 2-cm aneurysm at the splenic hilum with outflow vessels from the aneurysm to the upper and lower poles of the spleen. (**b**) Selective embolization of the aneurysm outflow vessels. (**c**) Embolization of the aneurysm and the splenic artery. At 1-month follow-up, the patient was pain-free and a CT demonstrated a partial splenic infarction and exclusion of the aneurysm

patients present with a "double rupture," where an initial contained rupture is followed by a free intraperitoneal rupture within 48 h. The mortality for ruptured aneurysms is at least 10% and often much higher: ruptured celiac and SMA aneurysms have mortality rates exceeding 70–80% in most series.

- Pregnancy is associated with a high rate of splenic artery aneurysm rupture, particularly in the third trimester, with maternal and fetal mortality rates approaching 90–100%.

Evaluation of Celiac and Superior Mesenteric Arteries

Duplex Ultrasonography

Advantages: safe, widely available, ability to assess blood flow velocity and waveforms

Limitations: highly operator-dependent, technically challenging because of bowel gas, obesity, and patient positioning

Tips on Ultrasound

- Peak Systolic Velocity >275 cm/s in SMA (sensitivity 92%) or >200 cm/s in celiac axis (sensitivity 87%) corresponds to >70% stenosis (accuracy is 96% for SMA and 82% for celiac axis).
- End Diastolic Velocity >45 cm/s in SMA or >55 cm/s in celiac correspond to >50% stenosis.
- The applicability of a mesenteric "stress-test" – duplex measurements before and after a meal, has not been determined.

CT Angiography

Advantages: excellent imaging of mesenteric arteries; can identify significant collaterals; can exclude alternate causes of abdominal pain

Limitations: image interpretation can be difficult with heavily calcified arteries; exposure to ionizing radiation and iodinated contrast; risk of contrast-induced nephropathy.

MR Angiography

Advantages: excellent imaging of the mesenteric arteries; can identify significant collaterals; no exposure to ionizing radiation or iodinated contrast

Limitations: gadolinium-based contrast is associated with nephrogenic systemic fibrosis in patients with moderate or worse chronic kidney disease; contraindications to MR include pacemakers, defibrillators, cochlear implants, spinal cord stimulators, etc; may not be tolerated by claustrophobic patients

Angiography

Advantages: Considered the "gold standard." Can evaluate for long segment stenosis and evidence of vasculitis; opportunity for intervention at the same time

Limitations: invasive, uses ionizing radiation and iodinated contrast

Treatment

Mesenteric Ischemia

- Patients with symptomatic mesenteric vessel stenosis should be treated because of the risk of acute mesenteric ischemia.
- Best medical therapy alone is not sufficient for symptomatic patients. Preventative therapy for atherosclerotic risk factors including aspirin, statins, blood pressure control, blood glucose control, smoking cessation, and exercise can help control disease progression.
- Patients are often dehydrated and malnourished. Aggressive fluid resuscitation, electrolyte correction, and possibly parenteral nutrition should be instituted prior to revascularization.
- Symptomatic disease is the indication for intervention. Options include balloon angioplasty vs. stent vs. open endarterectomy vs. open bypass graft.

- Short-segment stenosis (<2 cm) without eccentric plaque or thrombus is ideal for endovascular intervention.

Visceral Artery Aneurysms

- Because of a high risk of rupture, virtually all false aneurysms should be repaired.
- Several studies have suggested that stable true aneurysms have a low rate of rupture and can be observed. However, the relationship between growth rate and risk of rupture for visceral aneurysms is poorly understood. Given the high mortality rates associated with rupture, intervention is suggested for asymptomatic aneurysms that grow on serial imaging.
- Options include endovascular embolization vs. covered stent vs. open repair.
- Splenic artery aneurysms: all aneurysms in pregnant women or women of childbearing age should be repaired. Observation may be considered in patients with stable, small (<2 cm) aneurysms.
- Hepatic artery aneurysms: true aneurysms should be repaired if symptomatic, >2 cm in diameter, or if <2 cm but enlarging with serial imaging studies. Aneurysms in the common hepatic may be embolized if the gastroduodenal artery (GDA) provides adequate perfusion to the proper hepatic artery. Lesions in the proper hepatic artery often require arterial reconstruction. Intrahepatic aneurysms can usually be treated with embolization.
- SMA aneurysms: most are symptomatic at presentation and up to 60% are associated with an infectious etiology. Since aneurysm rupture is common (up to 50% of patients) and carries a high mortality rate (up to 90%), most SMA aneurysms should be repaired regardless of size. Care must be taken to tailor the intervention based on the anatomic and patient factors.
- Celiac artery aneurysms: symptomatic aneurysms and those >1.5 cm should be repaired. An open approach with arterial reconstruction may be required to preserve hepatic and splenic artery perfusion.

How I Do It

- Access: 5-Fr short sheath in either the femoral artery or left brachial artery is acceptable.
- A Pigtail or Omniflush catheter is positioned in the distal descending aorta at T12 for anteroposterior and lateral angiography using 10–15 mL of contrast. The celiac axis is just caudal to the diaphragm at the level of L1 and the SMA is a few centimeters caudal to the celiac axis. Both the celiac artery and SMA face inferiorly but the celiac axis comes off the aorta at a more acute angle than the SMA.
- Lateral projections are optimal as the SMA and celiac axis are typically projecting directly anterior or a few degrees lateral of anterior.
- The patient is heparinized and the short sheath is exchanged for a long (90-cm) 6-Fr guiding sheath positioned at the origin of the celiac artery or SMA.
- To cross the lesion, an angled-guide catheter and a 0.018 or 0.014-in. stiff wire is used. Care must be taken to position the end of the wire in the main trunk of the SMA or a large jejunal branch to avoid dissection or perforation. Similarly, for the celiac axis the end of the wire is carefully positioned in the splenic or hepatic artery. Alternatively, a 0.035-in. hydrophilic guidewire may be used if more support or better visualization is needed.
- Primary stenting of orificial lesions is preferred while balloon angioplasty with selective stenting can be performed for mid-vessel lesions. Pre-dilation is performed with a 2–3 mm balloon followed by placement of a 5–6 mm balloon expandable stent with minimal (1–2 mm) protrusion into the aortic lumen.
- For aneurysms, the access is similar, but the location and configuration of the aneurysm will determine the exact approach. Proximal aneurysms often can be treated with embolization coils and a stent or exclusion with a stent graft to maintain artery patency (see Fig. 15.5). For more distal aneurysms, the collateral flow is typically greater, thus the risk of end organ ischemia is lower. These aneurysms may be treated by embolizing the artery proximal and distal to the

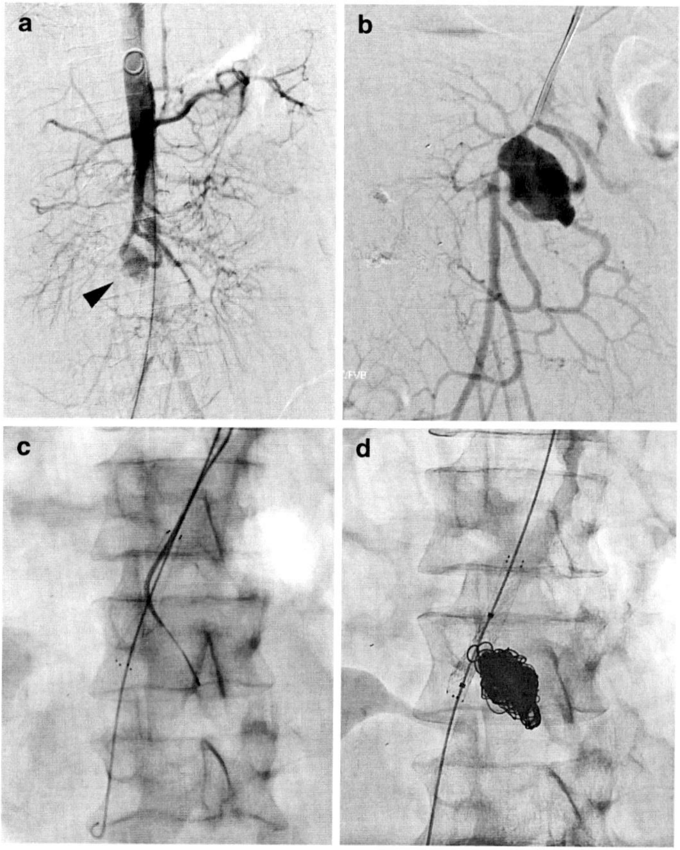

FIGURE 15.5 A 28-year-old man who sustained a gunshot wound to the abdomen requiring an exploratory laparotomy and left thoracotomy. Five months later, he was found to have an enlarging 2.8-cm pseudoaneurysm of the SMA. (**a**) Aortogram demonstrating an SMA pseudoaneurysm (*arrow*). (**b**) Selective catheterization of the SMA shows the neck of the pseudoaneurysm is broad, approximately 1–1.5 cm. (**c**) Placement of a bare metal stent across the aneurysm neck to provide a scaffold for embolization of the aneurysm. Notice that the guidewire has been placed through the struts of the stent into the pseudoaneurysm. (**d**) Successful embolization of the pseudoaneurysm with placement of an additional covered stent across the pseudoaneurysm neck for complete exclusion

aneurysm with coils or cyanoacrylate glue or both, thereby "trapping" the aneurysm. Saccular aneurysms with a narrow neck may be treated with coil or glue embolization alone.

Tips of the Trade

- The acute downward angle of the celiac axis and SMA off of the aorta can create difficulties in catheter pushability when femoral artery access is used. A left brachial artery approach provides better vectors for catheter control and stent placement.
- External compression of the celiac axis by the median arcuate ligament (median arcuate ligament syndrome) can be differentiated from an internal lesion by taking inspiratory and expiratory phase images.
- Typically the SMA is treated before the celiac axis and there is some data that multi-vessel intervention may improve outcomes.
- Undersize the balloon slightly for pre-dilation to avoid causing dissections.
- Flare the proximal stent in the aortic lumen to facilitate subsequent catheterizations.
- Selective, intravascular nitroglycerin can be administered for vasospasm of the celiac or SMA branches.

Potential Pitfalls

- Careful wire control is paramount to avoid perforation or dissection.
- Avoiding over-dilation is critical to avoid aortic, celiac, or SMA dissection.
- Acute bowel infarction from SMA emboli or unrecognized acute mesenteric ischemia is rare but associated with a 25% mortality rate.
- Splenic and hepatic infarcts as well as pancreatitis are possible from celiac emboli or ischemia.

Follow-Up

- Patients are started on clopidogrel (300 mg loading dose then 75 mg/day) and aspirin (81 mg/day) for 1 month and then switched to aspirin (325 mg/day).
- For mesenteric ischemia, a duplex ultrasound is performed before discharged home followed by serial duplex exams every 6 months for the first year and annually thereafter. Ultrasound may overestimate stenosis after stent placement (falsely high velocities); therefore the decision to proceed to a repeat angiogram is based on increasing velocities on serial ultrasound studies or the recurrence of symptoms.
- For aneurysms, follow-up imaging with CT to document exclusion of the aneurysm is done at 1, 6, and 12 months, then annually.

Equipment List

Sheaths

5 Fr standard short sheath

- Cordis

6 Fr long (90-cm) guiding sheath

- Cook Flexor (Shuttle, RAABE, Ansel)
- Cordis Brite Tip

Larger sheaths (7–8 Fr) may be used if larger catheters are going to be used.

Guiding Catheters

5–7 Fr catheters with varying shapes

- Multipurpose
- SOS Omni

Guidewires

Typically we use 0.014 or 0.018 in. wires, including:

- BMW (Abbott)
- Roadrunner (Cook)

Alternatively, 0.035 in. wires such as a Glidewire/stiff Glidewire (Terumo) can be used.

Balloons

There are many balloon choices.

Stents

Balloon expandable are recommended. Typically we use:

- Express (Boston Scientific)

Stent-Grafts

Balloon expandable are recommended. Typically we use:

- iCast (Atrium)

Embolization Coils

- Tornado, Nester (Cook)

Bibliography

1. Peck MA, Conrad MF, Kwolek CJ, LaMuraglia GM, Paruchuri V, et al. Intermediate-term outcomes of endovascular treatment for symptomatic chronic mesenteric ischemia. Journal of Vascular Surgery. 2010;51(1):140–7.e1.
   → *A report on the peri-operative and intermediate outcomes after visceral artery stenting for chronic mesenteric ischemia in 49 patients with a mean follow-up of 3 years. In this series, 30% of patients required a repeat intervention by 3 years.*
2. Armstrong PA. Visceral duplex scanning: evaluation before and after artery intervention for chronic mesenteric ischemia. Perspectives in Vascular Surgery and Endovascular Therapy. 2007;19(4):386–92.
   → *A review of duplex ultrasound for evaluation of the visceral arteries before and after intervention.*
3. Wyers MC, Powell RJ, Nolan BW, & Cronenwett JL. Retrograde mesenteric stenting during laparotomy for acute occlusive mesenteric ischemia. Journal of Vascular Surgery. 2007;45(2):269–75.
   → *A small case-series on endovascular therapy in the setting of acute mesenteric ischemia, including six cases in which open retrograde SMA stenting was performed.*
4. Tulsyan N, Kashyap VS, Greenberg RK, Sarac TP, Clair DG, et al. The endovascular management of visceral artery aneurysms and pseudoaneurysms. Journal of Vascular Surgery. 2007; 45(2):276–83.
   → *A case-series on the endovascular treatment of 48 patients with visceral artery aneurysms.*

Chapter 16
Aorto-Iliac Intervention

Edwin C. Gravereaux

Etiology/Pathology

Typical disease processes of aorto-iliac (AI) segment include atherosclerosis, aneurysmal degeneration, dissection, and embolism.

The typical atherosclerotic occlusive lesions can affect the terminal infra-renal aorta, iliac bifurcation, and the common, external, and internal iliac arteries. Multi-level disease (including common femoral, profunda femoral, and superficial femoral arteries is frequently present).

Risk factors include hypertension, hypercholesterolemia, diabetes, age, and smoking. Typical patients presenting with aorto-iliac disease are male smokers.

Clinical Manifestations

Aorto-iliac occlusive disease may be more disabling than pure infra-inguinal disease, given the increase in muscle groups affected. Proximal muscle symptoms (buttock, hip,

---

E.C. Gravereaux
Department of Vascular Surgery, Brigham and Women's Hospital, Harvard Medical School, Boston, MA, USA
e-mail: egravereaux@partners.org

C.D. Owens and Y. Yeghiazarians (eds.), *Handbook of Endovascular Peripheral Interventions*, DOI 10.1007/978-1-4614-0839-0_16,

thigh) give clinical clue to aorto-iliac disease. Isolated AI atherosclerotic occlusive disease typically presents with claudication.

Leriche Syndrome
Claudication of buttock, hip, thigh muscles; buttock and thigh muscle atrophy; impotence (in males); absent femoral pulses.

Typical isolated AI arterial occlusive disease rarely presents with critical limb ischemia (CLI), whereas combined AI and infra-inguinal arterial occlusive disease (multi-level disease), is often seen with CLI.

Less common clinical presentations

- "Blue toe syndrome": distal athero-emboli from diseased "shaggy aorta" or other proximal arterial plaque.
- Isolated internal iliac stenosis with buttock claudication
- Aortic dissections: can spiral into iliacs, causing lower extremity malperfusion symptoms.
- In-situ thrombosis of chronic AI lesions can lead to precipitous worsening of symptoms from stable claudication to acute limb ischemia
- Concurrent aneurysmal disease: can warrant treatment based upon size, can be encountered in aorta or iliacs with stenotic plaque
- Previous pelvic radiation arteritis
- External iliac artery endofibrosis: an uncommon condition affecting young endurance athletes, such as cyclists or runners.

A thorough history and physical exam, with complete pulse exam, auscultation for bruits, search for signs of chronic and acute limb ischemia and distal embolization can suggest proximal or AI disease. Unilateral leg symptoms with ipsilateral diminished femoral pulse suggest iliac disease, whereas bilateral symptoms with diminished femoral pulse bilaterally is found with distal aortic and bilateral iliac lesions.

Testing

Vascular Lab Testing

Segmental Doppler Pressures and pulse volume recordings can confirm inflow disease with pressure drops at high-thigh level. Exercise treadmill testing may provoke pressure drop in affected limb(s) if resting measurements are normal.

Imaging

Noninvasive imaging is helpful in assessing extent of atherosclerotic occlusive disease and planning interventional strategy. *Importantly, any common femoral disease can be noted, as severe common or profunda femoral occlusive disease may preclude successful and durable aorto-iliac percutaneous intervention.* This issue is best addressed with hybrid surgical/endovascular procedure (e.g., common femoral surgical endarterectomy and patch angioplasty, with subsequent proximal aorto-iliac intervention with sheath and wire access through the patch).

Computed Tomography Angiography

- Can demonstrate location and extent of mural atherosclerotic plaque, but calcified disease may render true vessel patency determination difficult.
- Contrast use often problematic for renal insufficiency patients.

Magnetic Resonance Angiography

- Widely used, helpful in locating lesions and planning for intervention.
- Artifact in previously stented vessels limits assessment of stent patency.

- Nephrogenic systemic fibrosis a risk for renal insufficiency patients with the required gadolinium-based contrast.
- Poorly tolerated by claustrophobic patients.

Contrast Catheter-Based Angiography

- The "gold-standard" for anatomic assessment, allows for oblique imaging, pressure measurements across lesions (with provocative vasodilator use, if needed), and intravascular ultrasound (IVUS) interrogation.
- Traditional angiography can serve as both diagnostic and therapeutic procedure, with appropriate catheter-based intervention performed simultaneously.
- Pre-procedural non-invasive imaging modalities above can allow for a targeted intervention, with minimized IV contrast use.

Treatment

Medical Optimization for all

HTN and glycemic control, antiplatelet agent and statin, exercise regimen and smoking cessation.

Post-intervention aspirin and statin are life-long medications, Clopidegril 75 mg daily is generally used for 30 days after aorto-iliac intervention.

ACC/AHA/SVS Collaborative Recommendations, Intervention for Treatment of Claudicants*

- A predicted or observed lack of adequate response to exercise therapy and claudication pharmacotherapies.
- Presence of a severe disability, either being unable to perform normal work or having very serious impairment of other activities important to the patient.

**From (Hirsch AT, et al. J Am Coll Cardiol. 2006; 47)*

- Absence of other disease that would limit exercise even if the claudication was improved (e.g., angina or chronic respiratory disease).
- The individual's anticipated natural history and prognosis.
- The morphology of the lesion (must be such that the appropriate intervention would have low risk and a high probability of initial and long-term success).

Provisional stent placement is indicated for use in iliac arteries as salvage therapy for suboptimal or failed result from balloon dilation (e.g., persistent gradient (≥10 mmHg), residual diameter stenosis >50%, or flow-limiting dissection). Class IB recommendation

Stenting is effective as primary therapy for common iliac artery stenosis and occlusions. Class IB recommendation

Stenting is effective as primary therapy in external iliac artery stenosis and occlusions. Class IC recommendation

Figure 16.1 lists the TASC classification on aorto-ilac lesions.

Angiography for Aorto-Iliac Lesions

65-cm pigtail, tennis racquet, or Omni-flush catheter positioned at T12-L1 interspace, DSA angiogram at 15 cc/s for 30 cc injection at 900 psi pressure. Lateral aortic views facilitate interrogation of posterior aortic wall plaque. Catheter can be repositioned above aortic flow divider for ilio-femoral imaging for a 10 cc/s for 20 cc injection, with 30° anterior-oblique imaging for full assessment of iliac anatomic detail, location of internal iliac origin, and extent of external iliac disease.

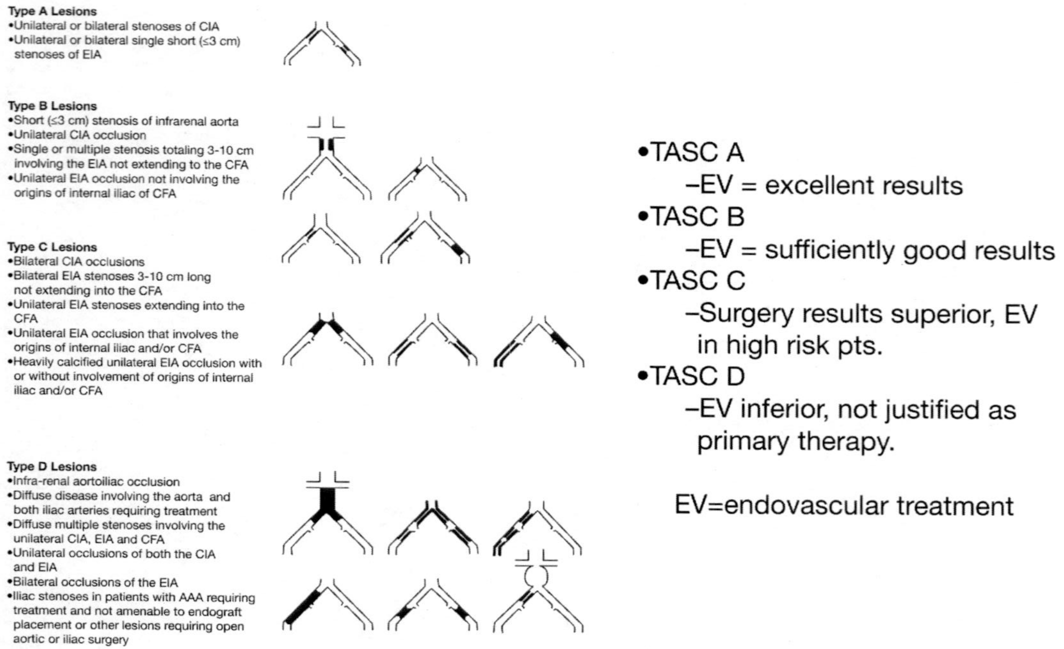

FIGURE 16.1 TASC II classification of aorto-iliac lesions

General Techniques/Tips of the Trade

Vessel Access

Selection of access site is determined by physical examination and subsequent non-invasive studies (SDP/PVR, CTA, MRA). For aorto-iliac lesions, retrograde femoral access via either one or both common femoral arteries is typical. Often, femoral access is made contralateral to the side of worse disease (or at side of strongest femoral pulse), to facilitate catheter placement for initial diagnostic aortography and iliac run-off. Brachial artery access can be utilized to image severe infra-renal occlusive disease or in the presence of extensive distal external iliac or common femoral disease. Pre-procedural MRA or CTA imaging can provide for a more targeted intervention, without need for more extensive diagnostic angiographic imaging (and can reduce contrast volume administered during intervention). US-guided needle entry helpful in the case of non-palpable femoral pulses.

Anticoagulation is initiated after wire and sheath access is obtained, with target ACT above 250. The patient should have also continued aspirin therapy the day of procedure.

Crossing Stenoses

- After arteriographic visualization, the uncomplicated iliac stenosis can often be crossed with the 0.035 J-wire or more steerable, and minimally traumatic, Wholey wire.
- For more complex lesions, a floppy-tipped hydrophilic wire and torque device can aid in maneuvering through lesion.
- A straight catheter over the guidewire provides additional support to steer and incrementally advance wire and catheter across lesion.
- Selective catheters can provide extra help in guiding wire across lesions in tortuous vessels.

- Road-mapping angiogram may provide better visualization for passing through the lesion-flow channel.
- Avoid excessive force or buckling of the wire to prevent dissection.

Crossing Total Occlusions

- Total occlusions can be challenging to cross with less reproducible results than stenoses.
- There is usually a critical lesion with adjacent accumulated organized thrombus. Diffuse lesions in a tortuous vessel may increase risk of vessel perforation or dissection during the intervention.
- Choosing an access site to minimize distance to the lesion is preferred, although sometimes a dual antegrade and retrograde approach to crossing occlusion can be required.
- Entering a subintimal plane may facilitate crossing, but re-entry into the true lumen may be challenging (especially at the aortic bifurcation) and must be ensured.
- First, thoroughly assess lesion angiographically to confirm lesion length and characteristics, with road-mapping a possible tool to ensure acceptable wire passage location.

Clinical Pointers

- Generally, the shorter and least calcified the occlusion, the easier it is to cross. The guidewire usually passes easily through the compacted thrombus, and meets resistance at the region of heaviest plaque.
- Hydrophilic wires supported by straight hydrophilic catheters can allow incremental advancement through the plaque.
- Most lesions can be crossed utilizing straight glidewire and 4 F glidecatheter.
- Once glidecatheter is advanced over wire across lesion, contrast can be carefully injected through the

catheter to ensure re-entry into the true lumen and no dissection.

- If the retrograde approach is not working, consider an antegrade approach to the lesion from a contralateral access. A snare will then be required to bring the wire out of the ipsilateral sheath, with passage of a crossing catheter back over this wire to cross lesion and obtain true-lumen entry.
- Once total occlusion is crossed, and true-lumen position beyond lesion is established; it is recommended to advance a long sheath across the lesion after predilation, to ensure that the balloon-mounted stent will not be dragged through the lesion and off the balloon.
- This is especially important for hand-mounted stents and available pre-mounted covered stents.
- Generally, 0.035 balloon and stent platforms are utilized for aorto-iliac intervention.

Adjunctive Measures

Pressure measurement across lesions can be performed to quantify physiologic significance of the stenosis. Dual pressure transducers can be arranged (one connected to the catheter, the second to the side-arm of sheath, as long as there is at least one French-size difference between the two) and vasodilators such as nitroglycerin administered distal to the lesion in question to exacerbate or provoke the pressure gradient by diminishing distal peripheral vascular resistance. This is best used for low resting-gradient lesions, or those of potential physiologic importance, to mimic an exertional state.

Mechanical thrombectomy devices can be employed to remove fresh thrombus in an "acute-on-chronic disease" clinical situation, unmasking the true lesion and reducing embolic potential of the fresh thrombus.

True-lumen re-entry devices may be of use for returning to intra-luminal position from a dissection plane established while crossing an iliac lesion in total occlusions.

Methods for Accurate Vessel Size Measuring
Intravascular ultrasound (IVUS) can be used for lesion interrogation (degree of calcium or soft plaque), and for more exact sizing of vessel diameters to aid in balloon and stent size selection. IVUS can be helpful in determining post-deployment stent apposition to vessel wall, and guide the need for further post-dilation.

Predilation with a purposefully lower-sized balloon can aid in visual estimation of the correct balloon/stent size for ultimate use.

Angiographic calibrated measurement software can often be made by referencing a known size in the image (sheath, marker pigtail catheter) to provide insight into correct vessel sizing.

How I Do It

Isolated aortic stenoses can be accessed via unilateral approach from either femoral artery. Angiography and calibrated measurement of nominal aortic diameters adjacent to the lesion are important assessments, as is characterization of the plaque. Pre-procedural non-invasive imaging (CTA, MRA), IVUS, calibrated angiography measurement, or purposefully pre-dilating with an undersized balloon can be utilized. Cautious, low-pressure balloon inflations should be employed in the aorta, with either self-expandable (SE) or balloon-expandable (BE) stents able to be placed. BE stents can often be more precisely placed than SE stents, and the higher radial force of a BE stent may be required for densely calcified aortic lesions. Expansion of the lesion to 10–12 mm (regardless of the pre and post-lesion aortic diameter) is

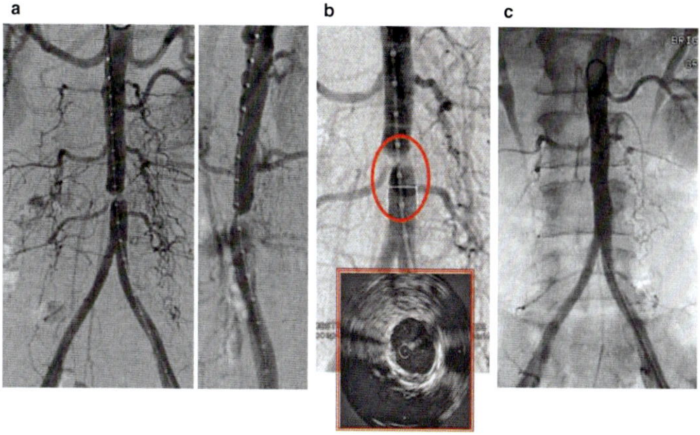

FIGURE 16.2 (**a**) Aortic lesion angiogram with calibrated pigtail catheter. (**b**) Size measurement of aorta using calibration or with IVUS (inset). (**c**) Completion angiogram

usually adequate clinically, despite imperfect angiographic appearance. Lesions of high concern for embolism can be primarily stented in an attempt to trap or "jail" plaque in the lesion (Fig. 16.2).

Potential Pitfalls

Balloon dilation of an occlusive lesion adjacent to a segment of aneurysmal dilation is contraindicated, unless preparation has been made to treat both pathologies with a covered stent-graft.

Aortic bifurcation lesions extending into the proximal iliac arteries are best managed with kissing balloon angioplasty +/– stenting, to avoid plaque shift which may compromise the other iliac orifice. BE stents provide the greatest radial force for typically calcified bifurcation plaque, and raising the aortic flow divider several centimeters is common. BE stents can be precisely placed more easily, and sizes from 7 to 8 mm diameter are sufficient, with post-dilation with larger balloons as necessary to optimize stent-vessel apposition. SE stents in densely calcified aortic bifurcation lesions may not provide sufficient radial force or one stent may collapse the other. In the presence of a more diffuse proximal aortic lesion, the aortic lesion can first be treated, with subsequent placement of the kissing bifurcation stents. Here, bilateral access is obtained, but remember to withdraw the contralateral wire before deploying the BE aortic stent, and then reinsert wire back through the aortic stent for subsequent kissing iliac stent placement (Figs. 16.3 and 16.4). Figure 16.5 shows a clinical case of a patient with acute limb ischemia (rest pain, paresthesias) with longstanding stable bilateral claudication history. An Angiojet percutaneous mechanical thrombectomy device was used to clear fresh thrombus, unmasking chronic distal aortic/bilateral CIA disease, which was treated with aortic and bilateral iliac stents.

Potential Pitfalls

Must ensure catheter true-lumen catheter re-entry into aorta, as it is not uncommon to have wire "spiral" in a dissection plane at aortic bifurcation with retrograde attempts at crossing long iliac occlusions.

For stenting of both aortic and common iliac diseases, be careful to ensure that the shoulders of the balloon the BE stent is mounted on treating an aortic lesion are above iliac origins, to avoid rupture of the iliac arteries.

Isolated common iliac lesions can be approached either retrograde from the ipsilateral femoral, or from an "up-and-over" contralateral approach, provided that the aortic bifurcation is not too "peaked," and there is sufficient nominal-sized

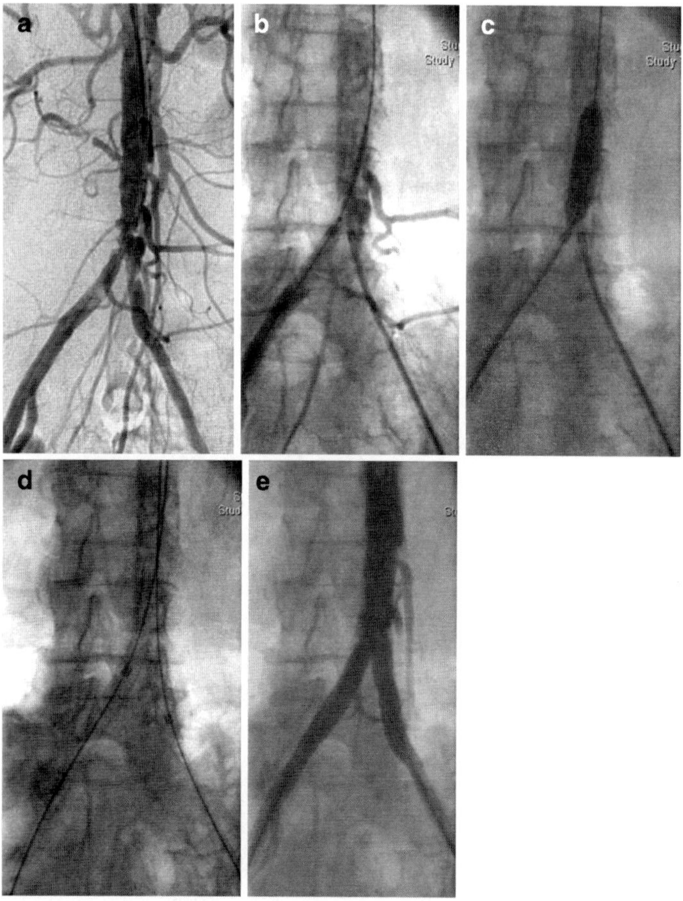

FIGURE 16.3 (**a**) Angiogram demonstrating distal aortic stenosis with bilateral common iliac disease (CIA) disease. (**b**) Bilateral sheath access, balloon expandable stent delivered for distal aortic stenting. (**c**) Aortic balloon expandable stent deployment (shoulder of balloon must be above iliac ostia). (**d**) Bilateral CIA "kissing" stents. (**e**) Completion angiogram of aorto-iliac reconstruction

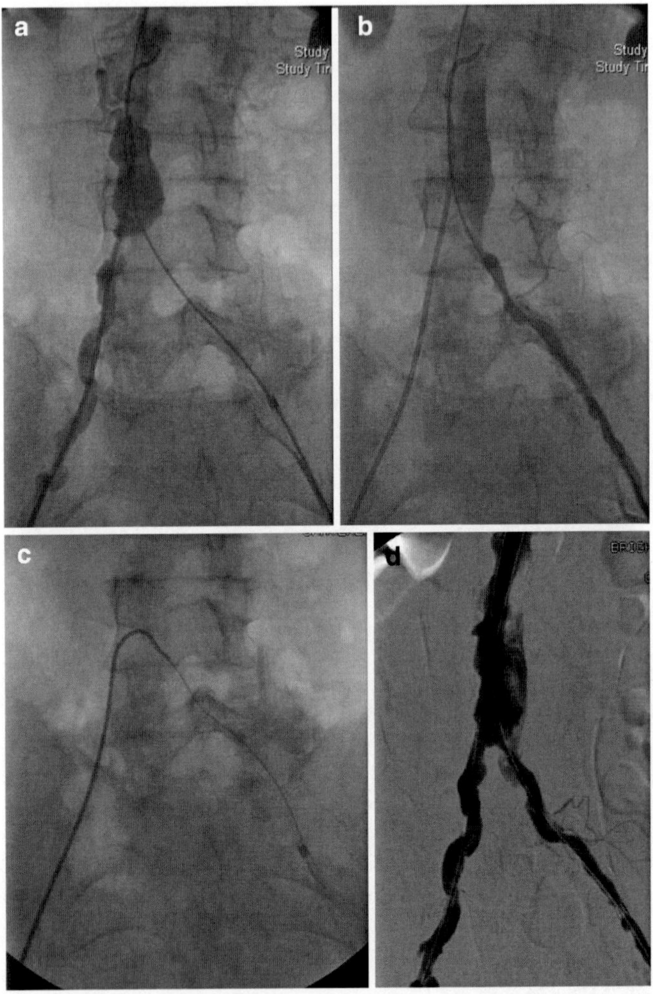

Figure 16.4 (**a**) Aortogram showing R CIA stenosis, L CIA occlusive disease. (**b**) L iliac retrograde sheath angiogram confirming aorto-iliac dissection and no true-lumen re-entry after L retrograde iliac crossing attempt. (**c**) Switch to antegrade wire passage. (**d**) Now true-lumen access confirmed for L sided wire (dissection still filling). (**e**) Kissing bilateral iliac stents placed. (**f**) Completion angiogram, with no further filling of dissection (contrast visible is retained contrast, CT scan following day confirmed no dissection)

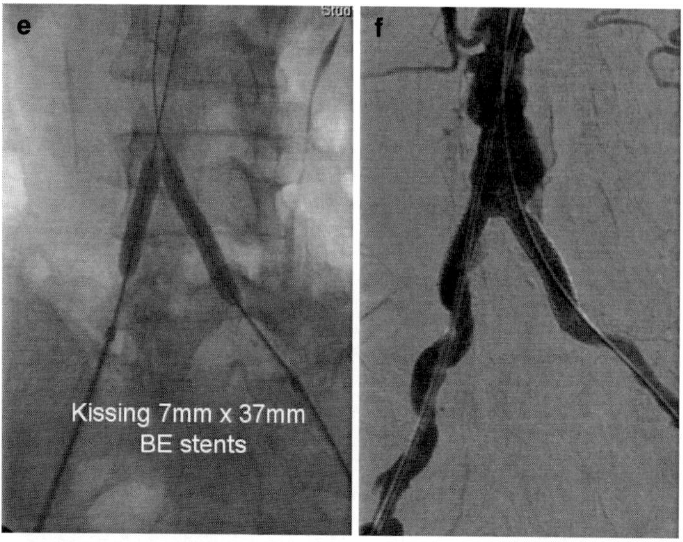

FIGURE 16.4 (continued)

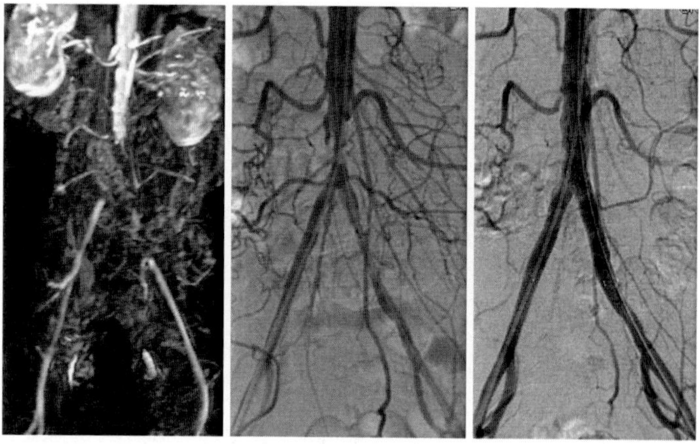

FIGURE 16.5 Clinical case of a patient with acute limb ischemia (rest pain, paresthesias) with longstanding stable bilateral claudication history. An Angiojet percutaneous mechanical thrombectomy device was used to clear fresh thrombus, unmasking chronic distal aortic/bilateral CIA disease, which was treated with aortic and bilateral iliac stents

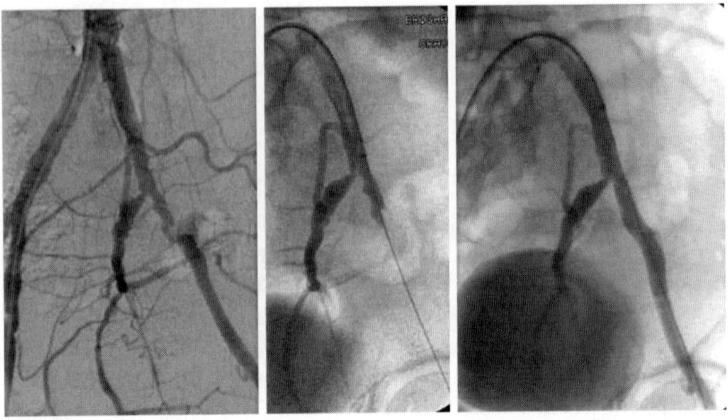

FIGURE 16.6 Focal L external iliac atherosclerotic lesion, treated from contralateral approach

proximal iliac artery to allow balloon/stent placement beyond the bifurcation. In cases of stenoses associated with distal post-stenotic dilation, stent sizing can be often kept to an 8-mm diameter, which will be well-engaged and held by the lesion, and judicious post-dilation with incrementally larger balloons can increase stent size to obtain wall apposition without over-dilating the original lesion. A covered stent can be used in this location if the lesion is excessively calcified and there is a concern for rupture or dissection.

Isolated external iliac artery (EIA) lesions can be approached from either retrograde or antegrade access, depending upon distal extent of disease. Up-and-over sheaths are utilized to facilitate angiographic interrogation to ensure precise placement as well as reduce bifurcation trauma with device exchanges. These sheaths aid in tracking the device to desired location, confirming placement, and the performance of completion angiography. SE stents are more easily placed in tortuous vessels. Pre-dilation with a 5–6 mm balloon, followed by SE stent placement and gentle post-dilation to 7 or 8 mm is often possible. Covered SE stentgrafts may have a role in reducing in-stent restenosis, particularly in the external iliac vessels. Care is taken to avoid jailing the hypogastric artery during stenting (Figs. 16.6–16.8).

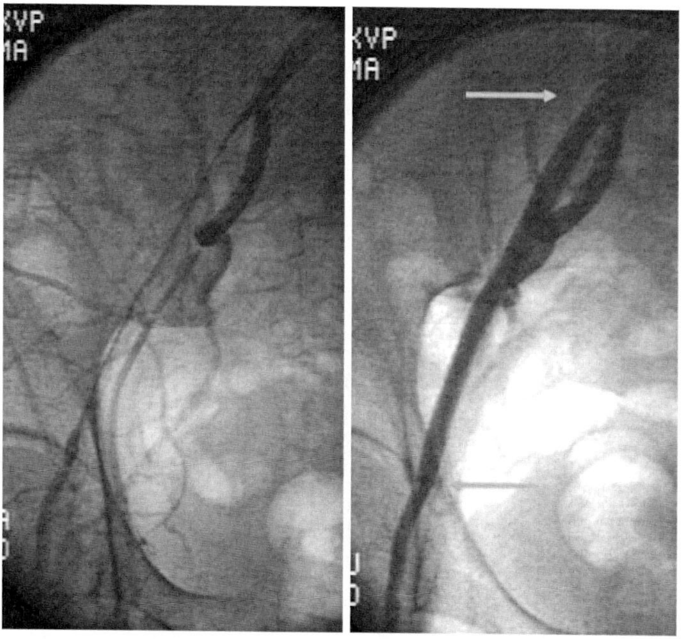

FIGURE 16.7 Diffuse R EIA stenosis, treated from contralateral approach. Completion angiogram shows SE stent distal to hypogastric artery origin, extending to just beneath inguinal ligament

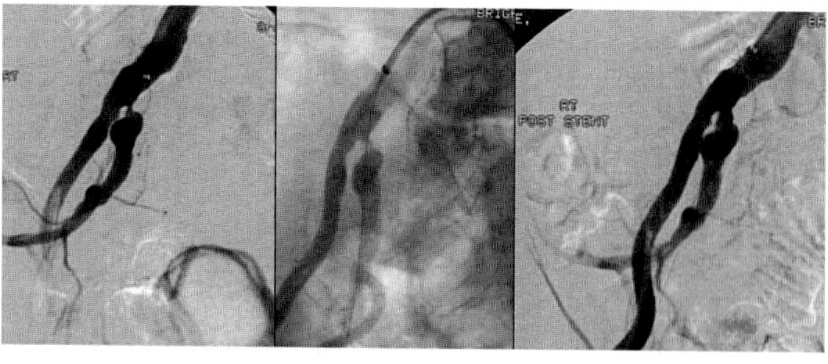

FIGURE 16.8 Patient with known PAD and with symptoms of severe and limiting R buttock claudication. R internal iliac lesion on angiogram, PTA and stenting from contralateral approach

Potential Pitfalls

Placing stents in treatment of proximal common iliac lesions (encroaching on aortic bifurcation) can be challenging with an antegrade approach. Advisable to access retrograde from contralateral approach.

External iliac vessels are relatively fragile vessels and are a common site of vessel rupture during intervention.

For diffuse or distal external iliac disease, consensus is to avoid placing SE stents distal to the inguinal ligament. If distal EIA or common femoral artery (CFA) disease is evident, then consider hybrid technique: surgical CFA endarterectomy and patch closure (which can be carried proximally into distal EIA, under the inguinal ligament), with subsequent sheath access and intervention through the patched femoral vessel. Stents can then be deployed to the proximal patch level.

Isolated internal iliac lesions are frequently most easily accessed and treated form of contralateral approach, given angle of vessel origin and take-off. The lesions are most often ostial, and often have post-stenotic dilation distal to this ostial lesion. Short BE stents (often 6–7 mm diameter) placed after predilation offer precision of placement, and should not be sized to the post-stenotic diameter. The 0.014 platforms allow for lower crossing profiles and shorter stents, which are useful for these lesions.

Hybrid surgical/endovascular cases are recommended for disease involving the common femoral (CFA) and profunda femoral arteries, which improves the outflow for the proximal aorto-iliac intervention. An open groin incision is employed, with common femoral endarterectomy and profundoplasty with prosthetic patch closure. The endarterectomy and patch are able to be extended into the distal external iliac artery (just proximal to the inguinal ligament). Then, under fluoroscopic guidance, the patch is accessed with arterial entry needle and wire and sheath passed, with proximal intervention performed. With extensive external iliac plaque contiguous with the common femoral disease, it may be helpful to first access the CFA with needle, wire, and sheath, obtain passage of the wire across the iliac disease into the aorta, and then proceed with the surgical endarterectomy. This pre-endarterectomy wire access avoids possible challenging wire crossing of the proximal "shelf" of distal external iliac post-endarterectomy divided plaque, thus minimizing the chance of external iliac dissection. Following patch angioplasty closure, the external iliac stent can be brought down to just under the inguinal ligament, avoiding the common femoral flexion site. There may be a benefit to limiting in-stent restenosis by using covered self-expanding stent-grafts in the heavily disease external iliac vessels.

Aorto-iliac restenoses can be treated with repeat PTA, and there may be a benefit to using covered stents in prevention of recurrence

Equipment

- *Arterial entry needle, micropuncture kit*
- *Starter 0.035 access wire* (J-wire, Benson wire, Wholey wire)
- *Selective wire* (Glidewire), with torque-control device
- *Exchange wire* (Stiff Glidewire or Amplatz Super-Stiff) to straighten tortuous anatomy or provide more support for passage of sheath/balloon/stent across bulky lesions or total occlusions
- *Flush catheter* for imaging, pigtail, tennis racquet, Omni-flush catheter also useful for obtaining "up-and-over" aortic bifurcation wire access
- *Exchange catheter* (4 F glidecatheter) for both wire support in crossing occlusions and wire exchange
- *Directional catheter* (Berenstein) for directional wire control, Sos-omni or RIM catheter for crossing over aortic bifurcation

- *Sheath:* Standard 5 F access sheath, long straight sheaths 6–9 F (23–35 mm with radio-opaque tip) for balloons and stents and retrograde vessel imaging, 6 F or larger cross-bifurcation sheaths (Ansel, Balkin) for contralateral iliac lesion treatment
- *PTA balloons* of various sizes and lengths (5–18 mm diameters, 2–4 cm lengths)
- *Aortic occlusion balloons:* When performing aortic intervention for emergent management of rupture
- *Balloon-expandable stents* (pre-mounted: 6–10 mm diameters, 17–59 mm lengths; unmounted Palmaz stents)
- *Self-expanding stents* (8, 10, 12, 14 mm diameters, 20, 40, 60 mm approximate lengths)
- *Covered stents* for bailout of vessel rupture, treatment of in-stent restenosis
- Both BE and SE covered stents helpful, I prefer to use the Atrium ICAST or the W.L. Gore Viabahn stent in these situations.
- *IVUS* for accurate vessel sixing and post-stenting result assessment.

Bibilography

1. ACC/AHA/SVS collaborative recommendations, Intervention for treatment of claudicants, Hirsch AT, et al. *J Am Coll Cardiol.* 2006;47.
   → *Comprehensive overview and treatment recommendations for PAD.*
2. Peter Schneider, Endovascular Skills: Guidewire and catheter skills for endovascular surgery, 3rd ed., New York, Informa Healthcare, 2008.
   → *Excellent and very detailed textbook covering the technical aspects of endovascular intervention. Well illustrated.*
3. Chang RW, Goodney PP, Baek JH, et al. Long-term results of combined common femoral endarterectomy and iliac stenting/stent grafting for occlusive disease. J Vasc Surg. 2008 Aug;48(2):362–7.
   → *The largest series reported of hybrid surgical/endovascular management of aorto-iliac with common femoral occlusive disease.*

Chapter 17
Femoropopliteal Percutaneous Interventions

Jeffrey M. Sparling and Andrew C. Eisenhauer

Etiology

Atherosclerosis (primary cause), thromboembolic disease, *in situ* thrombosis, vasculitidies, extrinsic compression, aneurysmal disease

Background

Atherosclerotic femoropopliteal peripheral arterial disease (PAD) is often discovered in the asymptomatic patient with routine non-invasive lower-extremity blood pressure measurement and in the symptomatic individual via a history of claudication or rest pain

J.M. Sparling
Cardiovascular Division, Brigham and Women's Hospital, Harvard Medical School, Boston, MA, USA
e-mail: jsparling@partners.org

A.C. Eisenhauer (✉)
Cardiovascular Division, Department of Medicine, Brigham and Women's Hospital, Harvard Medical School, Boston, MA, USA
e-mail: aeisenhauer@partners.org

C.D. Owens and Y. Yeghiazarians (eds.), *Handbook of Endovascular Peripheral Interventions*, DOI 10.1007/978-1-4614-0839-0_17,

Prevalence

High prevalence in those with traditional cardiac risk factors and with increased age (~30% of all patients older than 70 years and patients older than 50 years with cardiovascular risk factors) as identified by history and/or ankle-brachial index (ABI)

Clinical Presentation/Clues

- Accurate history and focused physical examination critical for distinguishing lower extremity arterial disease from venous and non-vascular etiologies (Table 17.1)
- Claudication from femoral and/or popliteal PAD usually presents as calf discomfort produced with effort and relieved with rest
- Critical limb ischemia (CLI) often results from occlusive disease at multiple orders of arterial distribution, including above-the-knee disease
- Acute limb ischemia is often caused by thrombosis or thromboembolism; the superficial femoral artery is a common site of involvement
- Non-invasive assessments can help localize and characterize the severity of disease

Screening

Ankle-Brachial Index (ABI)

- Can be performed at the bedside by calculating the ratio of highest dopplerable dorsalis pedis or posterior tibialis systolic pressure to highest brachial systolic pressure
- Values <0.9 are abnormal and consistent with PAD; values >1.4 are consistent with non-compressible arteries and have no negative predictive value

TABLE 17.1 Differential diagnoses of lower extremity discomfort

Diagnosis	Location of pain	Description	Effect of movement	Exam	Other hints
Intermittent claudication	Calf (for SFA/popliteal disease)	Cramping, aching, heaviness	Exacerbated by walking, quickly relieved with rest	Diminished popliteal and distal pulses	Presence of traditional CV risk factors
Neuropathic pain	Radiates down leg	Sharp, shooting, "like an electric shock"	Can occur at rest or while walking, often worse when sitting	Improves with position change	History of back or neck arthritis
Arthritic pain	Lateral hip and thigh	Aching	Worse throughout course of day	Discomfort with passive maneuvers	
Spinal stenosis	Buttocks, thigh	Weakness, heaviness	Better when leaning forward	Standing from sitting position and extension exacerbates pain	Often ambulates while leaning forward on assistive devices to aid in spinal flexion
Baker's cyst	Behind the knee	Swelling and tenderness	Worse with movement, not relieved with rest	Palpable mass in popliteal fossa, best visualized with knee fully extended	Ruptured cysts can mimic acute thrombophlebitis

- Should be performed on:
  - All patients with exertional leg discomfort
  - Patients between 50 and 69 years with at least one CV risk factor
  - All patients older than 70
  - All patients with Framingham risk score 10–20%
- *Strengths*: Simple, low-cost, no-risk, highly sensitive and specific and well-validated; can be used as a diagnostic modality or to follow efficacy and durability of therapy
- *Limitations*: Accuracy is compromised by calcific, incompressible arteries, resulting in supradiagnostic values; localization of disease is not possible

Segmental Pressure Examination

- Performed in a non-invasive vascular diagnostic laboratory
- Segmental systolic blood pressures on the thigh, calf, and ankle
- Often coupled with pulse volume recording (see below)
- *Strengths*: Simple, low-cost, no-risk; can be utilized to localize disease and predict level of healing as well as to follow efficacy and durability of therapy
- *Limitations*: As with ABI, accuracy compromised by calcific, incompressible arteries

Pulse Volume Recording (PVR)

- Performed in a non-invasive vascular diagnostic laboratory
- Graphical representation of limb volume
- *Strengths*: Simple, low-cost screening test that can be utilized to localized disease and predict outcomes pre- and post-revascularization; unlike ABI and segmental pressures, it can be utilized in patients with incompressible arteries
- *Limitations*: Does not provide vessel visualization; reliance can be affected by poor cardiac output (though leg pressures may be compared to brachial pressures as a control to minimize this bias)

Duplex Ultrasonography

- *Strengths*: Combined continuous wave Doppler imaging and 2D-ultrasound provides both quantitative and qualitative assessment of PAD in a low-risk, non-invasive manner
- *Limitations*: Usefulness in post-revascularization surveillance of PTA and surgical conduits (both vein and synthetic grafts) is of questionable significance

Tips of the Trade: Non-invasive Imaging

- Often advantageous to proceed with CT or MR prior to invasive angiography in patients with non-invasive studies suggestive of multi-segmental disease
- This allows pre-interventional planning for access (i.e., antegrade or retrograde), and planning (need for athterectomy devices, re-entry catheters, etc.)

Computed Tomographic Angiography (CTA)/Magnetic Resonance Angiography (MRA)

- *Strengths*: Useful in diagnosing the location and degree of arterial stenoses and occlusions in a non-invasive manner; significantly less ionizing radiation exposure than traditional angiography; allows planning of future methods of revascularization
- *Limitations*: Can underestimate or omit (in the case of CTA, particularly with single-detector studies) or overestimate (in the case of MRA) a non-occlusive stenosis; with MRA, metal objects in the body can cause significant artifact or (as with the case of implantable cardiac devices) be an absolute contraindication

Treatment

- Aggressive medical treatment of cardiovascular risk factors, with an emphasis on smoking cessation, should be encouraged

- Supervised exercise training should be the initial therapy for all patients with claudication, regardless of the decision for revascularization
- Aspirin (or clopidogrel as an aspirin alternative) should be administered for primary prevention of stroke, MI, or death in patients with established PAD
- Cilostazol can improve symptoms in claudicants without heart failure; pentoxifylline can be utilized in patients with PAD who are unresponsive to or not candidates for therapy for cilostazol
- Revascularization therapy (surgical or endovascular) can be employed based on symptom severity, lesion morphology, and favorable risk-to-benefit ratio (Table 17.2)

Femoropopliteal Percutaneous Revascularization: Methods

Diagnostic Angiography

Equipment

- 5 or 6 Fr 10-cm introducer
- Diagnostic non-selective angiography catheter (e.g., Omni Flush, straight pigtail, tennis racket)
- Diagnostic selective angiography catheter (e.g., LIMA, JR, MP, Teurmo Glidecath)
- Standard 0.035″ J wire
- Steerable 0.035″ guide wire (e.g., stiff angled Terumo Glidewire, Wholey Hi-Torque)
- Contrast power injector

Non-selective Angiography

- Access: 5 or 6 Fr introducer, typically in a retrograde fashion (though antegrade punctures are ideal in specific clinical situations as discussed below)
- Utilizing a J-wire, pass a non-selective catheter into the distal abdominal aorta just proximal to the aorto-iliac bifurcation

Table 17.2 TASC criteria for infrainguinal disease and recommendations for revascularization

TASC Type A	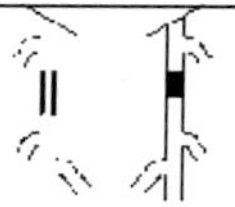	• Single stenosis ≤10 cm in length • Single occlusion ≤5 cm in length	Endovascular recommended
TASC Type B	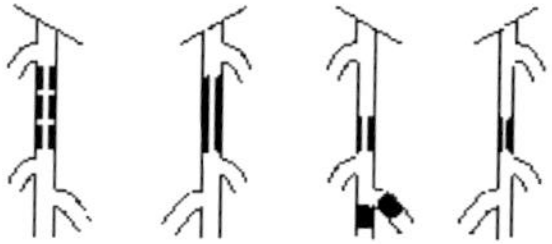	• Multiple lesions (stenoses or occlusions), each ≤5 cm • Single stenosis or occlusion not involving the infrageniculate popliteal artery • Heavily calcified occlusions ≤5 cm • Single popliteal stenosis	Endovascular recommended
TASC Type C	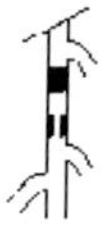	• Multiple stenoses or occlusions totaling >15 cm with or without heavy calcification • Recurrent stenoses or occlusions that need treatment after two endovascular interventions	Surgery recommended for good-risk profile patients; endovascular treatment may be considered when weighing risk/benefit
TASC Type D	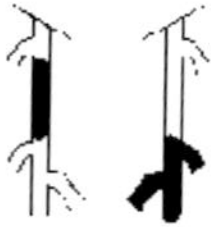	• Chronic total occlusions of the CFA or SFA (>20 cm, involving the popliteal artery) • Chronic total occlusion of the popliteal and proximal trifurcation	Surgery recommended

Adapted from the Inter-Society Consensus for the Management of Peripheral Arterial Disease – TASC II

- The bilateral femoropopliteal systems may then be imaged as a part of the overall lower extremity angiogram utilizing traditional "run-off" angiography or digital subtraction angiography (DSA) via the "bolus-chase" method in capable angiographic suites

Selective Angiography

- Select the contralateral common iliac with a steerable 0.035″ guidewire, then "hook" the bifurcation with the non-selective catheter by pulling catheter and wire as a unit and seating the wire distal into the iliofemoral system
- Exchange the non-selective catheter for the selective catheter of choice
- Runoff cine' angiography or digital subtraction angiography performed in segmental "stations" may then be performed in the limb contralateral from the access site
- Ipsilateral angiography may be performed in a similar fashion via injections directly into the arterial introducer
- The common femoral artery and the SFA/profunda bifurcation are often best imaged with 30–45° of ipsilateral angulation so as to minimize vessel overlap
- The remainder of the SFA and popliteal arteries may be imaged in an AP projection, with angulation as dictated to best visualize segments of interest

Percutaneous Revascularization of the Femoropoliteal Arteries: How I Do It

Equipment

- 6 or 7 Fr 40 cm introducer (e.g., Ansel, Balkan Contralateral, Pinnacle Destination) for contralateral limb access
- 6 Fr 11 cm introducer (in cases requiring ipsilateral retrograde access)
- Stiff 0.035″ guide wire (e.g., Rosen, Amplatz)
- Steerable 0.035″ guide wire (e.g., stiff angled Terumo Glidewire, Wholey Hi-Torque)

TABLE 17.3 Commonly used angioplasty balloons in femoropopliteal interventions

Company	Balloon	Minimum guidewire diameter (in.)	Minimum sheath size (Fr)	Available balloon diameters (mm)	Available balloon lengths (cm)
Abbott	Viatrac	0.014	4	4, 4.5	1.5, 2, 3, 4
			5	5, 5.5, 6, 6.5, 7	1.5, 2, 3, 4
	Agiltrac	0.035	5	4, 5, 6, 7	2, 4, 6, 8, 10
			6	6, 7, 8, 9, 10	2, 4, 6, 8, 10
	Agiltrac 0.018	0.018	5	4, 5, 6, 7, 8	2, 3, 4, 6
			6	8, 9, 10	2, 3, 4, 6
	Fox Plus	0.035	5	3, 4, 5, 6, 7, 8, 9, 10, 12	2. 3. 4. 6. 8. 10, 12
	Fox sv	0.018	4	2, 2.5, 3, 4, 5, 6	1.5, 2, 3, 4, 6, 8, 10, 12
	FoxCross	0.035	5	3, 4, 5, 6, 7, 8, 9, 10, 12, 14	2, 3, 4, 6, 8, 10, 12
Bard	Ultraverse	0.018	4	2, 3, 4, 5, 6, 7	2, 4, 6, 10
Boston Scientific	Sterling Monorail	0.014, 0.018	4	3, 3.5, 4, 4.5, 5, 5.5, 6, 6.5, 7, 8	1. 1.5, 2, 3, 4, 6
	Sterling OTW	0.014, 0.018	4	4, 5, 6, 7, 8	2, 3, 4, 6, 8
	Sterling ES	0.014	4	1.5, 2, 2.5, 3, 3.5, 4	2, 3, 4

(continued)

TABLE 17.3 (continued)

Company	Balloon	Minimum guidewire diameter (in.)	Minimum sheath size (Fr)	Available balloon diameters (mm)	Available balloon lengths (cm)
Cook	Advance 14LP	0.014	4	2, 2.5, 3, 4	2, 4, 6, 8, 12, 16, 20
	Advance 18LP	0.018	4	3, 4, 5, 6, 7	2, 4, 6, 8, 10
	Advance 35LP	0.035	5	3, 4, 5, 6, 7, 8	2, 3, 4, 6, 8, 10, 12, 14
Cordis	Savvy	0.018	4	2, 2.5, 3, 3.5, 4, 5, 6	2, 3, 4, 6, 10
	Savvy long				12, 15, 22 (Long)
	Sleek Rx	0.014	4	2, 2.5, 3, 3.5, 4	4, 8, 10, 12, 15, 22
Cordis	Opta Pro PTA	0.035	5	3–10, 12	1, 1.5, 2, 3, 4, 6, 8, 10
ev3	EverCross	0.035	5	3–10, 12	1.5, 2–6, 8, 10, 12, 15, 20
	NanoCross	0.014	4	1.5, 2, 2.5, 3, 3.5, 4	2, 4, 8, 12, 15, 21
Invatec	Ampherion Deep	0.014	4	1.5, 2, 2.5, 3, 3.5, 4	2, 4, 8, 12
	Admiral Xtreme	0.035	5	3–10, 12	2, 4, 6, 8, 12
	Submarine Plus	0.018	4	2–6 (with half sizes), 7	2, 4, 6, 8, 12

TABLE 17.4 Commonly used self-expanding stents in femoropopliteal interventions

Company	Stent	Minimum guidewire diameter (in.)	Minimum sheath size (Fr)	Available stent diameters (mm)	Available stent length (mm)
Abbott	Xpert	0.018	4	4, 5, 6	20, 30, 40, 60
			5	6, 8	20, 30, 40, 60
	Dynalink	0.018	6	5–10	28, 38, 56, 80, 100
	Absolute Pro	0.035	6	5–10	20–40, 60, 80, 100
Bard	Lifestent	0.035	6	6–10 (Lifestent)	20, 30, 40, 60, 80
	Lifestent XL			6, 7 (XL)	100, 120, 150, 170 (XL)
Boston Scientific	Wallstent	0.035	6	6–10	27, 29, 31, 33, 46, 50, 53, 54, 57, 67, 72, 77, 80, 83, 93, 100
Cook	Zilver 518 (Rx and OTW)	0.018	5	4–10	20–40, 60, 80
	Zilver 635	0.035	6	4–10, 12, 14	20–40, 60, 80
Cordis	S.M.A.R.T.	0.035	6	6–10	20, 30, 40, 60, 80, 100 (in 6–8 diam)
ev3	Protégé EverFlex	0.035	6	5–8	20–40, 60, 80, 100, 120; 150 (except in 5 diam)
	Protégé GPS	0.018	6	6–10	20–40, 60, 80

Tips of the Trade: Access for Interventions

- Most femoropopliteal interventions can be performed with a 6 Fr introducer
- However, if atherectomy or re-entry is contemplated, it may be advantageous to utilize a 7 Fr sheath for access
- Use of a sheath with a hemostatic valve rather than a Touhy may limit bleeding

- Variety of steerable 0.014″ guide wires (e.g., Balance Middle Weight, PT Graphix, Miracle Bros.) in cases of total occlusions
- Peripheral support catheter (e.g., Terumo Glide Catheter, Spectranetics Quick-Cross)
- Angioplasty balloon catheters (Table 17.3)
- Peripheral self-expanding stent catheters (Table 17.4)

Access

- *Contralateral (retrograde)*: The diagnostic introducer is exchanged over a stiff 0.035″ guide wire parked in the contralateral SFA for a long (40 cm) 6 or 7 Fr introducer. Care must be taken to observe the introducer pass over the aorto-iliac bifurcation, as the system can "push back" and disengage without adequate distal wire position
- *Ipsilateral (antegrade)*: May be utilized in patients with tortuous iliac vessels or proximal SFA disease (Fig. 17.1) that would prevent adequate introducer support from the contralateral approach. Care should be taken to utilize the micropuncture technique for access, to remove the sheath as soon as possible post-procedure, and to minimize bleeding complications. Standard 10 cm introducers are typically adequate

Anticoagulation

- Should be administered after introducer exchange or new antegrade access

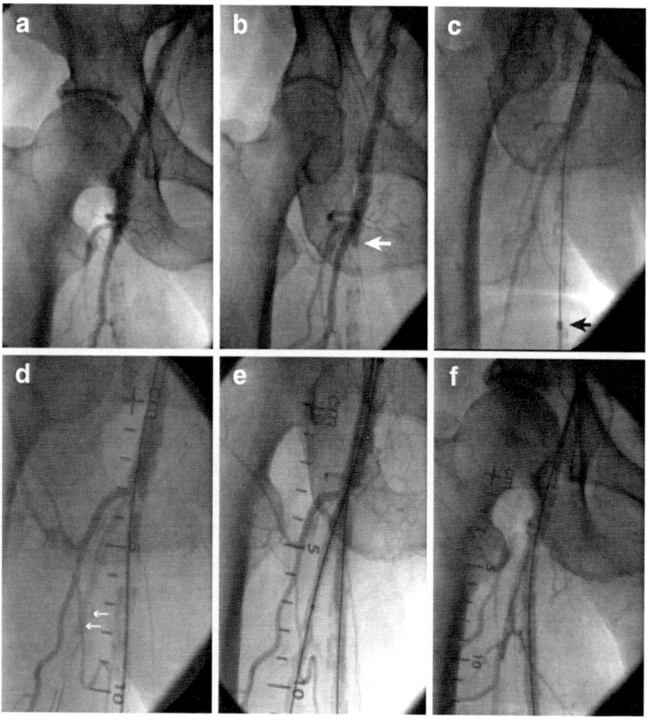

FIGURE 17.1 The proximal origin of the superficial femoral artery (SFA) is often heavily diseased and insufficient treatment of this segment is often a source of failure in endovascular approaches to the SFA. The patient illustrated above is a 61-year-old man with severe disabling claudication and proximal SFA occlusion. This AP view demonstrated an occluded and heavily calcified proximal SFA (**a**). An ipsilateral 20° oblique view demonstrates the proximal "nubbin" of the SFA (*white arrow*, **b**). After several unsuccessful attempts to cross the lesion via a contralateral approach, ipsilateral popliteal access was achieved and the lesion was crossed in a retrograde fashion. The *black arrow* indicates the tip of the sheath (**c**). A 0.014 wire was introduced from the contralateral groin and advanced into the profunda femoris artery (PFA) to protect its orifice and to prevent plaque shift (*double arrow*, **d**). A 6 mm by 10 cm Viabahn stent (W.L. Gore and Associates) was placed at the orifice of the SFA and a 4 mm by 4 cm Nanocross balloon (EV3) was placed in the orifice of the popliteal artery (**e**). The stent was deployed while the balloon was inflated in a kissing-style technique. Completion angiogram revealed widely patent SFA and PFA and the patient's severe claudication completely resolved (**f**)

- Target activated clotting time (ACT) of 250 s with unfractionated heparin
- Thienopyridine (e.g., clopidogrel) loading is usually accomplished post-procedure and daily dosing continued thereafter for a period of 3 months when peripheral nitinol stents are implanted (in the absence of a need for longer therapy, such as in the presence of a drug-eluting coronary stent)
- No role for glycoprotein IIb/IIIa inhibitors

Stenosis

- Non-occlusive stenoses are usually crossed with an 0.035 steerable guide wire with a support catheter or balloon catheter
- After lesion crossing, the stenosis is dilated with a balloon and dependent on the arterial distribution, angioplasty result, flow characteristics, and presence or absence of flow-limiting dissection, may or may not be stented (see below)
- Lesion characteristics may necessitate the use of adjunct therapies such as rotational atherectomy to facilitate angioplasty

Occlusions

- Often long and heavily calcified, particularly in the SFA
- An over-the-wire balloon catheter or a dedicated support catheter (e.g., Terumo Glidecath, Spectranetics Quick-Cross) is usually utilized
- Either 0.035″ stiff wires (e.g., Terumo stiff angled Glidewire) or extra-support 0.014″ coronary wires (e.g., Miracle Bros., Confienza) can be employed for lesion crossing
- The lesion is often traversed in the subintimal space, with re-entry into the true lumen at the distal end of the occlusion

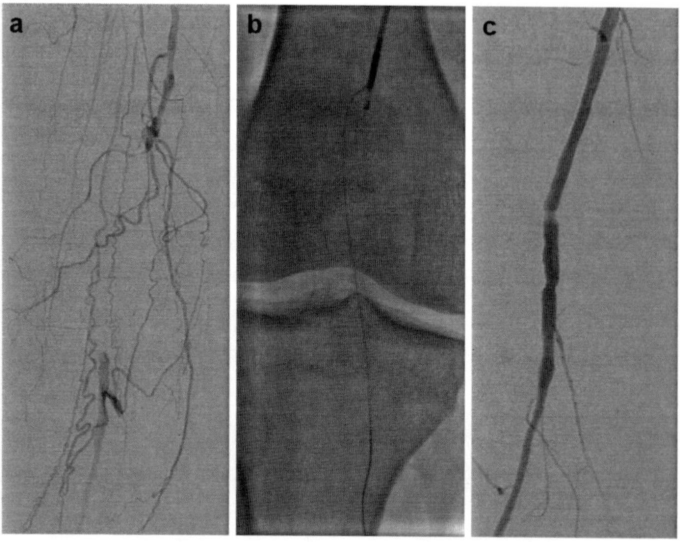

FIGURE 17.2 Use of an Outback LTD® luminal re-entry catheter during revascularization of an occluded distal right superficial femoral artery (pane **a**). The traditional techniques of wire re-entry described in the text were unsuccessful, so a 6 Fr Outback LTD® was passed into the sub-intimal space. Pane **b** illustrates the device with its re-entry needle extended at 9 o'clock, and a 0.014″ guidewire extended into the distal vessel. Intraluminal position was confirmed with contrast injection, and then the vessel repaired with self-expanding stents (pane **c**)

Tips of the Trade: Dissection After Balloon Angioplasty

- Because the SFA is often heavily calcified, dissection after even the most careful PTA is common
- However, dissections in the lower extremity are often not flow-limiting and thus not clinically significant
- If a dissection is apparent after PTA but does not appear severe or hemodynamically significant, consider accepting the balloon result alone
- It can be helpful to measure a pressure gradient across a dissection; the authors will typically accept <10 mmHg as satisfactory

- After lesion crossing and confirmation that the distal wire is intraluminal, balloon angioplasty +/– stent deployment occurs as with stenoses
- Lumen re-entry devices (Cordis Outback LTD, Medtronic Pioneer) are often utilized in situations where lumen re-entry from the subintimal space is challenging; these typically require gentle subintimal tract dilation with either a small caliber angioplasty balloon or passage of a guiding catheter prior to introduction of the re-entry catheter (Fig. 17.2)

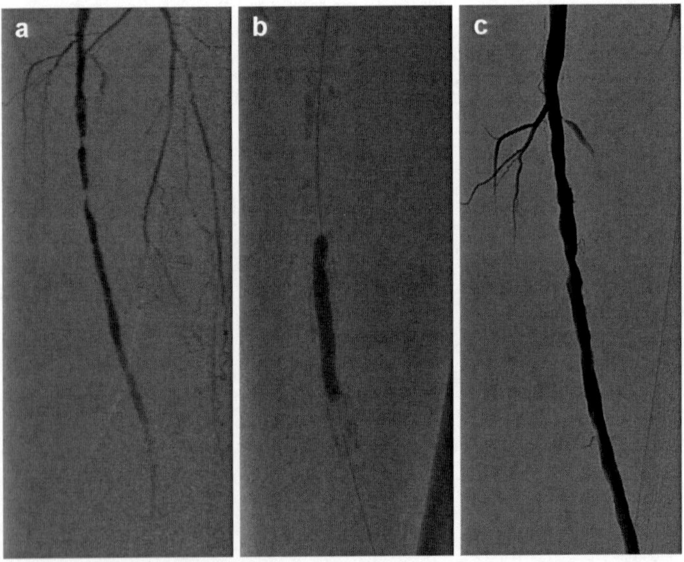

FIGURE 17.3 Percutaneous transluminal angioplasty as the primary treatment for discrete superficial femoral artery obstructive disease. The vessel in pane **a**, while heavily calcified, had two short, discrete obstructive lesions just prior to the adductor canal. These were treated by balloon angioplasty with 4 mm and 5 mm diameter balloons at nominal atmospheres for 3-min each inflation (pane **b**). Post-PTA angiography (pane **c**) revealed an excellent angiographic result with PTA alone; this was confirmed hemodynamically with near-complete resolution of measured trans-lesional gradients

Balloon Angioplasty: Special Considerations

- Balloon angioplasty alone is the therapy of choice in arterial beds where torsion (and thus the risk of stent fracture) is common, such as the common femoral and popliteal arteries
- Long, lower-pressure inflations of non-compliant peripheral angioplasty balloons are recommended to reduce the risk of dissection; the authors typically utilize nominal pressure inflations of 1–2 min in length
- Balloon angioplasty alone (particularly in discrete, short SFA lesions) often provides adequate and satisfactory results; stenting is not an absolute, particularly if the hemodynamic gradient is alleviated and no angiographic evidence of flow-limiting vessel trauma is evident (Fig. 17.3)
- Balloons are typically sized 1:1 with artery, though using a smaller initial size and progressively increasing balloon diameters may minimize arterial injury
- Pre-dilitations are usually performed prior to stent placement

Stenting: Special Considerations

- Direct stenting (without balloon predilitation) is rarely performed in the SFA
- Primary stenting of the SFA (after balloon predilitation) is a reasonable strategy that has been associated with increased patency at 6 months, and increased walking distance at 12 months when compared with PTA

Potential Pitfall: Nitinol Stent Undersizing

- Because of the shape memory characteristic of nitinol, stents are virtually impossible to post-dilate to a larger size than manufactured

- A stent undersized for artery will thus be at risk for migration and/or embolization
- Expanded nitinol stents are often too large to exteriorize percutaneously, requiring surgical removal
- Thus, stents should be oversized by at least 1 mm; because of nitinol's elasticity, perforation is rare

- Stenting of the CFA and popliteal arteries is traditionally avoided except in "bail-out" situations such as flow-limiting dissection; if stents are placed in these distributions, stiffer less-flexible balloon-expandable stents should be avoided to reduce fracture risk
- Stenting potential surgical anastamotic sites is typically avoided so as to preserve a surgical revascularization option in acceptable candidates
- Nitinol self-expanding stents are typically sized 1 mm larger than the reference vessel to ensure adequate expansion
- Non-compliant balloon post-dilitation is usually performed with both balloon-expandable and self-expanding stents to ensure the greatest acute lumen gain possible

Atherectomy: Special Considerations

- The use of atherectomy is typically reserved for lesion modification and debulking when adequate balloon and/or stent expansion is in question
- Multiple devices and modalities are available, including directional atherectomy (SilverHawk) and rotational atherectomy (Jetstream Pathway, CSI Diamondback)
- Many operators prefer to use atherectomy devices in conjunction with a distal filter embolic protection device to reduce the risk of distal particulate embolization
- Following atherectomy, it is standard to proceed with the primary therapy of choice (PTA or stenting)

Restenosis: Special Considerations

- Restenosis after intervention in the femoral and popliteal arteries remains a concern, occurring in 30–40% of interventions after 12 months
- Treatment of in-stent restenosis in the SFA is associated with a high failure rate
- Multiple modalities have been advocated as treatment, though there exists very little data investigating the treatment of ISR in the femoro-popliteal arteries
- IR-192 brachytherapy has shown promise in the prophylaxis of restenosis during primary treatment and by extension is advocated for treatment of ISR; its widespread use is limited by logistical difficulties in administering gamma radiation to long segments
- Other modalities for either the primary prevention of restenosis or its subsequent treatment (e.g., cryoplasty, laser atherectomy) have not been thoroughly evaluated in large controlled trials
- Early surveillance is critical to treat restenosis before it becomes a diffuse process

Thrombosis: Special Considerations

- Can occur either *de novo* or in the setting of previous stent placement
- Angiographically apparent as occlusion or near-occlusion with multiple filling defects; often very easy to traverse with a guidewire (as opposed to a calcific, stenotic occlusion)
- Catheter-based thrombolysis (with or without associated Angiojet rheolytic thrombectomy) can be very helpful
  - Angiojet with "pulse-spray" thrombolysis and subsequent thrombectomy is often utilized with large thrombotic burden
  - 10 mg of r-tPA is "sprayed" throughout the thrombosed vessel via the Angiojet catheter and allowed to dwell for 15 min prior to thrombectomy

  - Often, residual thrombus is present; an indwelling infusion catheter may be placed and r-tPA infused (typically 1 mg/h) for 12–18 h
  - Re-look angiography and intervention if necessary is typically performed the following day

Post-procedure Management and Follow Up

- Baseline ankle-brachial index
- Baseline duplex ultrasonography
- Follow-up visits with repeat ultrasonography and ABI at 6 months and 12 months post-procedure, then yearly thereafter for at least 2 years
  - Consider re-look angiography for ≥75% in-stent restenosis, reduction in ABI, or worrisome signs/symptoms
- Much of the data involving surveillance of balloon angioplasty and stents is extrapolated from experiences with surgical lower extremity bypass grafts
- The goal of surveillance and re-look angiography (if indicated) is assisted patency of previous interventions

Bibliography

1. ACC/AHA Guidelines for the Management of Patients with Peripheral Arterial Disease. J Am Coll Cardiol 2006;47(6): 1239–1312.
   → *ACC/AHA consensus document on the management of all aspects of peripheral arterial disease, including but not limited to options for revascularization.*
2. TASC II Document on the Management of Peripheral Arterial Disease. J Vasc Surg 2007;45 Supp S:S5-67.
   → *Intra-society consensus document on PAD with particular emphasis on methods of revascularization.*
3. Angioplasty vs. stenting for superficial femoral artery lesions. Cochrane Database of Systematic Reviews 2009:2.
   → *A thorough, evidenced-based review of the major trials examining stenting and PTA in the femoropopliteal system.*

4. Restenosis After Lower Extremity Interventions: Current Status and Future Directions. J Endovasc Ther 2009;16(Suppl I): 1170–1182.

→ *Excellent review of the ongoing problem of restenosis after percutaneous SFA interventions and possible treatment modalities.*

5. Endovascular Therapy for Superficial Femoral Arterial Disease. *In:* Manual of Peripheral Vascular Intervention. pp 225–251.

→ *An excellent in-depth chapter on the anatomy and techniques of SFA interventions.*

Chapter 18
Tibial Interventions

Warren J. Gasper, Christopher D. Owens, and Charles M. Eichler

Etiology

Atherosclerosis (most common), thromboangiitis obliterans (Buerger's disease), popliteal aneurysm, peripheral emboli, fibromuscular dysplasia, Takayasu's disease, arteritis, trauma, radiation injury, pseudoxanthoma elasticum.

Background

Tibial occlusions are more commonly associated with limb-threatening ischemia because of a lack of collaterals. Isolated tibial vessel occlusion is a pattern of disease frequently seen in patients with diabetes mellitus.

W.J. Gasper • C.D. Owens (✉)
Division of Endovascular and Vascular Surgery, Department of Surgery, University of California – San Francisco, San Francisco, CA, USA
e-mail: warren.gasper@ucsf.edu; christopher.owens@ucsfmedctr.org

C.M. Eichler
Division of Vascular Surgery, Department of Surgery, University of California – San Francisco, San Francisco, CA, USA
e-mail: charles.eichler@ucsfmedctr.org

C.D. Owens and Y. Yeghiazarians (eds.), *Handbook of Endovascular Peripheral Interventions*, DOI 10.1007/978-1-4614-0839-0_18,

Prevalence

PAD increases with age: the estimated prevalence is 1% among 40–44-year olds rising to approximately 7% of 70–74-year olds. The progression to critical limb ischemia (CLI) is uncommon, with an estimated annual incidence of 500–1,000 new cases per million in the general population.

Clinical Presentation

- Non-palpable pedal (dorsalis pedis and posterior tibial) pulses
- ABI < 0.9
- Intermittent claudication
- Ischemic rest pain
- Tissue loss – gangrenous toe(s) or non-healing ischemic ulcer (Table 18.1)

TABLE 18.1 Rutherford's classification of chronic limb ischemia (From Norgren et al. Journal of Vascular Surgery, 2007)

Grade	Category	Clinical description	Objective criteria
0	0	Asymptomatic	Normal treadmill test
I	1	Mild claudication	Complete treadmill, but AP >50 mmHg and at least 20 mmHg lower than at baseline
I	2	Moderate claudication	Between categories 1 and 3
I	3	Severe claudication	Cannot complete treadmill test; AP <50 mmHg after treadmill test
II[a]	4	Ischemic rest pain	Resting AP <40 mmHg, TP <30 mmHg

TABLE 18.1 (continued)

Grade	Category	Clinical description	Objective criteria
III[a]	5	Minor tissue loss	Resting AP <60 mmHg, TP <40 mmHg
III[a]	6	Major tissue loss	Resting AP <60 mmHg, TP <40 mmHg

Treadmill test 5 min. at 2 miles/h on a 12% incline. *AP* ankle pressure, *TP* toe pressure *Minor tissue loss* non-healing ulcer or focal gangrene with diffuse pedal ischemia, *Major tissue loss* extending above transmetatarsal level or foot no longer salvageable
[a]Grade II and III represent critical limb ischemia

Clinical Pointer: Lower Extremity Bypass Surgery Versus Endovascular Therapy for Tibial Disease

- At this point, we consider lower extremity bypass to be the standard of care for patients with peripheral arterial disease (PAD) affecting the tibial arteries.
- We reserve angioplasty of the tibial arteries for patients with critical limb ischemia who are unable to have a bypass due to a lack of appropriate target vessel, lack of vein for conduit, or patients who have a prohibitive operative risk.
- This opinion is based on a number of studies which have shown better long-term results for bypass, including the Bypass versus Angioplasty in Severe Ischaemia of the Leg (BASIL) trial, which remains the only randomized-controlled trial comparing lower extremity bypass versus endovascular therapy (angioplasty) for initial revascularization.
- There have been no trials that demonstrate stents are superior to balloon angioplasty. Therefore, we primarily treat with PTA and reserve stents for severe dissections or residual stenosis after PTA.

Clinical Pointer: Characteristics of Ulcers

- *Arterial (ischemic)*: typically painful with a pale, dry base; commonly on toes, heel, or ankle.
- *Venous*: mildly painful with an irregular border and pink, moist base; commonly on medial malleolus in the setting of venous insufficiency changes, e.g., edema, hemosiderin skin deposits.
- *Neuropathic*: typically not painful with a surrounding callous and often deep infection; commonly located on the plantar surface of the foot (weight-bearing surface), often with an underlying bony abnormality.
- *Mixed*: both venous and neuropathic ulcers can occur in the setting of arterial insufficiency and therefore revascularization may be necessary.

Evaluation

Vascular Lab

- *Ankle-brachial index (ABI)*: Measure the blood pressure in the dorsalis pedis (DP) and posterior tibial (PT) arteries with a blood pressure cuff at the ankle. Divide the highest ankle pressure by the highest blood pressure in the brachial artery (left or right arm).
  - An ABI <0.9 is diagnostic of PAD.
    - >1.3 – non-compressible
    - 1–1.29 – normal
    - 0.91–0.99 – borderline
    - 0.41–0.9 – mild to moderate PAD
    - <0.4 – severe PAD
  - Patients with severely calcified arteries (i.e., diabetics) may have non-compressible arteries (ankle pressure >250 mmHg or ABI > 1.3), in which case further testing (toe-brachial index, pulse volume recordings) is necessary.

- *Toe-brachial index (TBI)*: Special blood pressure cuff is placed on the first or second toe. Measure the toe blood pressure and divide by the highest blood pressure in the brachial artery (left or right arm).
  - Useful for patients with severely calcified, non-compressible vessels.
  - A TBI < 0.7 is diagnostic of PAD.

Duplex Ultrasound

- *Advantages*: non-invasive; no radiation exposure; can identify and characterize the extent of arterial lesions.
- *Disadvantages*: operator-dependent; imaging of the entire leg can be very time consuming; visualization of the tibial and crural arteries can be difficult, especially if the arteries are heavily calcified.

Magnetic Resonance Angiography (MRA)

- *Advantages*: non-invasive, no radiation exposure; no iodinated contrast exposure; no significant calcium artifact makes visualizing the lumen of small calcified vessels (i.e., tibials) easier.
- *Disadvantages*: no artifact from calcium make visualizing plaques difficult; stent artifacts cause a flow "drop-out"; gadolinium-based contrast associated with nephrogenic systemic fibrosis in patients with renal insufficiency; MRI contraindications (pacemakers, defibrillators, cochlear implants, and spinal cord stimulators); may not be tolerated by claustrophobic patients.

Computed Tomographic Angiography (CTA)

- *Advantages*: non-invasive; rapid exam; able to assess plaque morphology.

- *Disadvantages*: radiation exposure; iodinated-contrast exposure; calcium can cause a "blooming" artifact that makes assessing the lumen of small vessels (i.e., tibials) difficult.

Arteriography

- *Advantages*: "gold standard" for the diagnosis of PAD.
- *Disadvantages*: radiation exposure; iodinated contrast exposure; invasive technique.

Treatment

- Medical treatment of risk factors (antiplatelet therapy, smoking cessation, anti-hypertension therapy, statin therapy, blood glucose control)
- Invasive treatment is only reserved for critical limb ischemia/limb salvage therapy, not claudication. Bad result can convert claudication to a limb salvage emergency.
- "Limb salvage" procedure is either an amputation of part of the foot or surgical debridement after revascularization with the aim of preserving some or all of the foot. Typically the procedure is performed at least 3 days after revascularization to allow for demarcation to occur.
- Broad-spectrum antibiotics before and after the intervention are required in the setting of tissue loss

How I Do It

Access

- Antegrade puncture – easiest if pre-procedure imaging shows a patent SFA and popliteal artery or the patient has palpable popliteal pulse (see Fig. 18.1).
  - Place a long (55–90 cm) 5 or 6 Fr sheath (see equipment list) down to the distal popliteal artery. Extra sheath length extending from groin creates working space away from C-arm.

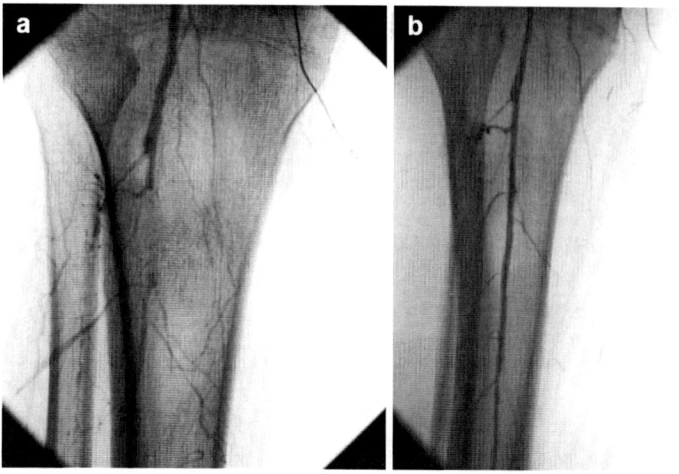

FIGURE 18.1 A 74-year-old man with right leg critical limb ischemia (<1/2 block claudication, a hallux blister, ABI of 0.33). A pre-operative angiogram showed a widely patent right common and external iliac arteries, an occluded SFA with reconstitution of the popliteal artery at the adductor canal via collaterals from the profunda femoris. Distally, however, the anterior tibial and tibioperoneal trunk arteries were occluded with distal reconstitution of the peroneal artery that fed the dorsalis pedis and posterior tibial arteries at foot. (**a**) Intraoperative angiogram after performing a right femoral to popliteal bypass. There is a chronic total occlusion of the anterior tibial artery and tibioperoneal trunk with distal reconstitution of the peroneal artery. (**b**) Successful crossing and angioplasty of the tibioperoneal trunk and peroneal artery with run-off to foot. Post-operatively, the patient's toe ulcer healed and his exercise tolerance increased to >8 blocks. (**c**) Surveillance ultrasound of the peroneal artery showing a PSV of 108 cm/s. Approximately 10 months after the initial intervention, the patient had a surveillance ultrasound and MRA that suggested a stenosis at the tibioperoneal trunk. (**d**) An angiogram confirmed a patent bypass graft and popliteal artery with two stenoses of the proximal peroneal artery (*arrowheads*). (**e**) Successful angioplasty of the stenoses (*arrowheads*)

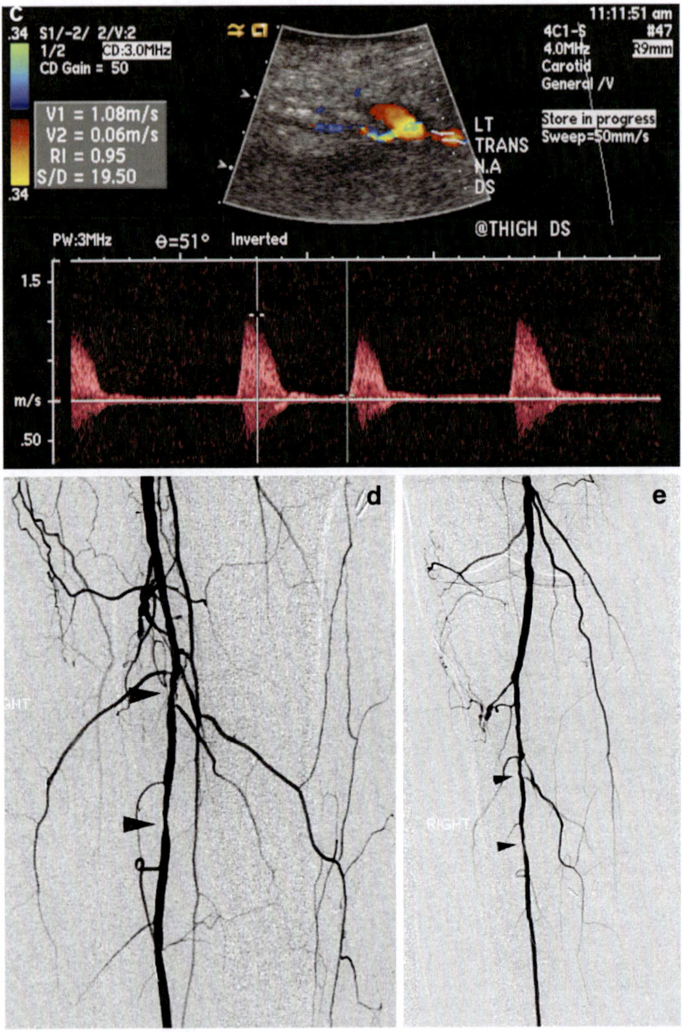

FIGURE 18.1 (continued)

  - The antegrade approach eliminates the up-and-over forces. In addition, even if treatment is all the way onto foot, there will never be problems with device length.
- Up-and-over (contralateral groin) – required when body habitus will not allow antegrade or treating concomitant SFA or popliteal disease.
  - Place a long (90 cm) 5 or 6 Fr sheath (see equipment list) down to the contralateral popliteal.
- Retrograde CTO crossing (see Fig. 18.2)
  - Patient supine, access foot or tibial vessel either with ultrasound, seeing calcification on flouro, or flouro fade/subtraction roadmapping.
  - 0.014 or 0.018-in. wire (see equipment list) through micropuncture catheter.
  - Snare from sheath placed as distal as possible.
  - Convert to wire from above and remove micropuncture catheter in distal artery to prevent injury to the foot vessel.

Tibial Stenosis and Occlusions

- Cross lesion intraluminal, do not go subintimal.
- Anticoagulate with heparin to an activated clotting time (ACT) >300 s.
- Get sheath close to tibial – both for support and better angiography.
- Use 0.035-in. Glidewire and 4 Fr angled glide catheter to get into tibials.
- Switch to 0.014-in. wire and catheter (see equipment list) for lesion crossing.
- After crossing, look for blood return in catheter and contrast injection to confirm position in artery distal to lesion.
- Plain old balloon angioplasty (POBA) if possible – use 0.014-in. base balloons (see equipment list). Try to completely treat

with single balloon – slow, steady inflation and keep inflated for 1–1.5 min.

- Stent only for a bad dissection or marked residual stenosis following PTA. Use a 4-mm self-expanding stent (see equipment list) and post dilate to 3 mm (see Fig. 18.3)
- Occlusions are very challenging, especially if the lesion is >5 cm in length. Use the telescoping technique for extra support.

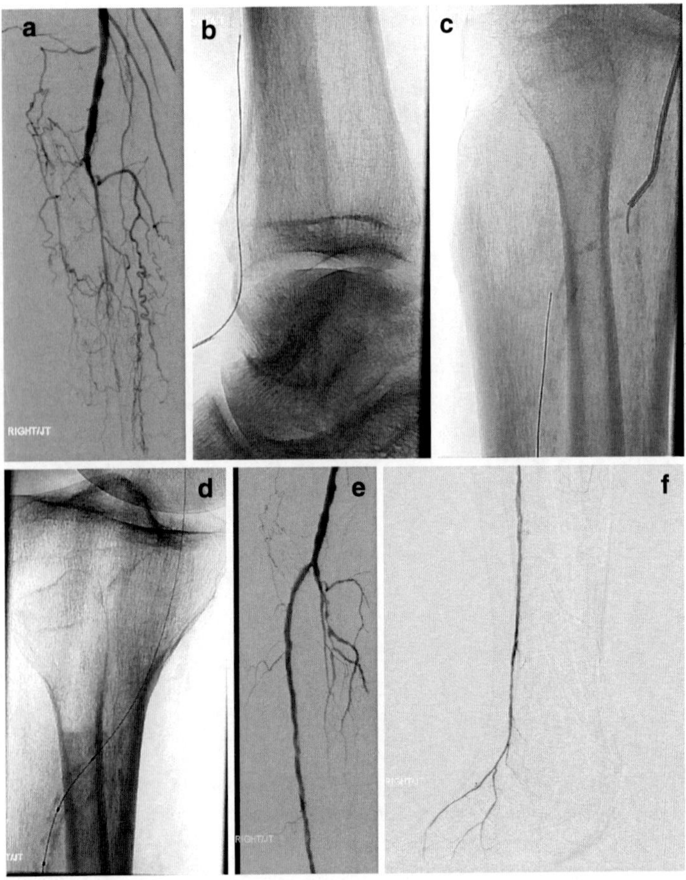

Tips of the Trade

- For added support through long tibial occlusions, use the telescoping technique:
  - Position the sheath in the distal popliteal artery.
  - Support your wire with a 0.014-in./150 cm Quick-Cross catheter inside a 0.035-in./135 cm Quick-Cross catheter.
  - Cross the lesion with 0.014-in. wire.
  - These telescoping catheters, combined with the sheath in popliteal artery, provide maximum pushability through tight arteries.
- An alternative for total occlusions is the Crosser (FlowCardia), which uses high frequency mechanical vibration to facilitate passage of the guidewire.

FIGURE 18.2 A 65-year-old kidney and liver transplant recipient with right leg critical limb ischemia (three gangrenous toes, foot cellulitis, ABI 0.58). (**a**) Angiogram via antegrade access of the right common femoral artery demonstrated patent femoral and popliteal arteries with occlusion of the infrapopliteal arteries. Distally, there was filling of the calcified dorsalis pedis in the foot. (**b**) The dorsalis pedis was accessed under ultrasound guidance with a 21-gauge Micropuncture needle and 0.018-in. wire. (**c**) A 0.014-in. Grand Slam wire was used to attempt a retrograde crossing of the anterior tibial artery. (**d**) Ultimately, the occlusion was crossed antegrade in a subintimal plane with assistance from the retrograde catheter. Intraluminal access was established from the right groin to the dorsalis pedal artery. (**e** and **f**) Completion angiogram after a successful subintimal angioplasty was performed the length of the anterior tibial artery with return of flow to the dorsalis pedis artery. Four days later the patient was taken to the operating room for a limb-salvage procedure which required amputations of the three gangrenous toes. After the procedure, the patient had a triphasic pulse in the dorsalis pedis artery and the amputation sites healed with local wound care and antibiotics

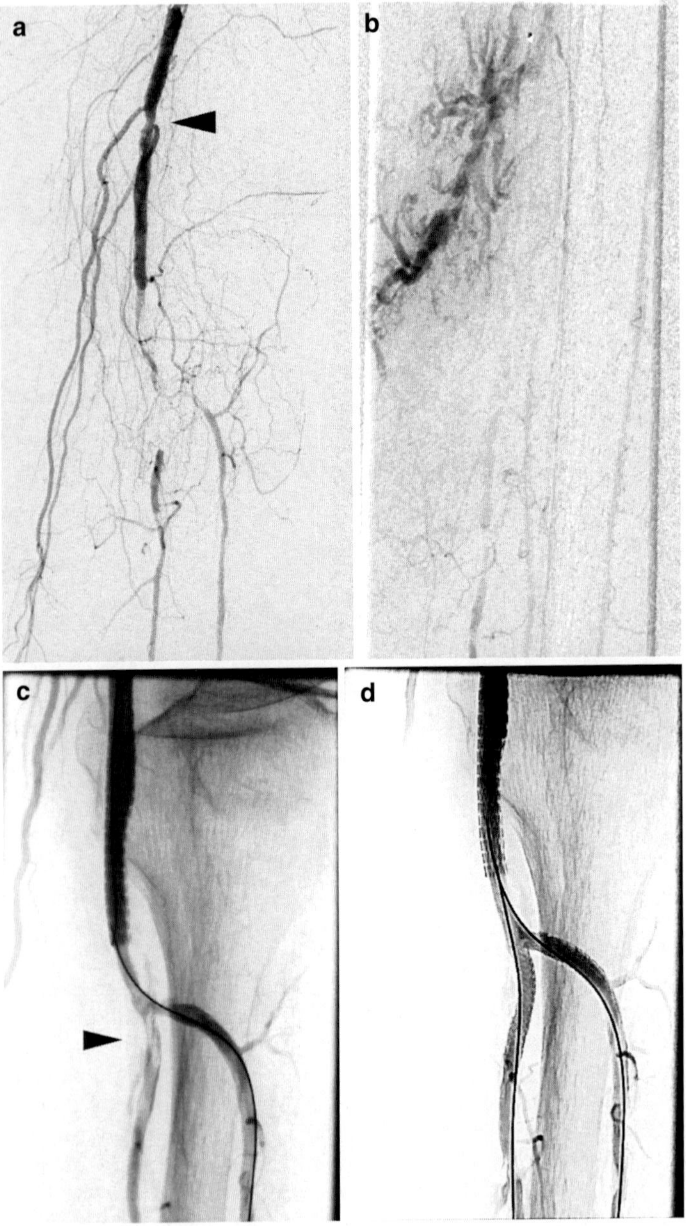
a
b
c
d

Potential Pitfalls

- Do not intervene on the tibial arteries unless critical limb ischemia is present. A bad result can convert claudication to a limb salvage emergency.
- In the event of extravasation, watch for tightness in the calf and signs of possible compartment syndrome. If suspected, compartment pressures should be assessed and the patient evaluated for four-compartment fasciotomy.

Tips of the Trade

- Tibial arteries are typically 2–4 mm in diameter.
- Local nitroglycerin (50–200 mcg) can be infused into a tibial artery both prior to an intervention as well as after in case of vasospasm (dilute 500 mcg NTG in 10 mL normal saline, infuse 1–4 mL). Must infuse directly into the appropriate artery, not into the sheath (proximal).

FIGURE 18.3 An 81-year-old diabetic woman with left leg critical limb ischemia (<1 block claudication, rest pain, ABI 0.59, toe brachial index of 0.28). (**a**) Angiogram showed widely patent iliac arteries, superficial and deep femoral arteries on the left. There was a 75% stenosis of the popliteal artery (*arrowhead*) and complete occlusion of the distal popliteal, anterior tibial, and tibioperoneal trunk with distal reconstitution of the anterior tibial and peroneal arteries. (**b**) Small amount of extravasation after an attempt to cross the occlusion to the peroneal artery. The calf remained soft and the extravasation was self-limited. (**c**) Successful crossing of the anterior tibial and peroneal occlusions. After angioplasty of the popliteal artery, anterior tibial, and tibioperoneal lesions, there was significant recoil in the popliteal artery stenosis and spiral dissections in the popliteal arteries and down the anterior tibial and peroneal arteries (*arrowhead*). (**d**) Successful stenting of the distal popliteal artery as well as stenting of the anterior tibial and peroneal arteries with drug-eluting stents using a kissing-stent technique. Post-operatively the patient had a palpable dorsalis pedis pulse, her exercise tolerance increased to >3 blocks and ABI increased to 0.86

Follow-Up

- Pre-treat with aspirin 325 mg.
- We do not pre-treat with clopidogrel (Plavix) because of the risk of excessive intraoperative bleeding if the patient requires an open bypass. If the intervention is successful, load the patient with clopidogrel 300 mg immediately post-op. Keep on dual anti-platelet therapy (clopidogrel 75 mg/day and aspirin 81 mg/day) for 1 month and then switch to aspirin 325 mg/day indefinitely.
- Surveillance ultrasounds at 1, 3, 6, 9, and 12 months then every 6–12 months thereafter.
- Consider repeat arteriography for increasing peak systolic velocities on ultrasound indicating a >50% restenosis (PSV >200 cm/s), recurrent tissue loss or symptoms. A drop in ABI of 0.2 or greater may also indicate restenosis but should correlate with an increase in duplex ultrasound velocity.
- MRA (or CTA) may help establish the presence of a stenosis before proceeding with angiography.

Equipment List

Sheaths

- 5 or 6 Fr long sheath (55–90 cm, long enough to reach the distal popliteal)
- Cook Flexor – Raabe, Shuttle Select
- Terumo Pinnacle Destination

Catheters

- 4 Fr angled catheters to engage the tibial vessel
- Straight support catheters once the vessel is engaged
- –0.035 and 0.014-in. Quick-Cross catheter (Spectranetics)

Guidewires

- For large (2.5–3 mm) tibial vessels
- –0.035-in. Glidewire (Terumo) (with a 0.035-in. Quick-Cross catheter)
- For smaller vessels
- –0.014-in. Asahi wire (Prowater, Confianza, Grand Slam, or Miracle Bros) (Abbott)
- Occasionally we try a slightly heavier wire
- –0.018-in. Platinum Plus (Boston Scientific) or 0.025-in. Glidewire (Terumo)
- Can also use the Crosser system (FlowCardia)

Balloons

- Use long true 0.014-in. balloons (120–200 cm) for easy passage and reduced risk of dissection. Use a slow and long (1–1.5 min) inflation time
- –0.014-in. Nanocross (ev3) or Amphirion (Invatec/Medtronic)

Stents

- Rarely used – only if there is a significant dissection or vessel recoil.
- No evidence that drug-eluting stents are better than bare metal.
- Use self-expanding stents: balloon expand at origin, self-expand for the rest of the artery
- 4 mm Zilver (Cook Medical)

Bibliography

Bradbury A W, Adam D J, Bell J, Forbes J F, Fowkes F G, et al. Bypass versus Angioplasty in Severe Ischaemia of the Leg (BASIL) trial: An intention-to-treat analysis of amputation-free and overall survival in patients randomized to a bypass surgery-first or a balloon angioplasty-first revascularization strategy. Journal of Vascular Surgery. 2010;51(5 Suppl):5-17S.

→ *The only randomized-controlled trial to compare surgical bypass versus balloon angioplasty revascularization strategies for severe limb ischemia due to infrainguinal disease (one third of the cohort had infrapopliteal disease). This final intention-to-treat analysis showed that there was no difference in amputation-free survival (AFS) or overall survival (OS) between interventions, but for patients who survived 2 years after randomization, there was a significant improvement in AFS and OS in the bypass-first group.*

Norgren L, Hiatt W R, Dormandy J A, Nehler M R, Harris K A, et al. Inter-Society Consensus for the Management of Peripheral Arterial Disease (TASC II). Journal of vascular surgery. 2007;45 Suppl S:S5-67.

→ *Trans-Atlantic Inter-Society Consensus statement (TASC II) on the diagnosis and management of peripheral arterial disease (PAD). Includes a comprehensive review of the natural history, diagnosis, and treatment of PAD.*

Romiti M, Albers M, Brochado-Neto F C, Durazzo A E, Pereira C A, et al. Meta-analysis of infrapopliteal angioplasty for chronic critical limb ischemia. Journal of Vascular Surgery. 2008;47(5):975–981.

→ *A meta-analysis of 30 studies assessing the outcomes after infrapopliteal angioplasty. Compared with the results of a similar meta-analysis of surgical bypass, the primary and secondary patency rates of angioplasty are lower, although limb-salvage rates are similar.*

Randon C, Jacobs B, De Ryck F, & Vermassen F. Angioplasty or primary stenting for infrapopliteal lesions: results of a prospective randomized trial. Cardiovascular and Interventional Radiology. 2010;33(2):260–9.

→ *A small (35 patients, 38 limbs) randomized, single-centered trial comparing angioplasty and bare metal stent placement of the tibial vessels for critical limb ischemia. Although the trial is small and may not be sufficiently powered, at 1 year there was no difference in patency rates, limb salvage, or survival for PTA vs. stent.*

Chapter 19
Venous Interventions for Thrombo-occlusive Disease

Robert K. Kerlan Jr. and Jeanne M. LaBerge

Overview

Venous intervention is a broad term covering a number of procedures used to treat a variety of disorders. In order to review venous interventions in an organized fashion the procedures will be separated into four groups: iliofemoral thrombosis, subclavian thrombosis, central venous obstruction, and vena cava filters.

Iliofemoral Thrombosis

Etiology

Multiple causes for iliofemoral thrombosis have been identified. These causes include extrinsic compression of the left common iliac vein by the right common iliac artery (May-Thurner Syndrome), external venous compression by

R.K. Kerlan Jr.(✉) • J.M. LaBerge
Interventional Radiology Division, Department of Radiology, University of California – San Francisco, San Francisco, CA, USA
e-mail: robert.kerlan@ucsf.edu; jeanne.laberge@ucsf.edu

C.D. Owens and Y. Yeghiazarians (eds.), *Handbook of Endovascular Peripheral Interventions*, DOI 10.1007/978-1-4614-0839-0_19,

retroperitoneal adenopathy, hypercoaguable states (factor V Leyden, anti-phospholipid antibody, oral contraceptives, malignancy, etc.), immobility, and thrombophilia. However, a substantial number of cases are idiopathic.

Background

The development of phlebothrombosis in the calf may propagate to involve the femoral and iliac venous systems. Progression of calf thromboses is more common in patients who are immobile or who have a hypercoagulable state.

Prevalence

Incidence of lower extremity deep venous thrombosis (DVT) has been estimated to approach 250,000 cases per year in the USA.

Clinical Presentations/Clues

- Unilateral calf and thigh edema
- Discoloration in severe cases
- Pain, improved with elevation
- Previous history of DVT

Clinical Pointers: Progression of Acute DVT to Chronic Venous Insufficiency

- Chronic venous insufficiency may develop in up to 75% of patients with iliofemoral DVT due to destruction of the valves.
- Early aggressive treatment is indicated to prevent chronic venous insufficiency.

Diagnosis

Ultrasound

- Ultrasound with graded compression is the primary test for infrainguinal thrombus
  - Acute thrombus is sonolucent and does not completely compress with the application of graded pressure.
  - Chronic thrombus is usually echogenic
- Proximal disease in the iliac vein or inferior vena cava (IVC) can be inferred from lack of respiratory variation in flow and lack of reversal of flow with the patient performing the Valsalva maneuver

Tips on Ultrasound: Acute Deep Venous Thrombosis
- Non-compressible
- Sonolucent thrombus (may not be visible)
- Vein is enlarged

Computed Tomography

- Contrast enhanced computed tomography (CT) is useful to show the extent of pelvic and abdominal thrombus.
  - Acute thrombus may completely occlude and distend the vein or have a small rim of flow peripherally.
  - Chronic thrombus is inferred from non-opacification and diminished vein size. Collateral veins are often visible.
- CT can reveal ancillary findings such as retroperitnoneal adenopathy and the presence of compression of the left common iliac vein by the right common iliac artery can be revealed.
  - Renal insufficiency is a relative contraindication for contrast-enhanced CT

Magnetic Resonance Venography

- Magnetic resonance venography (MRV) is useful to show the extent of pelvic and abdominal thrombus.

- MRV provides excellent depiction of the relationship of the left common iliac vein to the right common iliac artery.
- Since MRV does not expose patients to ionizing radiation, MRV is preferable to CT in younger patients.

- Contrast-enhanced MRV is contraindicated when the eGFR is less than 40
- The quality of the examination will be based on institutional expertise and patient factors including the ability to remain motionless.

Clinical Pointer: Should the Patient with Mildly Symptomatic Iliofemoral Thrombosis Be Simply Anticoagulated or Undergo Fibrinolytic Therapy?
In patients who have a good functional status there is a high likelihood of subsequently developing chronic venous insufficiency due to damage of the venous valves. Unless there is an underlying medical condition increasing the likelihood of a hemorrhagic complication, these patients should undergo fibrinolytic therapy.

Treatment

- Patients with acute iliofemoral DVT should be immediately anticoagulated with IV heparin.
- Subsequently, pharmacomechanical thrombectomy should be performed unless there is a contraindication to fibrinolytic therapy or the patient has a poor functional status.
- Patients with contraindications to fibrinolytic therapy (Table 19.1) should not undergo this procedure.

Procedure

- Under conscious sedation, the patient is placed prone on the angiographic table, and a patent segment of popliteal vein is punctured under real-time ultrasound guidance

TABLE 19.1 Contraindications to fibrinolytic therapy

• Absolute
Acute stroke
Active significant bleeding
CNS aneurysm or AVM
Recent brain or spinal cord surgery
• Relative
History of stroke
CNS tumor or metastases
History of significant GI bleeding
Uncontrolled hypertension
Advanced age (>80)
Recent thoracic, abdominal, or pelvic surgery

with a micropuncture (21-gauge) needle. A 0.018 in. guidewire is advanced into the vein with fluoroscopic confirmation of appropriate positioning.

- Using the conversion system, a 0.035 in. wire is placed.
- The conversion system is removed and a short 6-F sheath inserted over the 0.035 in. guidewire.
- A venogram is performed to confirm the extent of the thrombosis.
- A 5-F catheter is inserted and manipulated through the thrombus until a patent vessel is reached, usually at the junction of the common iliac vein and inferior vena cava. Either a straight catheter or curved catheter such as a Berenstein or Kumpe can be used. The operator should use the catheter that works best in their hands!
- After successful entry into the IVC, an inferior vena cavogram is performed.
- A decision is then made to perform a lytic infusion versus pharmacomechanical thrombolysis
  - If a simple infusion of fibrinolytic agent is desired, an infusion catheter is selected with an infusion length to

match the length of the thrombosed segment. The catheter is connected to an infusion pump and the agent is infused at the desired rate. The sheath is connected to a heparin drip. Both the catheter and sheath are secured and a sterile dressing is applied. The patient is then transferred to a continuously monitored care unit while the infusion proceeds. Arrangements are made for the patient to return in approximately 24 h for a follow-up venogram.

- Because of the time involved with infusion therapy alone, most operators elect to use a form of pharmacomechanical thrombolysis. Several devices are available for this purpose.
  - The Angiojet thrombectomy catheter (Medrad Interventional/Possis) is a rheolytic device that simultaneously uses high-power jets to macerate clot while aspirating clot debris through the central channel of the catheter. This catheter needs to be connected to a calibrated high-power pump for infusion of saline to operate. If a fibrinolytic agent is added to the saline, the efficiency of clot removal is enhanced. If the outflow is occluded, the clot can be effectively laced with a substantial amount of fibrinolytic agent.
  - The Trellis Catheter (Bacchus Medical) is a hybrid mechanical-aspirating dual balloon device designed for regional fibrinolytic infusion. The two balloons are separated by a variable distance that is selected to match the length of vessel to be treated. By isolating the region of fibrinolytic infusion, the systemic effects of the pharmaceutical agent can be reduced. Between the balloons the catheter can be angulated and rotated to macerate the clot.
  - The Trerotola device (Arrow Medical) is a mechanical thrombectomy catheter with a rotating basket that spins at relatively high velocity when attached to the disposable handle motor. There is extensive experience using this device in declotting dialysis access grafts. Reports of its safety in the native venous system are

limited; however, it does appear to be safe in limited applications. In treating iliofemoral DVT, this device should be used in conjunction with fibrinolytic therapy.

- Following mechanical thrombectomy, the venogram should be repeated through the insertion sheath to identify any obstructing lesions.
  - Obstructing lesions in the femoral venous system should be dilated with an angioplasty balloon.
  - Obstructing lesions within the iliac venous system should be dilated. These lesions are usually recalcitrant to simple balloon angioplasty and self-expanding stents are usually required to achieve a durable result (Fig. 19.1a–d).
- When satisfactory flow has been re-established, the sheath should be removed and the patient transitioned to oral anticoagulation for a minimum of 6 months.

Iliofemoral Thrombosis: How I Do It

- When patients are to undergo rheolytic thrombectomy, pre-hydration with IV saline and bicarbonate is performed.
- Venous access is achieved with the patient in the prone position. A careful real-time ultrasound examination of the tibial, sural, and popliteal vein of the involved extremity is performed. The preferable entry point is into a sural vein that drains into a patent segment of popliteal vein, as this minimizes traversing muscular tissue, diminishes damage to the popliteal vein, and avoids violating the nerves that are present adjacent to the popliteal vein. The vein is punctured with a 21-gauge echotip micropuncture needle using real-time ultrasound guidance. A 0.018 nitinol guidewire is advanced through the needle and successful entry is confirmed with ultrasound and fluoroscopy. The needle is removed leaving the guidewire in place and the conversion system is advanced over the guidewire. The guidewire and inner portion of the conversion system are removed. Two to 3 ccs of low-osmolar

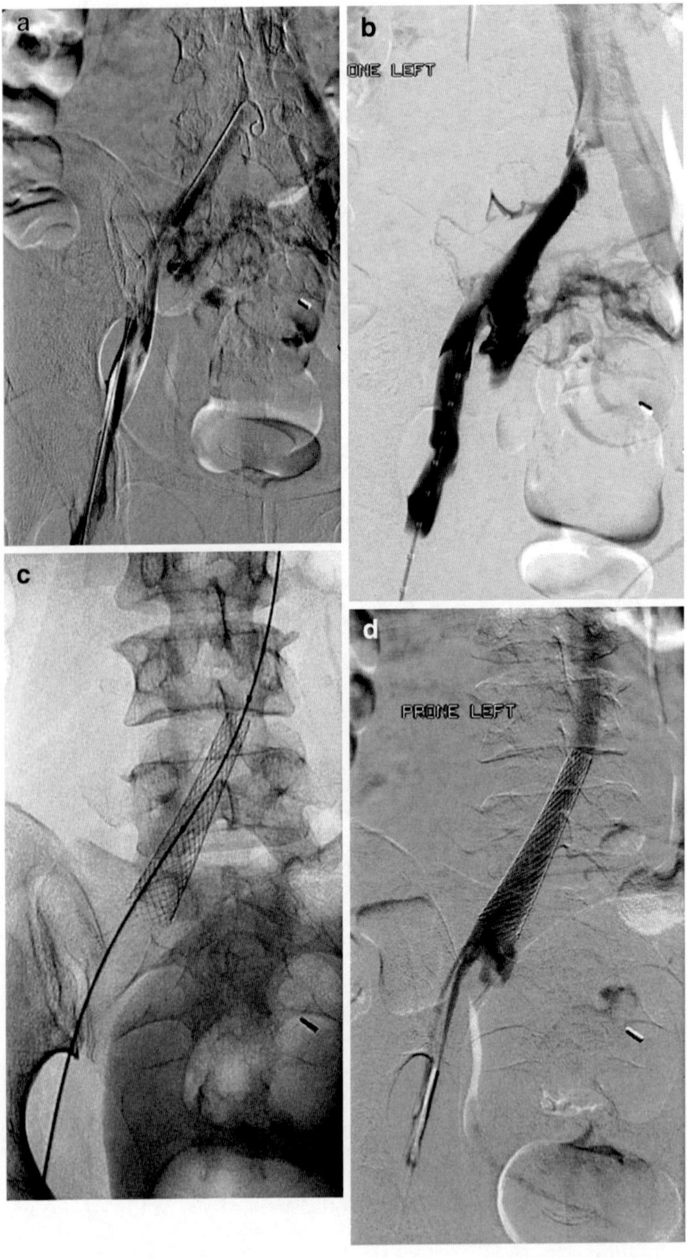
a
b
ONE LEFT
c
d
PRONE LEFT

FIGURE 19.1 A 36-year-old woman presented with massive left leg swelling secondary to iliofemoral thrombosis caused by compression of the left common iliac vein by the right common iliac artery (May-Thurner). (**a**) With the patient in a prone position, a guidewire has been advanced from the popliteal vein. Contrast injection confirms thrombus in the left iliac and femoral veins. (**b**) Following pharmacomechanical thrombolysis and overnight fibrinolytic infusion, the thrombus has been lysed but a high-grade stenosis of the medial left common iliac vein is present. (**c**) A 16-mm diameter, 60-mm length Wallstent (Boston Scientific) is deployed across the area of narrowing. (**d**) Venography following deployment of the stent confirms a widely patent lumen

contrast are injected to reconfirm appropriate entry. A LLT 15-J guidewire is inserted. The outer portion of the conversion system is removed and a short 6-F sheath is placed (Trerotola sheath, Arrow Medical).

- A venogram is then performed through the sheath to delineate the extent of thrombosis and assess for the presence of a duplicated femoral venous system.
- A 100-cm length Berenstein catheter (Cook) with angled tip hydrophilic guidewire (Terumo, Japan) is placed through the sheath. Under fluoroscopic guidance the catheter and guidewire are manipulated through the femoral and iliac veins into the inferior vena cava. The wire is removed and an inferior vena cavogram is performed through the Berenstein catheter by power injection of 20 mL of non-ionic contrast at a rate of 10 ccs/s.
- A 210-cm length 0.035 in. Rosen wire (Cook) is inserted through the catheter into the IVC and the catheter is removed.
- A 6-F Angiojet DVX thrombectomy catheter is prepped using 10 mg of tPA (Alteplase, Genentech, San Francisco, CA) into 200 cc of 0.9% normal saline.
- The Angiojet catheter is attached to the Angiojet Ultra thrombectomy pump system (Medrad Interventional/Possis) and is primed appropriately.
- The outflow of the pump is clamped.

- The catheter is advanced over the indwelling Rosen guidewire until its tip is in the most peripheral portion of the thrombus. The Possis pump is activated by the footswitch as the Angiojet catheter is slowly advanced along the total length of the thrombus to lace the clot with tPA. The guidewire is maintained motionless with its tip in the inferior vena cava.
- Wait for 20 min (by the clock!).
- The outflow of the pump is unclamped.
- The Angiojet catheter is then slowly (approximately 1 cm/s) advanced and withdrawn from distal to proximal over the entire length of the clot with the pump activated by the foot pedal.
- The total activation time of the Angiojet catheter should not exceed 10 min.
- The Angiojet catheter is removed leaving the guidewire in place.
- The venogram is repeated to assess the degree of clot clearing.
- Additional rheolytic thrombectomy is performed in areas that remain thrombosed.
- Though limited clot may be removed in a single setting using the rheolytic thrombectomy catheter, there is often residual substantial thrombus. When substantial thrombus persists, a 5-F fibrinolytic infusion catheter (Angiodynamics) is placed. The infusion length is selected to match the length of thrombus, and the patient is transferred to a monitored setting (ICU or step-down unit) for continued infusion of tPA at a rate of 1 mg/h. On the following day, the patient is returned to the angiography suite for a follow-up venogram.
- Once the iliofemoral venous system has been mostly cleared of thrombus, remaining areas of stenosis are dilated. The femoral vein usually requires balloons ranging from 8 to 12 mm in diameter. Iliac veins usually require balloons ranging in size from 12 to 16 mm in diameter. In most cases, self-expandable stents are needed to correct iliac vein stenoses. Either stainless steel Wallstents (Boston

Scientific) or nitinol Zilver stents (Cook) can be used. Wallstents are available in the 16-mm diameter to 20-mm diameter range for the larger diameter vessels. Zilver stents currently have a maximum diameter of 14 mm, so their use is limited to patients with smaller iliac veins.

- A final venogram is performed through the sheath to confirm an adequate technical result.
- The access sheath is removed and hemostasis is achieved by manual compression.

Tips of the Trade: Our Experiences

- Clearing of extensive clot burden requires a reasonably aggressive approach.
- Use tPA 10–20 mg in the saline bag used with the Angiojet thrombectomy catheter to lace the thrombus with fibrinolytic agent.
- Angioplasty balloons may be used to macerate residual resistant thrombus.
- Self-expandable stents may also be used to compress and macerate residual thrombus
- Stents are usually necessary to create durable patency in the iliac venous system.
- Stents are generally not used below the level of the lesser trochanter.
- Patients should be adequately anticoagulated before, during, and after the procedure.

Potential Pitfalls

- Prolonged activation of the rheolytic thrombectomy catheter (>10 min) has been associated with hemoglobinuria, renal failure, and death.

- Fibrinolytic therapy is safe but 1–2% of patients will have major bleeding complications
- Hematocrit and fibrinogen levels should be checked every 8–12 h
- Fibrinolytic infusion should be reduced if fibrinogen level falls below 150 mg/dL
- Fibrinolytic infusion should be stopped if fibrinogen level falls below 100 mg/dL
- Fibrinolytic therapy should be stopped and non-contrast cranial computed tomography obtained should be obtained immediately for any significant headache or neurologic change

Follow-Up After Reconstruction of Iliofemoral Thrombosis

- Intravenous bicarbonate infusion is continued for 6-h following the procedure.
- Anticoagulation therapy should be continued and the patient transitioned to coumadin. No level 1 evidence exists regarding the length of anticoagulant therapy; however, most investigators recommend a minimum of a year.
- Duplex ultrasound should be obtained the day following the procedure to serve as a baseline for future comparison.

Equipment List

This is a partial list as a variety of equipment can be successfully utilized.

Access

- 4 or 5 F micropuncture introduction system (multiple vendors)

Sheaths

- 6 F Trerotola sheath (Arrow)
- 9 to 11-F standard length sheaths for balloon and stent insertion (Cordis, Terumo, or Cook)

Catheters

- 5-F straight, 65 cm length (multiple vendors)
- 5-F Berenstein, Hockey stick, or Cobra, 65 cm length (multiple vendors)
- 5-F marking pigtail catheter, 65 cm length
- 6-F Angiojet DVX catheter (Possis)

Guidewires

- 0.035 in. angled glidewire (regular and stiff), 140 cm length (Terumo, Japan)
- 0.035 in. Rosen exchange wire, 210 cm in length (Cook).

Balloons

There are many balloon choices. Either a high-pressure or regular 0.035-in. system should be used and matched to an appropriately sized sheath. Balloons ranging in diameter from 8 to 20 mm should be available with a minimum length of 4 cm.

Stents

Self-expandable stents should be used. Diameters ranging from 10 to 20 mm should be available with a minimum length of 5 cm.

- Wallstent (Boston Scientific)
- Zilver (Cook)

Axillary-Subclavian Vein Thrombosis

Etiology

Axillary-subclavian thrombosis can be divided into two distinct groups: those related to catheters or pacemakers and those secondary to compression of the vein within the costoclavicular space. The latter has been termed "effort thrombosis" or the Paget-von Schroetter syndrome.

Background

It is critical to analyze patients with regard to the cause of axillary-subclavian vein thrombosis. Patients with catheter-induced thrombosis often have a limited life-span and multiple co-morbidities that may make aggressive treatment inappropriate. The current recommendation for patients with catheter-related subclavian thrombosis is anticoagulation, removal of the catheter, and 3–6 months of anti-coagulant therapy. Most of these patients are asymptomatic and very few develop a post-phlebitic syndrome. In contrast, the group of patients who develop "effort thrombosis" should undergo thrombolysis followed by surgical decompression of the costoclavicular space, usually requiring first rib resection. If left untreated, chronic problems with extremity edema and discomfort may develop and be associated with significant disability. This discussion will focus on "effort thrombosis."

Clinical Pointers: Axillary Subclavian Thrombosis

- Patients are usually in their early 30s and usually physically active
- Findings may be subtle without gross extremity edema

- Fatigue and "heaviness" with use of that extremity is usually reported
- Chest wall collaterals often visible

Prevalence

Incidence of axillary-subclavian "effort thrombosis" has been estimated to be 2 per 100,000 people in the USA.

Clinical Presentations/Clues

- Mean age at presentation is the early 30s
- Unilateral upper extremity and chest wall edema
- Discoloration of the arm in severe cases
- Multiple chest wall collaterals often visible in subacute cases
- Pain, improved with elevation
- Often associated with an episode of unusual activity requiring prolonged use of the involved extremity

Diagnosis

Ultrasound

- Ultrasound with graded compression for axillary thrombus
  - Acute thrombus is sonolucent and does not completely compress with the application of graded pressure.
  - Chronic thrombus usually echogenic
  - Ultrasound may not be able to visualize segments of the subclavian vein obscured by overlying clavicle
- Multiple collaterals on in surrounding tissue may be clue to occult thrombus in the subclavian vein.

Magnetic Resonance Venography

Magnetic resonance venography (MRV) is usually unnecessary as the combination of ultrasound and physical examination is generally diagnostic. If an MRV is performed, both abduction and adduction views should be obtained.

Contrast Venography

Contrast venography is the gold standard and is highly unreliable in establishing the diagnosis. However, it is also unnecessary as the diagnosis is usually made on the basis of the physical examination and ultrasound. Contrast venography should be reserved as part of the therapeutic thrombolytic procedure.

Treatment

- Patients with acute axillary-subclavian thrombosis should be immediately anticoagulated with IV heparin or enoxyparin. If IV heparin is used, infusion into the involved arm via a hand or a forearm vein is preferable.
- Subsequently, pharmacomechanical thrombectomy should be performed unless there is a contraindication to fibrinolytic therapy or the patient has a poor functional status.

Procedure

- Under conscious sedation, the patient is placed supine on the angiographic table with the upper extremity extended laterally and supported by an arm board.
- All access should be achieved with a 21-gauge micropuncture system under real-time ultrasound guidance.
  - A patent vein with direct communication to the basilic vein is selected with ultrasound.
  - If a tributary of adequate size (2–3 mm in diameter) cannot be located, puncture of the basilic vein is performed at a site peripheral to any visible thrombus.
  - If the basilic vein is too small, a brachial vein may be entered.

  - The cephalic vein should not be used because thrombus often extends peripheral to the cephalic subclavian junction.
- Using a conversion system (a 0.018 in. guidewire and coaxial catheter composed of an inner 3-F catheter and an outer 4 or 5-F catheter), a 0.035-in. wire is placed and a short 6-F sheath inserted.
- A venogram is performed to confirm the extent of the thrombosis
- The remainder of the procedure is extremely similar to the previous description of pharmacomechanical thrombolysis as described above for the treatment of ilio-femoral thrombosis.
- A 5-F catheter is inserted and manipulated through the thrombus until patent vessel is reached, usually at the junction of the subclavian vein and superior vena cava. Either a straight catheter or curved catheter such as a Berenstein or Kumpe can be used. However, due to scarring of the vein and web formation as the vein traverses the costoclavicular space, it may be more difficult to negotiate a wire into the superior vena cava.
- After successful entry into the SVC, a cavogram is performed.
- Pharmacomechanical thrombolysis is preferable in most cases because the amount of thrombus is usually less than that encountered with ilio-femoral thrombosis.
  - For fibrinolysis, a multi-side hole catheter is selected with an infusion length to match the length of the thrombosed segment. The catheter is connected to an infusion pump and the agent is infused at the desired rate. The sheath is connected to a heparin drip. Both the catheter and sheath are secured and a sterile dressing is applied. The patient is then transferred to a continuously monitored care unit while the infusion proceeds. Arrangements are made for the patient to return in approximately 24 h for a follow-up venogram.
- Because of the time involved with infusion therapy alone, most operators elect to use adjunctive mechanical thrombectomy along with pharmacologic lysis. The mechanical

thrombectomy devices were described previously. The two most common devices used are the Possis rheolytic thrombectomy catheter and the Trellis device. The Trerotola thrombectomy catheter is seldom used in the subclavian venous system but may be used in regions of focal residual clot.

- Following mechanical thrombectomy, a venogram is performed through the sheath to identify any obstructing lesions.
- It is important to recognize that surgical therapy is the treatment of choice for correction of the underlying venous obstruction causing "Effort Thrombosis." In contrast to iliofemoral thrombosis where angioplasty and stenting is often required, the underlying stenosis causing axillo-subclavian thrombosis should not be routinely stented.
- The underlying stenosis invariably occurs at the thoracic inlet and may be caused by a variety of pathologies at that location including connective tissue insertions of a thoracic rib, fibrous bands, aberrant muscular insertion from the scalenus anterior, or a congenitally small costoclavicular space. These abnormal external forces cause damage to the venous endothelium as a result of repetitive motion but due to the extrinsic compression do not respond to balloon angioplasty. Stent placement can provide temporary resolution; however, the motion of the structures in the medial subclavian vein will lead to stent occlusion in a very short period of time.
  - Because of the low durability of stents placed in the medial subclavian vein, virtually all patients with Paget-Schroetter should undergo open surgical decompression of the costoclavicular space.
  - The specific type of surgical intervention is dependent upon the encountered pathology.
  - Intraoperatively, balloon dilation of any residual stenosis is performed with a 10 or 12 mm diameter balloon.
  - Because balloon dilatation is performed intraoperatively, it is important that the patient remains anticoagulated until the time of the surgery.

Clinical Pointer: Should the Patient with Mildly Symptomatic Subclavian Thrombosis Be Simply Anticoagulated or Undergo Fibrinolytic Therapy?
In patients who have a good functional status there is a high likelihood of subsequently developing significant venous congestion due to chronic subclavian obstruction. Unless there is an underlying medical condition increasing the likelihood of a hemorrhagic complication, these patients should undergo fibrinolytic therapy.

Axillary-Subclavian Thrombosis: How I Do It

- Venous access is achieved with the patient in a supine position. The affected extremity is extended in a 90° position and supported with an arm board.
- A careful real-time ultrasound examination of the brachial and basilic veins of the involved extremity is performed. The preferable entry point is into a patent segment of basilic vein that is contiguous with the area of thrombosis.
- The vein is punctured with a 21-gauge echotip micropuncture needle using real-time ultrasound guidance. A 0.018 nitinol guidewire is advanced through the needle and successful entry is confirmed with ultrasound and fluoroscopy. The needle is removed leaving the guidewire in place and the coaxial conversion system (with an inner 3-F and outer 4 F catheter) is advanced over the guidewire. The guidewire and inner portion of the conversion system are removed. Two to 3 ccs of low-osmolar contrast are injected to confirm appropriate entry.
- A LLT 15-J guidewire is inserted. The outer portion of the conversion system is removed and a short 6-F sheath is placed (Trerotola sheath, Arrow Medical).
- A venogram is then performed through the sheath to delineate the extent of thrombosis.
- A 65 cm long Berenstein catheter with angled tip and hydrophilic guidewire (Terumo, Japan) is placed through

the sheath. Under fluoroscopic guidance, the catheter and guidewire are manipulated through the occluded axillary subclavian segment into the brachiocephalic vein. The brachiocephalic vein is invariably patent beyond the occlusion. The wire is removed and a venogram is performed through the Berenstein catheter to evaluate the appearance of the brachiocephalic vein and superior vena cava.

- A 210 cm long 0.035 in. Rosen wire is inserted through the catheter into the IVC and the catheter is removed.
- The Possis thrombectomy catheter is prepped using 10 mg of tPA (Alteplase, Genentech, San Francisco, CA) in 200 cc of 0.9% normal saline.
- A 6-F Expedior catheter (Possis) is attached to the Possis pump and is primed appropriately.
- The outflow of the Possis pump is clamped.
- The catheter is advanced over the indwelling Rosen guidewire until its tip is in the most proximal (central) portion of the thrombus. The Possis pump is activated by the footswitch as the Expedior catheter is slowly withdrawn along the total length of the thrombus to lace the clot with tPA. The guidewire is maintained motionless with its tip in the superior vena cava.
- Wait for 10 min (by the clock!).
- The outflow of the Possis pump is unclamped.
- The Expedior catheter is then slowly (approximately 1 cm/s) advanced and withdrawn over the entire length of the clot with the pump activated by the foot pedal.
- The Possis catheter is removed leaving the guidewire in place.
- The venogram is repeated to assess the degree of clot clearing.
- Additional rheolytic thrombectomy is performed in areas that remain thrombosed. The total activation time for the Possis device should not exceed 10 min.
- Although a limited amount of clot may be removed in a single setting using the rheolytic thrombectomy catheter, there is often some residual thrombus. When substantial thrombus persists, a fibrinolytic catheter is placed selected for the length of thrombus, and the patient is transferred to a monitored setting (ICU or step-down unit) for continued

infusion of tPA at a rate of 1 mg/h. On the following day, the patient is returned to the angiography suite for a follow-up venogram.

- Once the axillary subclavian venous system has been mostly cleared of thrombus the patient is systemically heparinized and arrangements are made for open surgical intervention to decompress the thoracic inlet.
  - An intra-operative venogram is performed that will usually demonstrate a residual stenosis at the thoracic inlet.
  - The stenosis is dilated with a 10–14 mm diameter balloon depending upon the size of the vein.
  - A follow-up intra-operative venogram is performed to assess the result of the balloon venoplasty.

Tips of the Trade: Our Experiences

- Use tPA 10–20 mg in the saline bag used with the Possis thrombectomy catheter to lace the thrombus with fibrinolytic agent.
- Balloon angioplasty and stents should not be used.
- The patient should undergo open surgical decompression of the thoracic inlet immediately after removal of the thrombus
- Intra-operative angioplasty should be used intra-operatively to correct residual stenosis in the vein following decompression of the thoracic inlet.

Potential Pitfalls

- If the subclavian vein is entered at the time of surgery, intraoperative angioplasty may extend the tear and lead to significant bleeding.
- Pleural effusions following surgery to correct thoracic inlet obstructions should be viewed with suspicion for bleeding as the cause of the effusion.

Follow-Up After Treatment of Axillary-Subclavian Thrombosis

- Anticoagulation therapy should be continued and the patient transitioned to coumadin. No level 1 evidence exists regarding the duration of anticoagulant therapy; however, most investigators recommend a minimum of a year.
- Duplex ultrasound should be obtained the day following the procedure to serve as a baseline for future comparison.

Equipment List

This is a partial list as a variety of equipment can be successfully utilized.

Access

- 4 or 5 F micropuncture introduction system (multiple vendors)

Sheaths

- 6 F short Trerotola sheath (Arrow)

Catheters

- 5-F straight, 65-cm length (multiple vendors)
- 5-F Berenstein, or Hockey stick (multiple vendors)
- 5-F marking pigtail catheter, 65-cm length
- 6-F Expedior rheolytic thrombectomy catheter (Possis)

Guidewires

- 0.035 in. angled glidewire (regular and stiff), 140-cm length
- 0.035 in. Rosen exchange wire, 210 cm in length (Cook).

Balloons

There are many balloon choices. Balloons ranging in diameter from 10 to 16 mm should be available with a minimum length of 4 cm. Either a high-pressure (inflation pressures up to 20–30 atm.) or regular-pressure balloon (inflation pressure up to 10 atm.) can be used. Balloons should be inserted through an appropriately sized sheath.

Central Venous Occlusions

Etiology

The term central venous occlusion refers to unilateral or bilateral occlusion of the brachiocephalic vein(s) with or without accompanying occlusion of the superior vena cava. The etiology of the occlusion may be central venous catheters, mediastinal malignancy, radiation, or sclerosing mediastinitis.

Clinical Pointers: Central Venous Obstruction Should Be Suspected in

- Dialysis patients with unilateral extremity swelling and visible chest wall venous collaterals.
- Patients with lung cancer who have facial swelling. The swelling can be severe leading to orbital edema with the eyes swollen shut.

Background

The most common cause of central venous occlusion is prior placement of long-term central venous catheters. Up to 60% of patients with long-term central venous catheters develop central venous occlusion. Most are asymptomatic and require no treatment. However, dialysis patients may develop unilateral extremity edema following placement of a hemodialysis access or graft in the involved extremity. These patients usually develop significant edema and frequently have recurrent thrombosis of their dialysis access.

The other group of symptomatic patients are those with mediastinal malignancy, usually related to metastases from lung carcinoma. When these patients develop occlusion of the superior vena cava they are often very symptomatic with facial swelling and dyspnea due to airway congestion.

Patients with fibrosing mediastinitis may also develop central venous obstruction and present with facial swelling and dyspnea. Fibrosing mediastinitis is often related to prior infection with histoplasmosis but it may be idiopathic.

Prevalence

Central venous occlusion occurs in 10–20% of hemodialysis patients. The majority of these patients have previously undergone a course of dialysis through a central venous dialysis catheter.

Clinical Presentations/Clues

- Unilateral or bilateral upper extremity edema
- Facial swelling in patients with superior vena caval obstruction
- Respiratory difficulty
- Swallowing difficulty
- Previous history of long-term central venous catheters
- History of lung cancer, particularly with prior radiation to the mediastinum

Diagnosis

Computed Tomography

- Contrast-enhanced computed tomography (CT) of the thorax generally shows compression or occlusion of the superior vena cava.

- Acute thrombus is usually not visualized.
- Multiple collateral veins are usually evident
- Enlargement of the azygos vein is often present
- Mediastinal mass or adenopathy is frequently present in patients with malignant obstruction of the superior vena cava

Magnetic Resonance Venography

- Magnetic resonance venography (MRV) of the chest can reveal findings similar to those observed with computed tomography.
- Contrast-enhanced MRV is contraindicated when the eGFR is less than 40.

Contrast Venography

- Central venous obstruction in the dialysis patient is usually diagnosed during pre-vascular access venography or dialysis fistulography.

Treatment

- Patients with central venous occlusion may be asymptomatic. Asymptomatic patients should not be treated.
- The vast majority of patients do not have fresh thrombus; therefore fibrinolytic therapy is not required.

Procedure

- All procedures are performed with conscious sedation.
- All access should be achieved with a 21-gauge micropuncture system under real-time ultrasound guidance.
  - Access for treatment of patients with brachiocephalic vein occlusion should be from the upper extremity on the involved side using either the basilic or brachial vein.

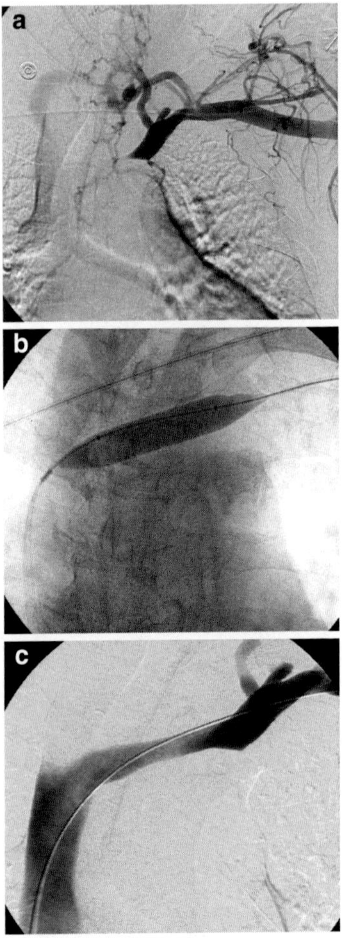

FIGURE 19.2 A 58-year-old dialysis patient developed left arm edema. Occlusion of the left brachiocephalic vein was identified during a left arm dialysis access fistulogram. (**a**) Venogram shows obstruction of left brachiocephalic ein. (**b**) A 14-mm diameter balloon is inflated in the left brachiocephalic vein. (**c**) Venography following balloon dilatation shows an excellent result

  – Access for treatment of superior vena cava occlusion should be from the right internal jugular vein. In some cases it may be necessary to obtain access from both the right internal jugular vein and the right femoral vein.
- Using the conversion system, a 0.035-in. wire is placed and a standard 6 or 7 F sheath is inserted.
- A venogram is performed to confirm the extent of the occlusion.

- A 5-F catheter is inserted and manipulated through the occlusion until patent vessel is reached. Either a straight catheter or curved catheter such as a Berenstein or Kumpe can be used.
  - Traversing chronic occlusions may be difficult. Replacing the standard vascular access sheath with a longer sheath that can reach from the access point to the area of obstruction may be extremely useful.
  - A variety of guidewires including angled-hydrophilic wires, a Rosen wire (Cook), or a Lunderquist-Ring torque guide (Cook) may be useful. Selection of the specific guidewire should be based on the specific experience of the operator.
- After successful entry into the SVC, a cavogram is performed.
- For patients with catheter-induced central occlusion, balloon dilatation of the obstructed segment should be performed with the appropriately sized balloon
  - A 4-cm long balloon with a diameter ranging from 10 to 16 mm is usually used to dilate the obstruction. The result of balloon angioplasty is evaluated by venography. A satisfactory result is obtained when there is brisk flow, minimal residual stenosis, and no evidence of collaterals.
  - If venography demonstrates a satisfactory result, the catheter and sheath are removed (Fig. 19.2a–c).
  - If the result is marginal, but improved, a stent should not be placed.
  - If the result is unacceptable, a self-expanding stent (Wallstent or Zilver stent) should be placed in the occluded segment (Fig. 19.3a–d).
- In patients with superior vena caval occlusion due to malignancy, primary stenting should be performed.
  - Self-expanding stents should be used. Either a nitinol stent (Zilver) or stainless steel stent (Wallstent) can be deployed.
  - Stent diameters usually range from 12 to 20 mm.
  - The stent length should be selected to cover the obstructed segment without significant extension into the right atrium.

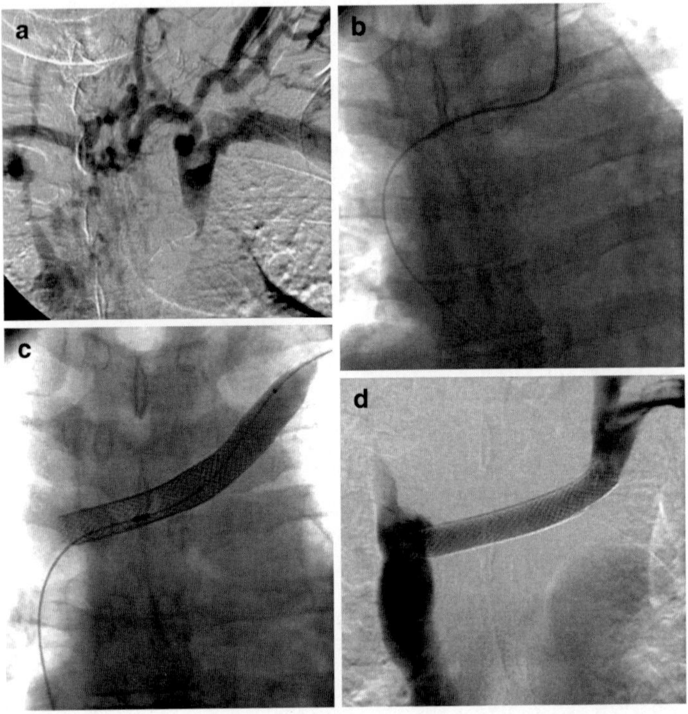

FIGURE 19.3 A 68-year-old dialysis patient presented with left arm edema. Occlusion of the left brachiocephalic vein was discovered during a left arm dialysis access fistulogram. (**a**) Venography shows obstruction of left brachiocephalic vein with multiple trans-mediastinal collaterals. (**b**) A guidewire is manipulated through the obstructed vein. (**c**) Two 12-mm diameter, 40-mm long Wallstents are deployed sequentially in the left brachiocephalic vein. (**d**) Venography following stent deployment shows an excellent result

- Following stent deployment, balloon dilatation is usually necessary to achieve the desired diameter.

Central Venous Occlusion: How I Do It

- Venous access is achieved with the patient in a supine position. The affected extremity is extended in a 90° position and supported with an arm board.

- A careful real-time ultrasound examination of the brachial and basilic veins of the involved extremity is performed. The preferable entry point for a dialysis-related brachiocephalic occlusion is through the venous limb of the dialysis access. The preferable entry point for a SVC stenosis or occlusion is the right internal jugular vein.
- The vein is punctured with a 21-gauge echotip micropuncture needle using real-time ultrasound guidance. A 0.018 nitinol guidewire is advanced through the needle and successful entry is confirmed with ultrasound and fluoroscopy. The needle is removed leaving the guidewire in place and the conversion system is advanced over the guidewire. The guidewire and inner portion of the conversion system are removed. Two to 3 cc of low-osmolar contrast are injected to reconfirm appropriate entry.
- A LLT 15-J guidewire is inserted. The outer portion of the conversion system is removed and a standard length 6-F sheath is placed (Cordis Bright – Tip).
- 5,000 U of heparin are given intravenously.
- A venogram is then performed through the sheath to delineate the extent of occlusion.
- A 65-cm length Berenstein catheter with angled tip and hydrophilic guidewire (Terumo, Japan) is placed through the sheath. Under fluoroscopic guidance the catheter and guidewire are manipulated through the occluded or stenotic segment into the patent vessel distally. Manipulation through an occluded segment of superior vena cava must be done with some care as inadvertent perforation into the pericardium could potentially lead to bleeding and pericardial tamponade. We prefer using an angled Berenstein catheter (Cook Inc., Bloomington IN) in combination with an angled glidewire (Terumo, Japan).
- Following successful traversal of the occluded segment, a 210-cm length 0.035 in. Rosen wire is inserted through the catheter into the right atrium and down the IVC. The Berenstein catheter is removed and replaced with a pigtail catheter with measuring gold markers (Cook incorporated, Bloomington, IN).
- The venogram is repeated with simultaneous injection of the sheath and pigtail catheter. Measurements are made

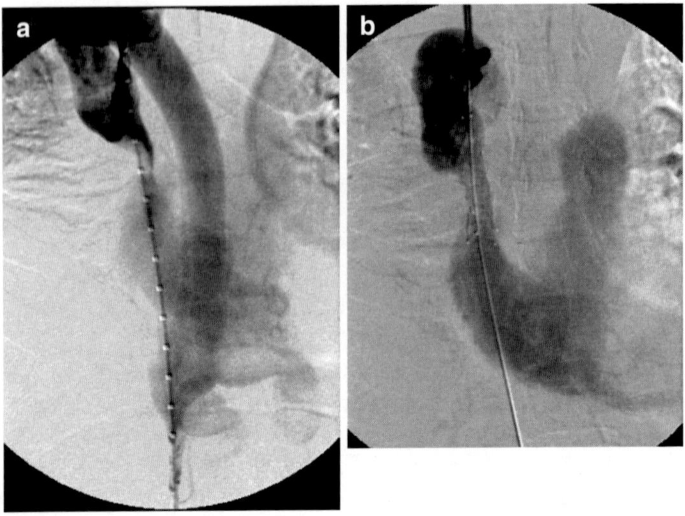

FIGURE 19.4 A 44-year-old woman presented with facial edema. She had a history of chronic central venous catheterization for the administration of total parenteral nutrition. (**a**) Superior venacavography following removal of the central line demonstrates a high-grade superior vena caval obstruction. (**b**) Superior venacavography following deployment of a 14-mm diameter Zilver stent (Cook) shows an improved luminal diameter

digitally after calibration with the marking catheter to ascertain the length of the occlusion and the diameter of the normal uninvolved SVC and adjacent brachiocephalic vein.

- For occlusions of the superior vena cava, a self-expanding Wallstent is selected with a diameter 3–5 mm larger than the measured diameter of the SVC or adjacent brachiocephalic vein. The stent length should be approximately 2 cm longer than the measured length of the venous occlusion.
- The 6-F access sheath must then be replaced with a sheath large enough to accommodate the selected stent. In most cases, a stent ranging from 14 to 20 mm in diameter and 6 cm in length are used. Such stents usually require sheaths ranging in size from 9 to 12 F, but the selected sheath must be matched to the selected stent.

- When deploying stents in the SVC (Fig. 19.4a, b), only a minimal amount of stent should extend into the right atrium. If excessive stent protrudes into the atrium, the possibility of atrial perforation and lethal pericardial tamponade exists.
- Following stent deployment, balloon dilatation is performed. The balloon should be slightly undersized in diameter to leave a minimal "hourglass appearance" that will stabilize the stent position.
- A follow-up venogram is performed through the sheath to confirm patency.
- For occlusions of the brachiocephalic veins, balloon dilatation should be attempted, and stents placed only if the result of the dilatation is inadequate.
- Following successful recanalization, the sheath is removed and hemostasis is achieved by manual compression.

Tips of the Trade: Our Experiences

- For treatment of brachiocephalic vein occlusion, access should be established in an ipsilateral arm vein. For treatment of SVC occlusion, access via the internal jugular vein is preferred.
- Use of a long sheath that extends all of the way from the venous entry to the occlusion will help facilitate traversal of the occluded segment.
- Stent placement is recommended for treatment of malignant central venous occlusion. Angioplasty alone may be sufficient to treat patients with catheter-induced occlusion.

Potential Pitfalls

- Aggressive manipulation of guidewires in the superior vena cava should be avoided due to the possibility of perforation into the pericardium

- Hypotension during the course of SVC recanalization should immediately lead to an evaluation for hemo-pericardium.

Follow-Up After Treatment of Central Venous Occlusions

- Anticoagulation therapy is usually not continued if flow is adequate.
- Routine imaging follow-up is usually not performed, as recurrence or occlusion is usually clinically apparent.

Equipment List

This is a partial list as a variety of equipment can be successfully utilized.

Access

- 4 or 5 F micropuncture introduction system (multiple vendors)

Sheaths

- 6 F short Trerotola sheath (Arrow)
- 9 to 12-F standard length sheaths for balloon and stent insertion (Cordis, Terumo, or Cook)

Catheters

- 5-F straight, 65-cm length (multiple vendors)
- 5-F Berenstein, Hockey stick, or Cobra 65-cm length (multiple vendors)
- 5-F marking pigtail catheter, 65-cm length

Guidewires

- 0.035 in. angled glidewire (regular and stiff), 140-cm length
- 0.035 in. Rosen exchange wire, 210 cm in length (Cook).

Balloons

There are many balloon choices. Either a high-pressure or regular 0.035-in. system should be used and matched to an appropriately sized sheath. Balloons ranging in diameter from 10 to 20 mm should be available with a minimum length of 4 cm.

Stents

Self-expandable stents should be used. Diameters ranging from 10 to 20 mm should be available with a minimum length of 6 cm.

- Wallstent (Boston Scientific)
- Zilver (Cook)

Vena Cava Filters

Background

Placement of inferior vena cava filters is an extremely common procedure. Placement of superior vena caval filters is seldom indicated clinically. The traditional indications for inferior vena cava filter placement are listed in Table 19.2.

Placement of superior vena cava filters is quite unusual and only performed in patients with documented pulmonary emboli from a subclavian source in patients with a contraindication to anticoagulation.

Filters can be permanent or retrievable. A retrievable filter that does not get retrieved becomes a permanent filter.

TABLE 19.2 Indications for IVC filter placement

1. Recurrent pulmonary embolization in a therapeutically anticoagulated patient
2. Free-floating thrombus within the inferior vena cava
3. A patient with an iliac, femoral, or popliteal thrombus and a contraindication to anticoagulation
4. A patient with an iliac, femoral, or popliteal thrombus and has a complication related to anticoagulation
5. A patient with an iliac, femoral, or popliteal thrombus who requires cessation of anticoagulation for a surgical procedure
6. A patient with an iliac, femoral, or popliteal thrombus who is non-compliant or has a risk of falling making long-term oral anticoagulation dangerous
7. A patient requiring prolonged immobilization (such as pelvic fracture or other significant trauma) and a contraindication to anticoagulation. In this circumstance a prophylactic IVC filter may be placed, but this therapeutic strategy is controversial

In general, retrievable filter designs are preferred over permanent filter designs because with retrievable filters, removal is always an option.

Prevalence

In the USA, 600,000–1,000,000 patients per year are treated annually for deep vein thrombosis. More than 50,000 IVC filters are placed annually in the USA.

Diagnosis

The diagnosis of deep venous thrombosis of the lower extremities is routinely made with graded compression ultrasound. The diagnosis of iliac thrombosis or free-floating thrombus within the inferior vena cava is usually made by contrast-enhanced computed tomography (CT). CT pulmonary angiography has become the most common modality to diagnose pulmonary embolism. Obviously, the initial treatment of phlebothrombosis and pulmonary embolism is anticoagulation, and filters are only placed for the indications outlined above.

Procedure

- IVC filter placement can be performed with local anesthetic alone. Conscious sedation can be used when patients who are anxious or cannot cooperate.
- IVC filters can be placed from either a jugular or femoral approach. Access should be achieved with a 21-gauge micropuncture system under real-time ultrasound guidance.
- Using the conversion system a 0.035 in. wire is placed and a standard 5-F sheath inserted.
- A wire is advanced into the inferior vena cava and a 5-F graduated measuring pigtail catheter is inserted positioned with its tip in the caudal IVC.
- A venogram is performed to confirm absence of thrombus within the IVC and to ascertain the level of the renal veins.
- Measurements are made to determine the diameter of the IVC. Most filters are approved for caval diameters up to 28 mm in diameter.
- Next, the filter is selected. The specific filter selected will dictate the remaining steps of the procedure. A list of filters currently approved in the USA by the Food and Drug Administration is listed in Table 19.3. There is no scientific evidence to date that documents the superiority of one type of filter design over another. The majority of filters are packaged with the appropriate insertion sheath. The majority of filters are deployed through a sheath that has

Table 19.3 US approved IVC filters

Non-removable

- Stainless steel Greenfield (Boston Scientific)
- Titanium Greenfield (Boston Scientific)
- 12-F stainless steel Greenfield (Boston Scientific)
- Vena-Tech LGM (Braun)
- Vena-Tech LP (Braun)
- Simon nitinol (Bard)
- Bird's nest (Cook)
- TrapEase (Cordis – Johnson & Johnson)

Removable

- G2 recovery (Bard)
- Recovery (Bard)
- Gunther Tulip (Cook)
- Celect (Cook)
- OptEase (Cordis – Johnson & Johnson)
- Option (Angiotech)

been appropriately positioned with its tip in the immediate infrarenal IVC. The filter is advanced through the sheath and is deployed by retracting the sheath while maintaining the filter in position with the filter stabilizer.

- Some filters require pressing a release button on the insertion apparatus to deploy the filter.
- Superior vena caval filters are deployed in an identical fashion, but the filter is released in an inverted position so that emboli coming from a cephalic direction can be captured. In many cases, deployment in the brachiocephalic vein is preferred over deployment in the SVC to avoid penetration of the segment of the SVC within the pericardial reflection.

IVC Filter Insertion: How I Do It

- Venous access is achieved via the right internal jugular vein with the patient in a supine position. The right neck is first prepped and draped.
- The right internal jugular vein is punctured with a 21-gauge echo-tip micropuncture needle using real-time ultrasound guidance. A 0.018 nitinol guidewire is advanced through the needle and successful entry is confirmed with ultrasound and fluoroscopy. The needle is removed leaving the guidewire in place and the conversion system is advanced over the guidewire. The guidewire and inner portion of the conversion system are removed. Two to 3 cc of low-osmolar contrast are injected to reconfirm appropriate entry.
- A LLT guidewire is inserted. The outer portion of the conversion system is removed and a standard length 5-F sheath placed (Cordis Bright – Tip). A venogram is then performed through the sheath to delineate the extent of occlusion.
- The LLT guidewire is manipulated through the right atrium and into the caudal aspect of the inferior vena cava.
- A 65-cm length graduated marking pigtail catheter is advanced over the guidewire into the caudal IVC and the guidewire is removed.
- An inferior vena cavogram is performed. The level of the confluence of the renal veins with the IVC is marked on the image intensifier.
- The width of the inferior vena cava is measured digitally to ensure it does not exceed 28 mm.
- A 145-cm long, 0.035 in. Amplatz exchange guidewire (Cook Inc., Bloomington IN) is advanced through the pigtail catheter and the pigtail catheter is removed.
- The Gunther Tulip filter package is opened and its contents placed on the angiographic table. All catheters are flushed with heparinized saline.
- The 11-F dilator is advanced over the wire and withdrawn after the venotomy has been enlarged.

- The Gunther Tulip insertion sheath with dilator is advanced into the caudal IVC and the dilator removed.
- The sheath is positioned with its tip approximately 3-cm below the entry of the lowest renal vein.
- The filter insertion assembly is then loaded into the sheath and advanced to the tip of the sheath.
- When the caudal aspect of the filter reaches the tip of the sheath, the sheath is retracted allowing the filter to expand within the caval lumen.
- The filter is deployed by depressing the release button on the deployment device while maintaining gentle traction on the deployment catheter.
- An angiographic image is exposed in order to document the filter position.
- The sheath is removed and hemostasis is achieved by manual compression.
- An air-occlusive dressing is applied to the venotomy site.

Tips of the Trade: Our Experiences

- We prefer to insert IVC filters from a right IJ approach. In patients with recent neck surgery or tracheostomy, a femoral vein approach can be used.
- Retrievable filters are used in almost all cases. They can function as permanent filters if removal is not desired.
- If a retrievable filter is noted to be in a poor or inappropriate position after deployment, it can easily be retrieved and repositioned.

Follow-Up After IVC Filter Insertion

- Orders are written to observe the puncture site for bleeding or hematoma.
- No additional routine follow-up is performed.

Equipment List

This is a partial list as a variety of equipment can be successfully utilized.

Access

- System 4 or 5 F micropuncture introduction (multiple vendors)

Sheaths

- 5 F standard access sheath (multiple vendors)
- Filter insertion set (multiple vendors)

Catheters

- 5-F Berenstein (multiple vendors)
- 5-F marking pigtail catheter 65 cm length

Guidewires

- 0.035 in. 145 cm length LLT (multiple vendors)

IVC Filter Kits

- See Table 19.3

Bibliography

Iliofemoral Thrombosis

Comerota AJ, Gravett MH. Iliofemoral venous thrombosis. J Vasc Surg. 2007;46(5):1065–76.

→ *Comprehensive review of the management of iliofemoral thrombosis.*

Vedantham S, Millward SF, Cardella JF, Hofmann LV, Razavi MK, Grassi CJ, Sacks D, Kinney TB. Society of Interventional Radiology position statement: treatment of acute iliofemoral deep vein thrombosis with use of adjunctive catheter-directed intrathrombus thrombolysis. J Vasc Interv Radiol. 2009;20 (7 Suppl):S332-5.

Wicky ST. Acute deep vein thrombosis and thrombolysis. Tech Vasc Interv Radiol. 2009;12(2):148–53.

→ *Excellent review of technical aspects of procedure.*

Subclavian Vein Thrombosis

Illig KA, Doyle AJ. A comprehensive review of Paget-Schroetter syndrome. J Vasc Surg. 2010;51(6):1538–47.

→ *Superb review of subclavian thrombosis.*

Molina JE, Hunter DW, Dietz CA. Paget-Schroetter syndrome treated with thrombolytics and immediate surgery. J Vasc Surg. 2007;45(2):328–34.

Shah AD, Bajakian DR, Olin JW, Lookstein RA. Power-pulse spray thrombectomy for treatment of Paget-Schroetter syndrome. AJR Am J Roentgenol. 2007 May;188(5):1215–7.

→ *Description of technical aspects of the procedure.*

Urschel HC Jr., Patel AN. Surgery remains the most effective treatment for Paget-Schroetter syndrome: 50 years' experience. Ann Thorac Surg. 2008 Jul;86(1):254–60

Central Venous Stenosis and Occlusion

Bakken AM, Protack CD, Saad WE, Lee DE, Waldman DL, Davies MG. Long-term outcomes of primary angioplasty and primary stenting of central venous stenosis in hemodialysis patients. J Vasc Surg. 2007;45(4):776–83.

→ *Comparative trial of balloon venoplasty versus stent placement.*

Lanciego C, Pangua C, Chacón JI, Velasco J, Boy RC, Viana A, Cerezo S, García LG. Endovascular stenting as the first step in the overall management of malignant superior vena cava syndrome. AJR Am J Roentgenol. 2009 ;193(2):549–58.

Rajan DK, Saluja JS. Use of nitinol stents following recanalization of central venous occlusions in hemodialysis patients. Cardiovasc Intervent Radiol. 2007;30(4):662–7.

Vena Cava Filters

Ingber S, Geerts WH. Vena caval filters: current knowledge, uncertainties and practical approaches. Curr Opin Hematol. 2009;16(5):402–6.

→ *Excellent literature review.*

Owens CA, Bui JT, Knuttinen MG, Gaba RC, Carrillo TC. Pulmonary embolism from upper extremity deep vein thrombosis and the role of superior vena cava filters: a review of the literature. J Vasc Interv Radiol. 2010;21(6):779–87.

→ *Assessment of superior vena caval filters.*

Tschoe M, Kim HS, Brotman DJ, Streiff MB. Retrievable vena cava filters: a clinical review. J Hosp Med. 2009;4(7):441–8.

Chapter 20
Endovascular Therapy for Venous Insufficiency

Kristian Ulloa, S. Marlene Grenon, and Rajabrata Sarkar

Essential Anatomy and Physiology of Veins

A thorough understanding of the venous anatomy and physiology in the lower extremity is essential for diagnosis and treatment of venous insufficiency.

- The venous anatomy of the thigh and leg consists of three components:
  - The superficial venous system (greater saphenous and lesser saphenous veins)
    - Greater saphenous vein: The greater saphenous vein originates from the dorsal venous arch in the foot and passes anterior to the medial malleolus as it courses in the medial leg and thigh, where it eventually perforates the deep fascia at the fossa ovalis to

K. Ulloa • R. Sarkar (✉)
Division of Vascular Surgery, Department of Surgery,
University of Maryland,
Baltimore, MD, USA
e-mail: kulloa@smail.maryland.edu; rsarkar@smail.maryland.edu

S.M. Grenon
Division of Vascular Surgery, Department of Surgery,
University of California – San Francisco,
San Francisco, CA, USA
e-mail: marlene.grenon@ucsfmedctr.org

C.D. Owens and Y. Yeghiazarians (eds.),
Handbook of Endovascular Peripheral Interventions,
DOI 10.1007/978-1-4614-0839-0_20,

enter the common femoral vein at the saphenofemoral junction. The vein ascends in the space between the deep and superficial fascial compartments of the lower extremity and can be found approximately 1 cm posterior to the tibia (Fig. 20.1). There are multiple tributaries to the greater saphenous vein. These tributaries arise in the superficial compartment and pierce the superficial fascia to enter the greater saphenous vein. Named tributaries include the posteromedial, anteromedial, posterolateral, and ascending superficial (vein of Giacomini) thigh veins. *These tributaries are responsible for the majority of clinically evident varicosities.*

    - Lesser saphenous vein: The small saphenous vein is typically responsible for focal varicosities in the posterior calf as opposed to the more extensive varicosities noted with greater saphenous vein incompetence. The dorsal venous arch gives rise to the small saphenous vein on the lateral aspect of the foot, where it begins its ascent in the midline of the posterior leg to join the popliteal vein in the popliteal fossa. Of note, isolated lesser saphenous reflux is responsible for 5% of venous stasis ulcers.
  - The perforator venous system.
    - These veins penetrate the deep fascia and connect the deep and superficial venous systems. Like the deep and superficial veins, the perforator veins have valves which may become incompetent and contribute to varicosities. There are several levels of perforators in the leg, each of which has the potential to become incompetent and contribute to venous insufficiency (Fig. 20.1).
  - The deep venous system.
- All of the disorders of the venous system leading to venous insufficiency arise from failure of the valves to prevent venous reflux, or occasionally, obstruction of the deep venous system from scarring after deep venous thrombosis. More rarely, arteriovenous malformations and congenital disorders may lead to venous insufficiency.

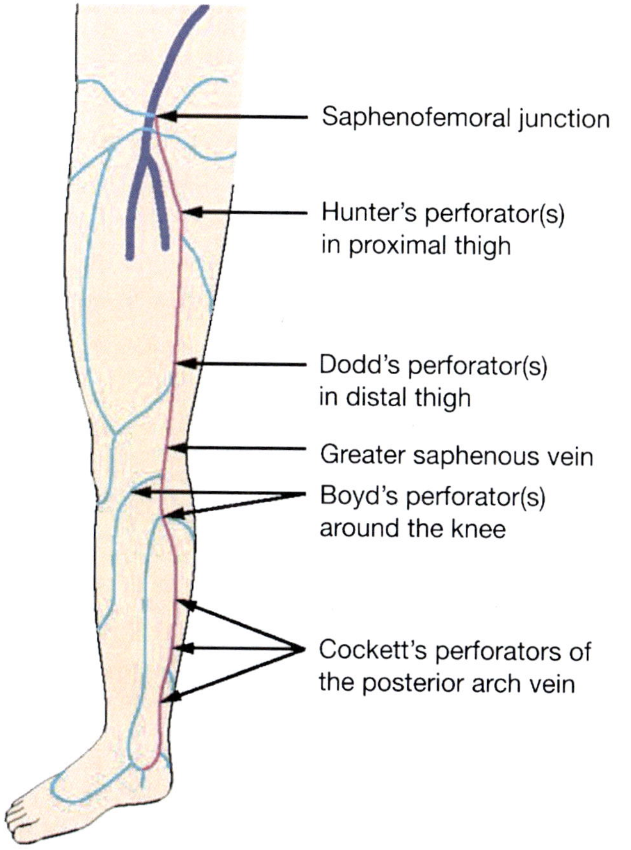

FIGURE 20.1 Diagram of superficial venous system and perforator veins of the lower extremity

- It is useful to refer to the following definitions:
  - Telangiectasias: a confluence of dilated intra-dermal venules of less than 1 mm in caliber.
  - Reticular veins: dilated bluish sub-dermal veins usually from 1 mm in diameter to 3 mm in diameter.

– Varicose veins: subcutaneous dilated vein equal to or more than 3 mm in diameter measured in the upright position.

Clinical Pointers
1. GSV tributaries are responsible for varicosities
2. Incompetent perforator valves contribute to venous insufficiency
3. Small saphenous vein reflux contributes to 5% of venous insufficiency

Clinical Features and Diagnosis

- Risk Factors: The risk factors for development of chronic venous disease are multifactorial but include heredity, race, gender, height and weight, occupation (prolonged standing), hormones including estrogen, progesterone, and pregnancy.

Prevalence of venous disease in men and women

Types	Men (%)	Women (%)
Venous disease (all types)	40–50	50–55
Visible varicose veins	20–25	20–25
Chronic venous insufficiency	3–5	1–1.5
Leg ulceration	0.5–1	1–1.5

- Symptoms: Patients with venous insufficiency often complain of pain and fatigue in the lower legs particularly after prolonged standing and toward the end of the day. They may also complain of swelling in the legs which also tends to occur in the evenings. Tenderness over the varicosities may indicate local superficial phlebitis. Discoloration of the skin is due to extravasation of blood cells which may also cause pruritis.
- Classification: Patients diagnoses with venous insufficiency should be classified according to the CEAP classification:

CEAP Classification of Chronic Venous Insufficiency
C: *Clinical* C1-spider telangiectasia, C2 varicose veins, C3 edema, C4 lipodermatosclerosis (pigmentation changes), C5 healed ulcer, C6 active ulcer.
E: *Etiology*: congenital, primary, or secondary
A: *Anatomic*: superficial, deep, or perforator
P: *Pathophysiology*: reflux, obstruction, or both

Clinical Pointers

- Essential to the successful performance of any endovenous procedure is a thorough preoperative venous duplex accurately delineating the anatomy and physiology of an individual's venous insufficiency.
  - GSV reflux is usually demonstrated by reversal of flow (blood flow back toward the feet) lasting longer than 0.5 s following a provocative maneuver such as a Valsalva maneuver. True reflux is usually documented from the saphenofemoral junction to the ankle.
  - It is also important to identify reflux in the LSV and in the perforators.
- An experienced and knowledgeable vascular ultrasound technician should work in concert with the endovenous surgeon in order to preoperatively effectively identify pathological vein segments.
- It is also our practice to perform an intra-operative ultrasound of the greater and lesser saphenous veins as well as perforator veins immediately prior to the procedure to confirm the preoperative exam. Others have advocated the use of preoperative marking immediately before the procedure by an ultrasound technologist of access sites for the greater or small saphenous vein, to guide the surgeon.

Treatment

- Indications: Treatment for venous reflux is usually offered for two main indications: symptoms of venous insufficiency (i.e., pain, tenderness, fatigue, or edema affecting quality of life which may be coupled with skin changes including hyperpigmentation, atrophy, ulceration, edema) and/or cosmesis (patient's concerns with the appearance of their veins). Duplex ultrasound findings of greater saphenous or small saphenous venous reflux must then be documented against patients presenting complaints.
- Our practice is to preferentially use radiofrequency ablation over laser ablation, as recent randomized prospective studies have definitively shown improved outcomes with this modality in comparison to laser ablation [3]. A complete list of equipment and supplies required for basic ablation of the greater saphenous vein is listed in Table 20.1.

Preprocedural Instructions

- No restriction on drinking before the procedure
- No food 2 h before the procedure
- Arrange for transportation home
- Patients should not be home alone the night after the procedure
- Wear loose fitting clothing and shoes
- Stop vitamins C and E, garlic and ginkgo 7 days before procedure
- Take routine medication as prescribed
- Anesthesia choice is between physicians and patient: we generally suggest pre-operative PO valium, short-acting IV versed, and a generous amount of local anesthetic. Lidocaine toxicity could occur at 7 mg/kg body weight. Never use more than 500 mg!

TABLE 20.1 Equipment list for radiofrequency ablation of the greater saphenous vein

Equipment list for radiofrequency ablation of the greater saphenous vein
Radiofrequency generator
Radiofrequency catheter
Sterile drapes
Ultrasound machine with 8 MHz (or greater) probe
Sterile probe cover
7 Fr sheath (either 7 or 11 cm in length)
Micropuncture set
Large (30 cc) syringes with 22–25 G needles to infiltrate tumescent solution
Tumescent solution: 1% lidocaine with epinephrine 1:100,000 diluted 1:10 in sterile saline
Steristrip for puncture site coverage
Optional Equipment and Supplies
Infusion pump to inject tumescent solution
Angled glide catheter and 0.008–0.025 wire for difficult access

How I Do It

- Set up and patient preparation: We use a well lit, warm procedure or operating room. If the patient is awake, we have soothing music available. The entire affected extremity is prepped with a chlorhexidine solution. A sterile tray is available with all dilators, sheaths, tubing, and local anesthetic that is anticipated to be needed, Fig. 20.2 (Table 20.1).
- A high-frequency linear array transducer is used with a sterile probe cover and acoustic gel to scan from the saphenofemoral junction to the medial malleolus. The leg is scanned with the probe in a transverse orientation using B-mode ultrasound to begin. The course of the vein is marked on the patient's skin.

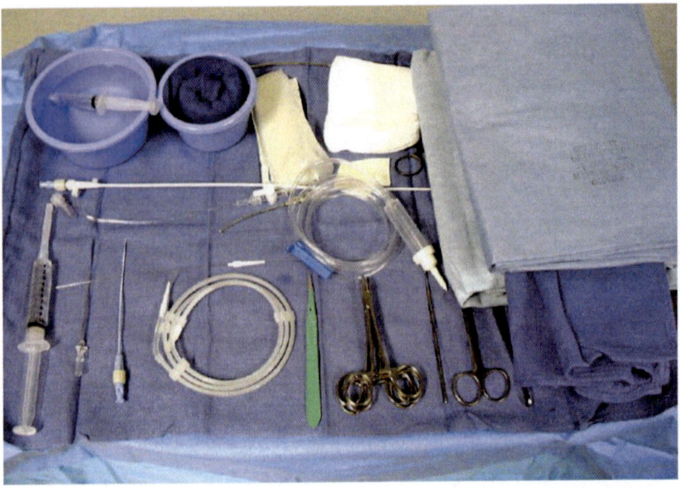

FIGURE 20.2 This is an example of the sterile tray set-up used at our institution for performing venous RF ablation. Local anesthetic, micropuncture introducer sheaths, 11 blade, small snaps, sterile drapes, etc., are prepared prior to the procedure, also see Table 20.1 for equipment list

- Compression with the probe, which should demonstrate apposition of the vein walls, is performed every 3 or 4 cm. Color Duplex imaging is then employed with proximal augmentation in order to assess for reversal of flow, which is demonstrated by flow toward the probe.
- When an ablation is performed for greater saphenous vein insufficiency, a segment of the vein no more distal than 10 cm below the knee should be chosen for access. The saphenous nerve runs in close proximity to the vein from the mid-calf to the ankle, thus ablation procedures more distal than 10 cm from the knee are associated with a greater risk of nerve injury.
- The transducer should be held in a transverse orientation to the vein.
- Using a micropuncture needle, the vein should be accessed under ultrasound guidance until return of blood is noted from the needle (Fig. 20.3).

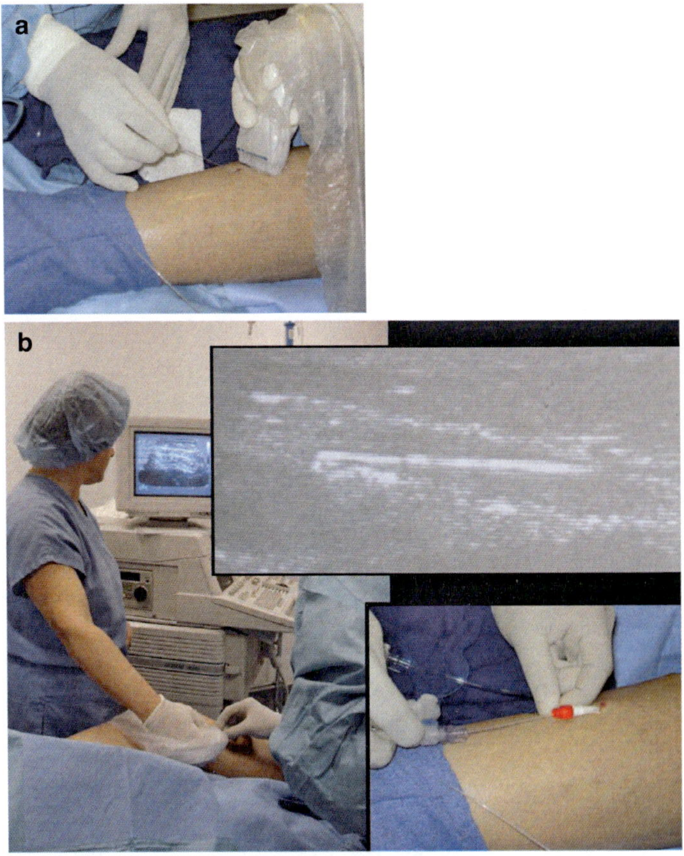

FIGURE 20.3 Ultrasound-guided needle insertion into the GSV (**a**). Correct needle position is confirmed by blood return as well as ultrasound confirmation of the needle in the vein. A wire is advanced into the vein via Seldinger technique (**b**)

- An echogenic needle (either commercially available or made by cross-serrating the distal 1 cm of the needle with a scalpel) is useful for less experienced operators or when dealing with a small or deep vein. Next, a micro access wire is placed through the needle and imaged within the vein. The microdilator is then placed over the micro wire, followed by an appropriately sized short sheath. At this point, the ultrasound transducer should be used to visualize the saphenofemoral junction.

- The radiofrequency or laser catheter is placed alongside the thigh from the sheath to the location of the saphenofemoral junction in order to determine roughly the distance of catheter that will be placed within the vein. The bumper on the RF catheter shaft should be moved to the point where the catheter will be at the required distance, thus helping to prevent advancing the catheter inadvertently into the deep venous system.
- *The critical step for safely performing an endovenous ablation is accurate identification of the saphenofemoral junction, and placing the device tip at the appropriate distance from this structure.* The ultrasound probe should be oriented slightly obliquely so that the greater saphenous vein, common femoral vein, and inferior epigastric vein can be viewed in a single image. We refer to this view when teaching these procedures as the "Mickey Mouse" view because of the appearance of the three circular structures: the "head" being the common femoral vein and the "ears" representing the femoral artery and greater saphenous veins (Fig. 20.4a). This view clearly identifies the saphenofemoral junction. Then the longitudinal view of the junction (Fig. 20.4b) is used to position the endovenous ablation device at the proper distance from the most caudal edge of the saphenofemoral junction. For example a radiofrequency ablation catheter is placed with the tip no closer than 2 cm from the saphenofemoral junction. *This distance is critical in order to decrease the risk of thrombus extension to the deep system and provide a complete ablation of the GSV.*

FIGURE 20.4 The transverse or "Mickey Mouse" view of the saphenofemoral junction. "Mickey's" face is the common femoral vein, and his "ears" are the saphenous vein and the femoral artery (**a**). The longitudinal view of the saphenofemoral junction. The change in the direction of the saphenous vein as it enters the femoral vein is evident. Note that the distal femoral vein is not seen as it does not run parallel to the saphenous vein and is thus out of the frame of the ultrasound transducer (**b**)

- In order to prevent thermal injury to adjacent structures and to compress the vein wall onto the catheter, the fascial compartment surrounding the vein to be ablated should be infiltrated with tumescent solution. We prefer a mixture of

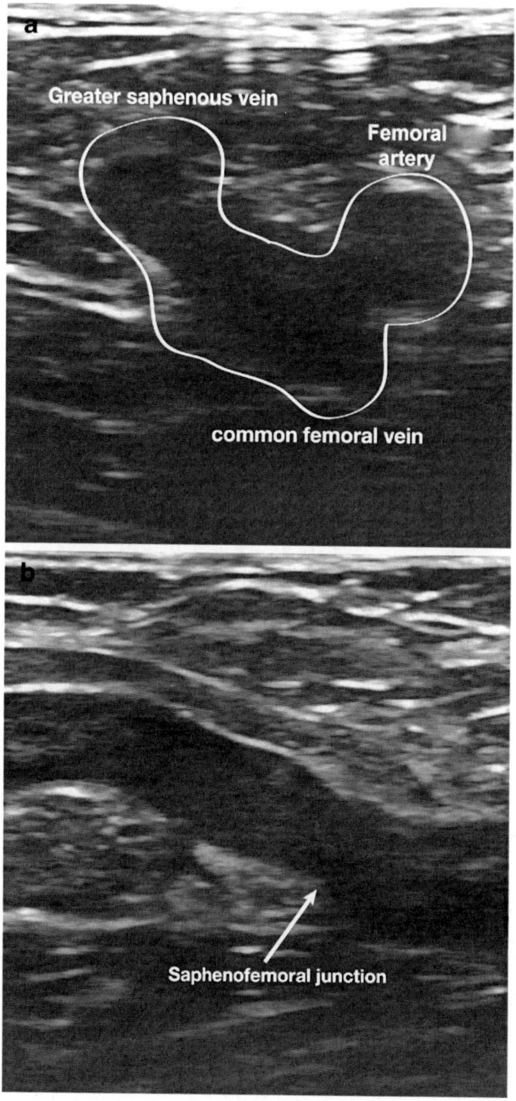

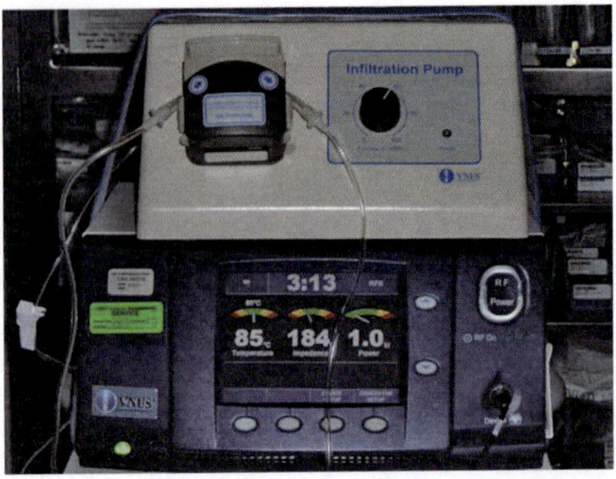

FIGURE 20.5 Radiofrequency generator in use displaying temperature, impedance, and power delivery. Note placement of tumescent infusion pump above generator on cart. How it works: During the procedure an electric current flows between bipolar electrodes at the tip of the catheter in the vein. This will generate heat from 85°C to 90°C. The heat causes physical shortening of collagen fibers of the vein wall in the subendothelial layers

1% lidocaine with 1:10,000 mg/mL epinephrine and sodium bicarbonate 8.4% solution. This solution is further diluted 1:10 with injectable saline to increase volume and dilute the pharmacologic agents. The tumescent solution is injected with 30 cc syringes or using an injector pump with the needle oriented at a right angle to the ultrasound probe. The fascial envelope should be infiltrated with enough tumescent solution to create a 1–2 cm separation between the vein and surrounding structures such as nerves, arteries, and skin. The entire segment of vein to be ablated should be infiltrated in this fashion. It is critical to recheck the catheter tip position after tumescent administration as the catheter tip tends to migrate proximally as the tumescent solution compresses and straightens the vein.

- Radiofrequency ablation is done at a temperature of 120°C for treatment of greater and short saphenous vein insufficiency. The radiofrequency generator provides continuous information regarding the temperature at the tip of the catheter, as well as the power being delivered and the impedance (which reflects tissue resistance) (Fig. 20.5). The vein should be ablated under ultrasound guidance, with the ultrasound probe compressing the vein in order to further bring the endothelium into close apposition with the heating element of the catheter. Usually, small bubbles can be seen within the vein on ultrasound as the ablation is performed. *It is recommended to perform the ablation of the segment of greater saphenous vein nearest the saphenofemoral junction twice in order to achieve a higher procedural success rate.* Radiofrequency ablation is done at a treatment rate of 20 seconds for every 7 cm of vein. Laser ablation rates are variable and dependent on wavelength and laser fiber. Once the catheter has been withdrawn to the level of the sheath, the sheath should be pulled back slightly so that the heating element of the catheter is not within the sheath.

- Following ablation, the ultrasound examination is repeated to ensure no thrombus in the common femoral vein and a successful seal of the greater saphenous vein. It is common to see a residual lumen in the treated saphenous vein, although there is usually no flow detectable within the vein. The leg is wrapped with a compressive dressing which is left in place for 48 h. A duplex scan is performed within 72 h to detect deep venous thrombosis and to check the seal of the treated vein. Patients can resume normal activity and are encouraged to ambulate immediately. We discourage vigorous exercise, airline travel, or swimming for 2 weeks after vein ablation.

Post-Operative Care Instruction

- Mobility
  - First 48 h, relax, keep leg elevation
  - Try to walk every hour some
  - Return to work in 3 days
  - Avoid strenuous exercise for 3 weeks

- Avoid long periods of immobility, e.g., air flight or car ride
- Dressing
  - Keep dressing/compression bandages on for 48 h
  - Wear compression hose for next 2 weeks
- Analgesia
  - Motrin 600 mg t.i.d. for 1 week
  - Zantac 150 mg b.i.d.

- Although we generally perform phlebectomy of varicosities at the same setting as endovenous ablation, roughly 60% of varicosities subside with saphenous ablation alone to the point where further therapy is not needed [1].
- We often will do two legs in the same setting if there is not extensive phlebectomy involved.
- The main contraindications when considering this procedure are: (1) acute phlebitis of the target vein (e.g., thrombus in the GSV) and (2) less than 2 mm distance between the GSV and skin. Superficial GSV can lead to postoperative hyperpigmentation. Arterivenous malformation, restricted mobility, and deep venous obstruction are also contraindications and should be documented on the preoperative duplex examination.

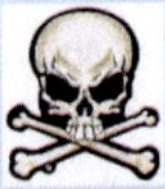

Potential Pitfalls

The incidence of asymptomatic deep venous thrombosis detected after radiofrequency or laser ablation is low (generally <5%) but it is of great concern to the patient should this be diagnosed post-operatively. We educate patients that 1–3% of post-operative scans will show some protrusion of thrombus from the saphenous orifice into the lumen of the common femoral vein, and that treatment with 7–10 days of therapeutic low molecular weight heparin will resolve this. Other complications include tenderness, phlebitis of branch varicosities, paresthesia, and the rare hyperpigmentation of the overlying skin from thermal injury (Fig. 20.2) which occurs in patients with saphenous veins close to the skin. Diligent application of tumescent anesthesia to create space between the vein and the skin can reduce, but not eliminate, the potential for this complication.

Laser ablation of the saphenous vein is another viable option for the treatment of varicose veins and saphenous vein reflux. The advantages of the laser over radiofrequency include cheaper disposable cost for the laser fiber in comparison to the radiofrequency catheter, and a slightly lower incidence of late recanalization [2]. *A prospective, randomized trial of 67 patients undergoing either endovenous laser ablation or radiofrequency ablation of the greater saphenous vein demonstrated improved quality of life and less complication at 2 weeks post-op in the radiofrequency ablation group* [3]. *Both techniques are associated with higher up-front costs than conventional high ligation and stripping, but the long-term costs when considering productivity losses are similar.*

Potential Pitfalls

An important consideration is the relationship between the saphenous nerve and greater saphenous vein, as they run parallel and in close proximity from a few centimeters distal to the knee to the level of the medial malleolus. The saphenous nerve may be injured during both open and percutaneous interventions in the leg. Although this is a sensory nerve, injury to this nerve from either surgical stripping or endovenous ablation of the greater saphenous vein below the knee can result in bothersome sensory parasthesia or anesthesia.

Potential Pitfalls

It is important to note that the small saphenous vein may enter the deep venous system anywhere from the middle third of the leg to the popliteal fossa or even higher in the thigh. Accurate identification of the site of entry of the small saphenous vein into the deep system is relevant to the treatment of reflux in this vessel, as endovenous ablation of this vein in the posterior thigh can cause thermal damage to adjacent motor nerves. Post-operative deep venous thrombosis is more common after ablation of the short saphenous vein and thus we place the tip of the radiofrequency catheter further away (3–4 cm) from the junction of the short saphenous vein with the popliteal vein.

Potential Pitfalls

Caution should be used in ablation of greater saphenous veins that are close (<3 mm) to the skin. Even with adequate tumescent anesthesia to create 1 cm of space between the vein and the skin at the time of ablation, permanent hyperpigmentation of the overlying skin (Fig. 20.5) may occur.

Bibliography

1. Welch HJ: Endovenous ablation of the great saphenous vein may avert phlebectomy for branch varicose veins. J Vasc Surg 2006;44:601–605.

   → *This study examined the incidence of subsequent phlebectomy for varicose veins after an initial saphenous ablation only. This study and others indicate that roughly one half of patients with varicosities will not need a subsequent phlebectomy. This does NOT mean however that the varicosities dissapear or become asymptomatic as this was not assessed.*

2. Gale SS, Lee JN, Walsh ME, Wojnarowski DL, Comerota AJ: A randomized, controlled trial of endovenous thermal ablation using the 810-nm wavelength laser and the closureplus radiofrequency ablation methods for superficial venous insufficiency of the great saphenous vein. J Vasc Surg;52:645–650.
   → *Randomized prospective study of laser vs. radiofrequency ablation for greater saphenous vein ablation demonstrating improved short-term outcomes with radiofrequency and higher seal rates with laser.*
3. Almeida JI, Kaufman J, Gockeritz O, Chopra P, Evans MT, Hoheim DF, Makhoul RG, Richards T, Wenzel C, Raines JK: Radiofrequency endovenous closurefast versus laser ablation for the treatment of great saphenous reflux: A multicenter, single-blinded, randomized study (recovery study). J Vasc Interv Radiol 2009;20:752–759.
   → *Randomized prospective study of laser vs. radiofrequency ablation for greater saphenous vein ablation demonstrating improved short-term outcomes with radiofrequency using a number of outcome measures.*

Chapter 21
Dialysis Access Intervention

Jong-Ping Lu and Charles M. Eichler

Background

End-stage renal disease (ESRD) affects over half a million Americans and the prevalence is increasing as the population ages. Hospitalizations for dialysis access and its associated problems cost over a billion dollars per year. Dialysis access is the lifeline for patients with ESRD, yet durable long-term outcomes are difficult to achieve.

Patency

- Primary patency is defined as the time interval in which a fistula is functioning without any need for intervention. The 1 year primary patency rate for arteriovenous fistulas (AVFs) is around 55%. It is 38% for arteriovenous grafts (AVGs).

J.-P. Lu
Department of Surgery, University of California – San Francisco, San Francisco, CA, USA
e-mail: jipperlu@gmail.com

C.M. Eichler (✉)
Division of Vascular Surgery, Department of Surgery, University of California – San Francisco, San Francisco, CA, USA
e-mail: charles.eichler@ucsfmedctr.org

C.D. Owens and Y. Yeghiazarians (eds.), *Handbook of Endovascular Peripheral Interventions*, DOI 10.1007/978-1-4614-0839-0_21,

- Assisted primary patency refers to the time interval that a fistula is functioning with the assistance of interventions without thrombosis.
- Secondary patency is defined as the time interval in which a fistula is functioning despite thrombosis because it was successfully salvaged.

Preoperative Evaluation

In addition to the physical examination of a patient's extremities, the veins of the patient are studied either by ultrasonography or by venography.

Ultrasonography-Vein Mapping

- *Strengths*: safe, non-invasive, avoids use of contrast in pre-dialysis patients, thus avoiding risk of renal toxicity
- *Limitations*: difficult to study central veins, dependent on operator expertise, limited by technical challenges related to obesity and arm position

Clinical Pointers

- Ultrasound vein mapping is the study of choice for pre-dialysis patients undergoing evaluation for dialysis access
- Use venography even in pre-dialysis patients if any of the following are present:
  - History of intravenous drug use
  - History of central lines or peripherally inserted central lines (PICC)
  - History or pacemakers, ports

We recommend veins to be a minimum of 3-mm diameter by ultrasound. It is doubtful that a smaller vein will mature well (Fig. 21.1).

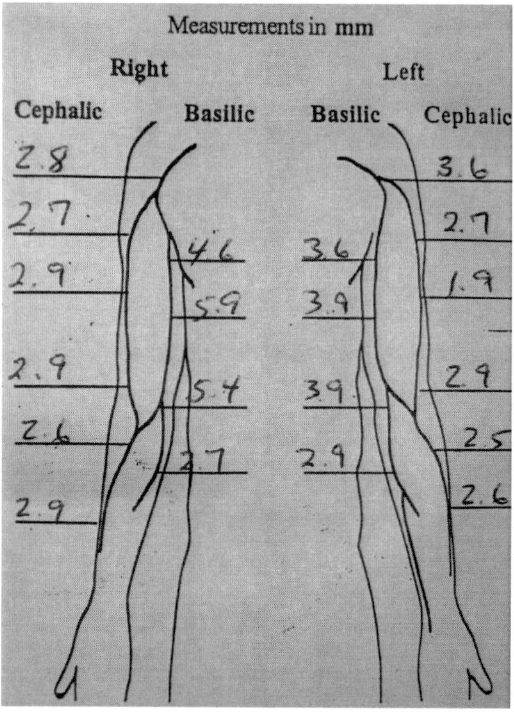

FIGURE 21.1 This is an example of pre-operative vein mapping in a patient with ESRD

Venogram

- *Strengths*: Excellent images can be obtained, detailed evaluation of central veins,
- *Limitations*: Involves the use of ionizing radiation and nephrogenic, iodinated contrast medium
- *How to perform a venogram* (Fig. 21.2):
  - Position the arm in anatomical position
  - Place a peripheral IV in the hand of the arm under evaluation
  - Place a tourniquet in the upper arm as proximal as possible

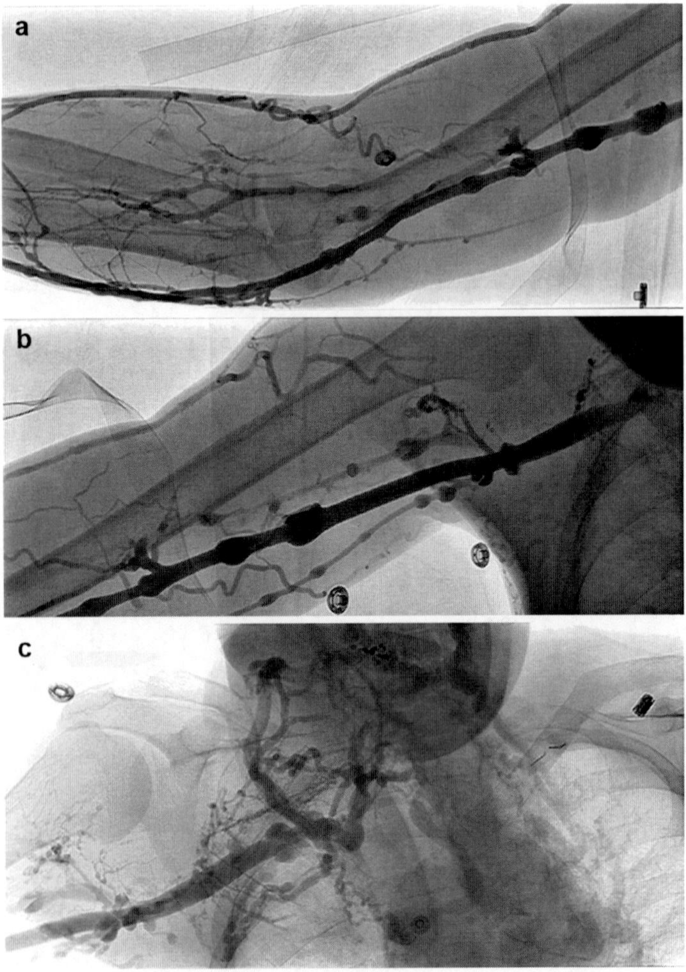

FIGURE 21.2 (**a**) Right upper extremity venogram of a 38-year-old man with a failed arteriovenous graft. The patient had an ultrasound that demonstrated a patent basilic vein. Venography is essential for workup of patients with failed access. Figures (**a**) and (**b**) would suggest that this patient is a candidate for basilic vein transposition; however Fig. (**c**) demonstrates central vein occlusion that could not be imaged by ultrasound

Potential Pitfalls

- Avoid placing the IV in the forearm cephalic vein
- Keep the arm in anatomic position throughout the venogram

- Inject 10 mL of Visapaque contrast
- Perform fluoroscopy sequentially moving up the arm
- Release the tourniquet
- To evaluate central veins, inject 20–30 mL of contrast into the arm, and perform run under fluoroscopy, using 20 mL saline flush to watch contrast move through central veins

Tips of the Trade

- If the basilic or the cephalic vein is not initially visualized, you can manually occlude the brachial vein and inject more contrast to encourage flow to these veins.
- If the patient has very small veins, it will take a slow, steady push of contrast to fill them. Be patient.

Clinical Pointer: Creating a Fistula

Identify the single best vein and create an arteriovenous fistula whenever possible. This strategy will lower rates of non-maturing fistulas and other complications.

Indicators of a Failing Dialysis Access

Evidence of 50% stenosis AND at least one of the following:

- Decreasing flow rates during dialysis (<600 mL/min)
- Arm swelling

- Elevated venous pressure or more than 0.4 ratio graft/systolic pressure
- Decreased dialysis dose (Kt/V)
- Prolonged bleeding after decannulation
- Increased urea recirculation (>10%)
- Aneurysm and pseudoaneurysm
- A history of previous thrombosis

Current State of Affairs

Recent emphasis as outlined in the National Kidney Foundation Dialysis Outcomes Quality Initiative (NKF KDOQI) guidelines on construction of arteriovenous fistulas (AVFs) over arteriovenous grafts (AVGs) has improved dialysis access outcomes. These guidelines urge prompt evaluation of an AVF that fails to mature, early evaluation and treatment of a failing AVF, and immediate intervention for a thrombosed AVF. Similar guidelines exist for AVGs. Many problems that have traditionally been treated surgically now have as-good percutaneous equivalents which we will discuss in this chapter. For all the procedures described below, we do not routinely systemically anticoagulate for the procedure, nor do we recommend post-procedural systemic anticoagulation apart from aspirin therapy. All patients who present with failing access or thrombosed access are initiated on aspirin therapy as this has been shown to increase patency.

Diagnosing the Problem

The first step in evaluating a failing or failed AVF or AVG is to perform a physical exam. Evaluation of thrill and pulsatility can be as good as imaging in detecting flow abnormalities, especially in the hands of an expert. Understanding the causative lesion will help guide treatment and many of these lesions can be identified by ultrasonography. Nonetheless, dialysis access angiography is the gold standard. Since it can be easily combined with a therapeutic intervention, most often times, it is the diagnostic test of choice.

Fistulogram (Use Same Technique to Evaluate an AVG)

How to Perform a Fistulogram

- Puncture fistula with direct access antegrade (toward the venous outflow) with a micropuncture set or a 19-gauge needle approximately 2 cm from the arterial anastomosis
- Pass a 0.035″ glidewire across entire fistula
- Place 4 Fr short sheath
- Inject 10 mL of Visapaque contrast under flouroscopy to evaluate fistula.

Potential Pitfalls

- DO NOT inject contrast into clot if the fistula under evaluation is a thrombosed fistula. This traps the contrast and eliminates your ability to interpret the images

- Move centrally, performing fluoroscopy to evaluate entire venous outflow track to the heart
- Once venous outflow evaluation is complete, occlude the venous outflow manually
- Inject 10–20 mL of Visapaque which will reflux to demonstrate arterial anastomosis.

Tips of the Trade

- If you suspect an arterial anastamotic stenosis or have evidence of this on preprocedural ultrasound evaluation, puncture retrograde at the venous end of the fistula and perform a fistulogram. This sets you up to intervene at the arterial end without performing a second puncture. To study the venous outflow, simply occlude the fistula, inject, and image proximally.

- If the fistula is too immature for puncture, it can be accessed through the radial artery and 4 Fr sheath can be placed safely.

Non-maturing Fistula

This problem is also called primary failure defined as a fistula that never provided reliable access for hemodialysis. On evaluation, the vein remains non-dilated and often there is a stenotic lesion present. Depending on the location of the fistula, rates largely range from 9% to 36%, though rates up to 60% have been reported in certain populations.

Treatment of Non-maturing Fistula

In the absence of a stenotic lesion, balloon-assisted maturation (BAM) can help bring a fistula to maturation. It is comprised of sequential, long-segment angioplasties and is successful in over 80% of cases. Overall, it appears to be safe and effective.

How to Perform BAM

- Puncture fistula antegrade approximately 2 cm from the arterial anastomosis
- Perform a fistulogram with imaging of central veins, studying the anastomoses
- Pass 0.035″ guidewire to level of central veins
- Treat stenotic lesions (see below)
- Select a non-compliant balloon that is 20–30% larger that the vessel (usually start with 4–6 mm)

Potential Pitfalls

- BAM is relatively difficult technique with steep learning curve and remains controversial
- Logistically difficult as patients need to return every 2 weeks
- This procedure is essentially equivalent to controlled dissection. Extravasation is a relatively common complication and will require manual compression

- Select non-compliant balloon with long balloon lengths (120–200 mm, i.e., EV3 everflex)
- Balloon entire length of fistula. Inflation times should be 2–3 min.
- Repeat every 2 weeks, increasing balloon size by 2–3 mm each visit until fistula progresses to a usable size (may need to use up to 16-mm balloon)

Fistula/Graft Stenosis

Stenosis is the most frequent causative lesion and venous outflow problems are much more common than arterial inflow problems. These lesions are usually due to neointimal hyperplasia and usually respond to percutaneous transluminal angioplasty (PTA) although recurrence is common. Nonetheless, PTA is minimally invasive, well-tolerated and does not carry the risk of losing the access site when compared to surgical revision. Stents have also been used to treat recurrent stenotic lesions but the current NFK KDOQI recommendations are to reserve stent placement for those who have lesions NOT amenable to surgical treatment.

Treatment of Fistula/Graft Stenosis

PTA is the standard first-line approach for a stenosis that is >50% and clinically symptomatic.

How to Perform PTA

- Puncture the fistula/graft and place a 6–8 Fr sheath
- Perform fistulogram with imaging of the central veins
- Pass 0.035″ guidewire to level of central veins. We start with glidewire and exchange to a stiffer wire (i.e., Supracore, Amplatz)
- Select a non-compliant balloon that is 20–30% larger than the vessel (usually 6–7 mm)
- Pass angioplasty balloon catheter to most proximal peripheral lesion visible
- Balloon sequentially up to 10, 15, or 20 atm

Potential Pitfalls

- Cutting balloons should not be used beyond the fistula. Not for use in central veins as any bleeding there is difficult to control.
- Be wary that the sheath can actually occlude a stenotic lesion.

- Consider an ultrahigh pressure (30+atm) balloon for a resistant lesion (i.e., Conquest, Dorado)
- Consider 6–8 mm cutting balloon for a recurrent, resistant lesion
- Repeat until radiographic result is achieved or if radiographic result cannot be achieved, consider stenting option (see below)
- Perform completion angiogram, assessing flow of radiocontrast visually
- Repeat the physical exam to assess flow

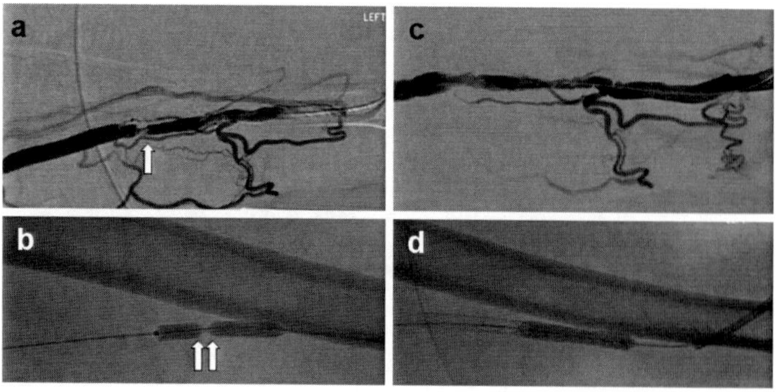

FIGURE 21.3 Fistulogram of a 52-year-old man with a non-maturing brachiocephalic fistula 3 months after creation. (**a**) A fistulogram was obtained using a 5 Fr sheath access into proximal portion of fistula and demonstrates focal stenosis in the vein with multiple venous collaterals (*white arrow*). (**b**) Percutaneous transluminal angioplasty using 6 mm × 4 cm EV3 EverFlex balloon (*double white arrow*). (**c**) Completion fistulogram showed marked recoil and small dissection. (**d**) This was treated with placement of a 7 mm × 50 mm EV3 Protégé self expanding nitinol stent. Completion angiogram demonstrated brisk flow through the vein and disappearance of the venous collaterals (not shown)

- Remove wire and sheath and apply manual pressure to obtain hemostasis with optional placement of skin closure stitch

Stent placement is still controversial at this point in time but many centers have used self-expanding stents to treat recurrent, resistant lesions. Self-expanding stents, either of stainless steel or of nitinol alloys, are the stents of choice as they are more flexible in comparison to balloon-expandable stents. Balloon-expandable stents are subject to deformation and fracture in the superficial position and therefore not suitable for use in dialysis access intervention. Recently stent grafts (covered stents) have also been used with seemingly improved results (Fig. 21.3).

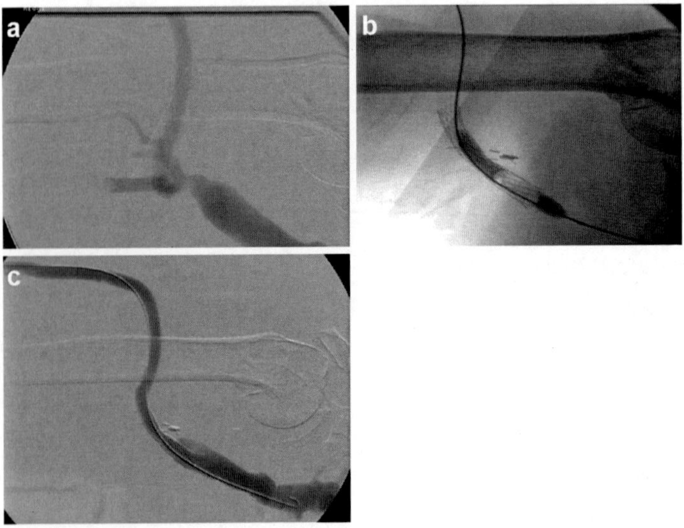

FIGURE 21.4 This patient is an 80-year-old woman with a brachial artery to axillary vein arteriovenous graft. She has had recurrent graft thrombosis secondary to venous anastomotic stenosis. (**a**) Fistulogram was performed though an 8 Fr sheath in the proximal portion of the graft, directed distally. This demonstrates persistent venous anastomotic stenosis. Balloon angioplasty using a 6 mm × 4 cm Dorado balloon failed to improve radiographic appearance. (**b**) An 8 mm × 4 cm Fluency stent graft was placed across the venous anastomosis and ballooned with an 8 mm × 4 cm Dorado balloon. (**c**) Completion angiogram shows resolution of stenosis

How to Perform Stent Placement

- Select self-expandable stent that is oversized by approximately 20%
- Deploy stent/stent graft such that the area of stenosis is covered (expect 10% shortening upon deployment when using stainless steel stents; nitinol stents do not shorten)
- Post dilate stent – use a balloon size that is 1 mm under bare metal size or in the case of a stent graft, use a balloon size that is the exact size of stent graft
- Perform fistulogram, evaluate central veins, and treat accordingly (Fig. 21.4)

Potential Pitfalls

- Do not use balloon-expandable stents. They are too rigid and subject to deformation
- If possible, avoid placing stents across joints as the movement in it may deform and/or fracture the stent
- Undersizing stents too much results in bad apposition and increases both risk of thrombus and of migration
- Oversizing stent grafts too much results in pleating of the stent which acts as nidus for future thrombus formation

Clinical Pointer: Utilizing the Stent Graft

- Stent grafts require a larger sheath size than bare metal stents
- Stent grafts placed in AVGs must be of the same size as the existing AVG, otherwise the stent graft will not expand completely
- You can use a stent graft to extend the venous limb of a GRAFT across a venous anastomotic stenosis.
- Always deploy a stent graft over a relatively stiff 0.035″ wire

Central Vein Stenosis (CVS) or Occlusion

This is a common complication of long-standing placement of tunneled dialysis catheters (TDCs) although it can be seen in patients with short-term temporary dialysis catheters as well. As high as 50% of hemodialysis patients have central vein stenosis on angiography, though many of these radiologic lesions will not cause any clinical symptoms. The etiology is presumed to be related to mechanical injury of the venous endothelium. The diagnosis must be entertained in a patient with a failing fistula/graft but found to have a normal fistulogram.

Clinical Clues to CVS

- Arm swelling and arm pain in a patient with or without a fistula
- Strongly pulsatile fistula
- Decreased flow in fistula
- Increased bleeding after needle removal following dialysis, secondary to high venous pressures.
- Fistula thrombosis without obvious fistula dysfunction
- Pleural effusion

Angiographic Clue to CVS

- Multiple collateral veins often despite mild appearing stenosis

Treatment of CVS

In an asymptomatic patient, observation is not only reasonable but may be the preferred approach as many patients may never develop symptoms, even in the setting of high grade CVS. PTA is the first-line treatment and is initially successful though results are not very durable. Therefore, stent-graft placement has become the treatment of choice for resistant and recurrent lesions.

How to Perform PTA for CVS

- Place 0.035″ glide wire to level central veins
- Exchange to glide wire for a stiff wire
- Position wire into inferior vena cava for additional support
- Select a non-compliant ultra high-pressure balloon that is 20–30% larger than the vessel (usually 10–12 mm for the subclavian, 16–18 mm for superior vena cava)
- Balloon sequentially to 10 atm or higher in order to break the lesion

Potential Pitfalls

- Cutting balloons should not be used in central veins as any bleeding here is difficult to control.

- Repeat until radiographic result is achieved or if radiographic result cannot be achieved, consider stenting option (see below)
- Perform completion angiogram

Stent placement may be a more durable option in symptomatic, recurrent CVS. Since the central veins change caliber with respirations, balloon expandable stents can migrate and therefore are not suitable for use in CVS. Stent grafts have also been used with apparent success although there are no studies to date evaluating their use.

How to Perform Stent Placement for CVS

- Choose a stent/stent graft as you would for peripheral venous stenosis

Potential Pitfalls

- Do not put a stent at the junction of the first rib and the clavicle as it may become deformed with time. A lesion here may actually require surgical thoracic outlet decompression

- Deploy stent under flouroscopy
- Perform completion angiogram (Fig. 21.5)

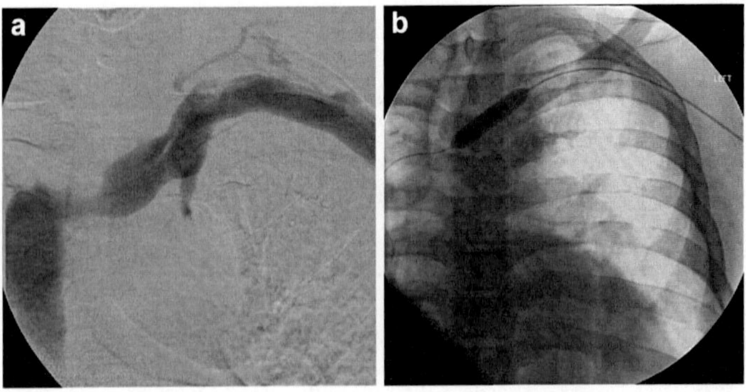

FIGURE 21.5 A 48-year-old man with a loop forearm graft on the left who presented with left arm swelling for 1 month. Workup of arm swelling requires a fistulogram to delineate arterial and venous anatomy. (**a**) Fistulogram performed through an 8 Fr sheath placed in the venous limb of the graft shows significant stenosis of the left innominate vein. (**b**) After passage of 0.035″ Supracore wire, the L innominate vein was dilated with a 12 mm × 4 cm Dorado to 20 atm for 3 min with successful relief of the stenosis

Aneurysmal and Pseudoaneurysmal AVFs

This occurs in approximately 5% of patients and carries the risk of rupture. Risk factors for developing an aneurysm are thin-walled veins, repeated puncture, and central vein stenosis. Traditionally, these aneurysms are managed surgically by resection, interposition grafting, placation, or ligation. However, covered stenting may be a reasonable option as long as the aneurysm is not so large and so degenerative that it is not amenable to hosting a stent.

Treatment of Aneurysmal AVFs

Percutaneously, covered stents may be an option to prolong the life of a fistula although data for this is lacking. The reported cases suggest that these stents can be accessed safely though the durability of the stents is not known.

How to Perform Covered Stent Placement for Aneurysm

- Access the fistula/graft with a 6–8 Fr sheath
- Perform fistulogram with imaging of the central veins
- Pass 0.035″ guidewire to level of central veins. We start with glidewire and exchange to stiffer wire (i.e., Supracore, Amplatz)
- Select a stent graft that will cross and exclude entire aneurysm
- Post dilate with a balloon that is the same size as the stent graft

Tips of the Trade
- If using multiple stents, large amount of overlap is required (5 cm)

Thrombosed Graft

An all too common problem, thrombosed grafts are now being treated percutaneously, as the superiority of surgical management is being challenged. Many studies show no difference in the two methods of treatment with the advantage of avoiding overnight hospital stays with the former.

Treatment of Thrombosed Grafts

This problem is usually treated with a combination of chemical and mechanical thrombolysis. There are many approaches that involve the instillation of a pharmacological lytic agent into the graft followed by use of the many devices available for mechanical thrombectomy.

Ways to Perform Chemical Thrombolysis

- The "lyse and wait" technique calls for instillation of TPA directly into clotted fistula and then performing a fistulogram after 20–30 min. Observe relative and absolute contraindiactions of TPA as described in Chap. 8 of this book.

- The pulse-spray technique requires the placement of a multi-side-hole catheter into the fistula and instilling TPA through it. We describe this technique below
- The cross-catheter technique is a variation of the pulse-spray technique utilizing two catheters in the fistula directed in opposite directions

Most often chemical thrombolysis is followed by mechanical thrombolysis. There are many devices available to assist with mechanical thrombectomy such as the Angiojet and the Trerotola. Post-procedure, there is no role for anticoagulation other than aspirin.

Interventional Graft Thrombectomy: How I Do It

- Access the graft antegrade with a 19-gauge needle 1 cm from the arterial anastomosis
- Pass glidewire through the clotted graft to the central veins
- Exchange for stiff wire
- Consider performing PTA of venous anastomosis
- Position a multi-side-hole catheter into the graft and begin instillation of 2 mg of TPA mixed with 3,000 U of heparin at approximately 1 mL/10 s.
- Perform fistulogram
- Repeat TPA instillation if a significant amount of thrombus remains (>20%)
- Next perform mechanical thrombectomy with your choice of device. We commonly utilize the Angiojet.
- Generally a 6 Fr sheath is adequate to accommodate the device.
- Put the device over a stiff wire (i.e., Amplatz or stiff Terumo)
- Make 1–3 passes with the device
- Once clot cleared, puncture the graft retrograde closer to the venous anastomosis and place a wire across the arterial anastomosis
- Perform embolectomy of the arterial anastomosis utilizing a Fogarty balloon as this area was not previously treated pharmacologically and usually, there will be an arterial plug to dislodge. Repeat sweep one to two times.
- Perform fistulogram, evaluate central veins, and treat any areas of stenosis

Tips of the Trade: Our Experiences

- For a patient who has a contraindications to TPA, can use heparinized saline through multi-side-hole catheter followed by mechanical thrombectomy
- Can implement the crossed-catheter technique in the setting of a loop graft where the length of graft to be treated is more than the length of a single multi-side-hole catheter
- Limit use of mechanical thrombectomy device to <10 min as there can be a significant amount of hemolysis.
- Will often perform PTA of venous anastomosis at beginning of procedure

Thrombosed Fistulas

Thrombosed fistulas are often difficult to salvage as the vein can become quite large and carry a large volume of thrombus. They require immediate intervention yet even so, the success rate is still significantly lower when compared to salvaging thrombosed grafts.

Treatment of Thrombosed Fistulas

This is a much more variable procedure compared to a graft thrombectomy given the variability of fistula anatomy but the principles are the same.

How to Perform Thrombectomy of Fistula

- Puncture the fistula antegrade just beyond the arterial anatomosis
- Utilize either chemical or mechanical thrombectomy or both to recannulize fistula
- Perform fistulogram, evaluate for any underlying causative lesions, and treat accordingly

Clinical Pointer: Always Utilize the Current Procedure to Identify the Next Access Site

- When performing an intervention to salvage access, it is time to think about the need for a new access site. Be prepared to perform bilateral upper extremity venograms.
- For example, if a forearm access site is thrombosed, access the vein and pass a wire and catheter into the antecubital region to identify the outflow vein in preparation for an upper extremity fistula
- Always be on the lookout for central vein stenosis

Follow-Up and Screening Dialysis Access

- Surveillance is not standardized and its role remains unclear
- Some centers perform duplex ultrasound which is non-invasive every 3–6 months which may help identify a problem early

Equipment List

This is a partial list as a variety of equipment can be successfully utilized.

Sheaths

4–6 F standard short sheath

- Terumo Pinnacle
- Cordis Brite Tip

If stent grafts are to be used, then larger sheaths (7–8 F) are needed.

Guidewires

We recommend 0.035″ wires. There are many wires that can be utilized. Commonly, we use one of the following:

- Glidewire (Terumo)
- Amplatz Super Stiff (Cook)
- Supracore (Guidant)

Balloons

There are many over the wire balloon choices.

- EverFlex (EV3)
- Conquest (Bard)
- Dorado (Boston Scientific)
- Cutting Balloon (Boston Scientific)

Stents

Self-expandable stents are recommended. We typically use one of the following:

- Zilver (Cook)
- Protégé (EV3)
- Smartstent (Cordis)

Stent Grafts

Self-expandable stents are recommended. We typically use one of the following:

- Viabahn (Gore)
- Fluency (Bard)

Bibliography

1. 2009 Annual Report United States Renal Data System. Available at http://www.usrds.org/adr.htm.
   → *This is a national site to find comprehensive data including incidence, demographics, and cost.*
2. KDOQI™ Guidelines and Commentaries. Available at http://www.kidney.org/professionals/kdoqi/guidelines_commentaries.cfm.
   → *This is a comprehensive the national evidence-based clinical practice guidelines and standard of care.*
3. Voormolen EH, Jahrome AK, Bartels LW, Moll FL, Mali WP, Blankestijn PJ. Nonmaturation of arm arteriovenous fistulas for hemodialysis access: A systematic review of risk factors and results of early treatment. J Vasc Surg. 2009 May;49(5):1325–36. Review. PMID: 19394557.
   → *This review of 33 studies conclusively shows that many non matured AVFs can be salvaged although techniques vary.*
4. Haage P, Günther RW. Radiological intervention to maintain vascular access. Eur J Vasc Endovasc Surg. 2006 Jul;32(1):84–9. Epub 2005 Nov 16. Review. PMID: 16297644 *renal angiography at the time of cardiac catheterization.*
   → *A comprehensive review from Germany author presenting common dialysis problems and suitable approaches to treating them.*
5. Gelbfish GA. Surgical versus percutaneous care of arteriovenous access. Semin Vasc Surg. 2007 Sep;20(3):167–74. Review.PMID: 17884618.
   → *This is an expert opinion piece that provides an excellent overview of dialysis access problems and how to approach them.*
6. Haskal ZJ, Trerotola S, Dolmatch B, Schuman E, Altman S, Mietling S, Berman S, McLennan G, Trimmer C, Ross J, Vesely T. Stent graft versus balloon angioplasty for failing dialysis-access grafts. N Engl J Med. 2010 Feb 11;362(6):494–503.PMID: 20147715.
   → *The trial is the first of its kind as it is a randomized trial of 190 patients, suggesting stent grafts may be superior to simple balloon angioplasty in treating AVG stenoses.*

Chapter 22
Nutcracker Syndrome

Matthew T. Menard and Richard Bafford

Background

- Nutcracker syndrome refers to the compression of the left renal vein (LRV) between the superior mesenteric artery (SMA) and the aorta (Fig. 22.1)
- It is a relatively uncommon entity predominately affecting young men and middle-aged women, often seen in association with a thin body habitus
- Symptomatic patients may present with left flank pain, hematuria, and associated symptoms of pelvic congestion
- Treatment usually consists of open surgical venous decompression
- Percutaneous intervention is being used with increasing frequency

M.T. Menard (✉)
Division of Vascular and Endovascular Surgery, Brigham and Women's Hospital, Harvard Medical School,
Boston, MA, USA
e-mail: mmenard@partners.org

R. Bafford
Division of Vascular Surgery,
University of Maryland School of Medicine,
Baltimore, MD, USA
e-mail: rbafford@smail.maryland.edu

C.D. Owens and Y. Yeghiazarians (eds.),
Handbook of Endovascular Peripheral Interventions,
DOI 10.1007/978-1-4614-0839-0_22,

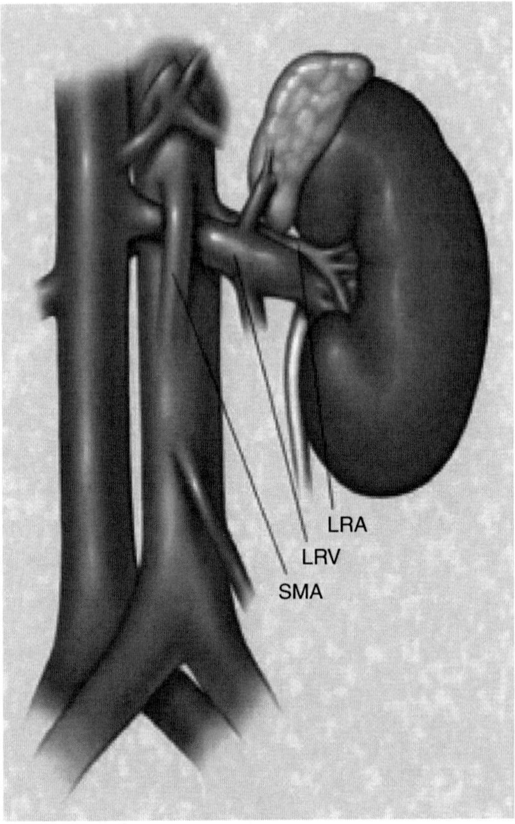

FIGURE 22.1 Anatomy of nutcracker syndrome. Superior mesenteric artery (*SMA*) drapes over the left renal vein (*LRV*). *LRA* left renal artery

Epidemiology

- Relatively uncommon condition, with true incidence and prevalence difficult to ascertain
- Wide spectrum of disease severity, from incidentally discovered asymptomatic left renal vein compression to severe manifestation of both nutcracker syndrome and associated pelvic congestion

Clinical Pointers: The Other Nutcracker Syndrome

- Aortomesenteric compression of the third part of the duodenum
- Also referred to as SMA syndrome or more properly, vascular compression of the duodenum
- Symptoms include nausea, bilious vomiting, abdominal pain, and weight loss

Etiology/Pathophysiology

- Narrowed aortomesenteric angle (normal 35–40°, less than 16° in nutcracker syndrome)
- Left renal vein compression results in renal venous hypertension leading to secondary development of thin-walled venous sinus collaterals that communicate with renal calyces
- Extravasation of red blood cells from venous sinuses into renal calyces results in hematuria
- Frank rupture of venous sinuses can result in brisk bleeding, formation and passage of blood clots through ureter, and associated flank pain
- Dorsal ptosis of the left kidney seen in some cases
- Poorly characterized genetic factors may predispose individuals with anatomic evidence of left renal vein compression toward symptom development
- Hormonal factors likely increase susceptibility to pelvic congestion during pregnancy and in the premenopausal individual

Clinical Signs/Symptoms

- Left flank pain
- Hematuria
- Orthostatic proteinuria
- Associated with left-sided varicocele
- Pelvic congestion – dyspareunia and dysuria

- Vulvar/scrotal varices
- Left-sided vaginal tenderness
- Lower extremity varicosities can be seen as a secondary manifestation of severe pelvic congestion
- Exacerbation of symptoms during pregnancy

Diagnosis and Imaging

- History and physical exam
- Clinical suspicion
- Cystoscopy – left ureteral orificial bleeding
- Retrograde urography – scalloping of renal pelvis or ureter from associated varicies
- Computed tomography angiography
- Magnetic resonance angiography
- Transvaginal ultrasound – document pelvic varices
- Duplex ultrasound
- Venography

Tips on Imaging

- Contrast-enhanced cross-sectional imaging can document degree of LRV compression by the SMA as well as extent of associated gonadal and pelvic venous involvement.
- Normal supine studies may underestimate venous dilation secondary to reduced venous filling when compared to upright position.
- Duplex ultrasound can provide hemodynamic correlates – elevated peak systolic velocity at point of LRV compression compared to hilar renal vein and inferior vena cava (IVC).
- Venography is definitive confirmatory diagnostic test – it provides renocaval pressure gradient data (normal 0–3 mmHg) and anatomic correlates.

Evolution of Open Surgical Treatment

- Pastershank 1974 – left renal vein venolysis
- SMA transposition
- Nephropexy
- Expansion of aortomesenteric angle
- Autotransplantation of left kidney to pelvis
- Nephrectomy
- External stenting of LRV with ringed polytetrafluoroethylene (PTFE)
- Resection of dilated left gonadal vein and associated varices
- Gonadal caval H-graft bypass
- Left renal vein bypass
- Left renal vein transposition

Treatment

- Conservative
- Surgical – mainstay is venous decompression by transposition of left renal vein to more distal point on IVC
  - Endovascular – endovenous stenting of LRV; while endovenous stenting is an acceptable treatment option, preliminary experience to date would suggest that durability is compromised compared to open surgical repair. As such, we favor an operative approach for younger patients and those without prohibitive surgical risk or contraindications. With further refinement in minimally invasive technology, endovascular treatment may evolve to become the treatment of choice.

- Coil embolization of pelvic varices for associated symptoms of pelvic congestion
  - Patients often require adjunctive treatment of dilated ovarian veins and pelvic varices for full symptomatic relief. This additional therapeutic step can be undertaken concurrently with endovascular treatment of left

renal vein constriction or can be addressed in a staged fashion if flank or pelvic symptoms persist following isolated left renal vein decompression. Treatment of pelvic varices also serves to prevent recurrence of lower extremity varicose veins associated with pelvic reflux and has replaced retroperitoneal surgical division of the refluxing pelvic veins connecting with extrapelvic varices.

Endovascular Approach: How I Do It

- Common femoral venous access with 5 F sheath inferior vena cavogram.

Potential Pitfalls: Endovascular Treatment
- Stent migration/embolization
- In-stent restenosis
- Stent thrombosis (see Fig. 22.2)

- Selective catheterization of left renal vein with an angled glide wire and Berenstein or Cobra catheter.
- Selective left renal venography to assess degree of renal vein stenosis.
- Additional views as appropriate to assess presence and degree of collaterals, with selective cannulation and venography of left ovarian vein as appropriate.
- Pull-back left renal vein to IVC pressure-gradient determination. A gradient >3 mmHg in the appropriate clinical setting is supportive of diagnosis of nutcracker syndrome.
- If diagnosis confirmed, upsize sheath to accommodate desired balloon and stent. Administer intravenous heparin to maintain an ACT >250 s.
- Predilate lesion with non compliant balloon(s) to facilitate stent delivery and accurate assessment of appropriate stent choice.

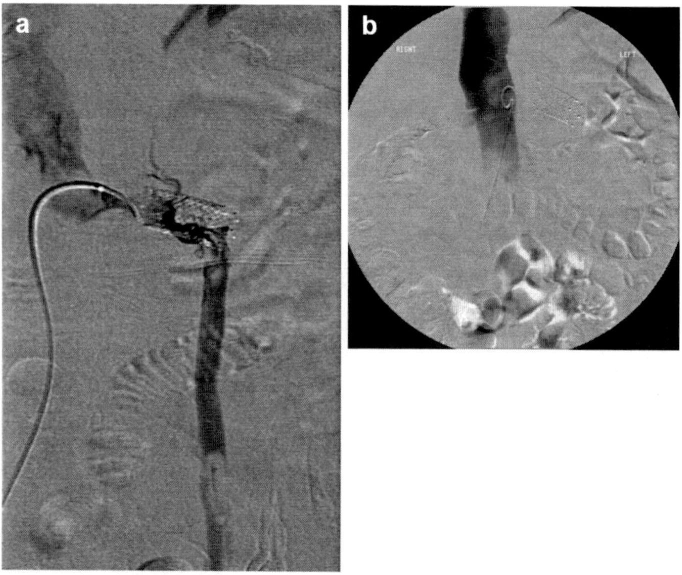

FIGURE 22.2 (**a**) In-stent restenosis. (**b**) Stent thrombosis of stent poorly positioned too distally in left renal vein. Note dilation of left ovarian vein in **a**

- Deploy 16–20 mm Wallstent or analogous self-expanding nitinol stent of appropriate length (Fig. 22.3c). Stent should protrude several millimeters into the IVC to maximize stent stability.
- If difficult to track stent into renal vein, a stiff guidewire can be advanced distally into the gonadal vein.
- Once the stent is successfully delivered into proximal left renal vein, the wire can be withdrawn from the gonadal vein and advanced more distally into the left renal vein. Post-dilate stent with appropriately sized non-compliant balloon.
- Confirm successful deployment with completion venogram (Fig. 22.3) and repeat pressure assessment to confirm obliteration of the renocaval gradient.
- Dual platelet therapy with aspirin 325 mg daily and clopidogrel 75 mg daily for minimum of 30 days.

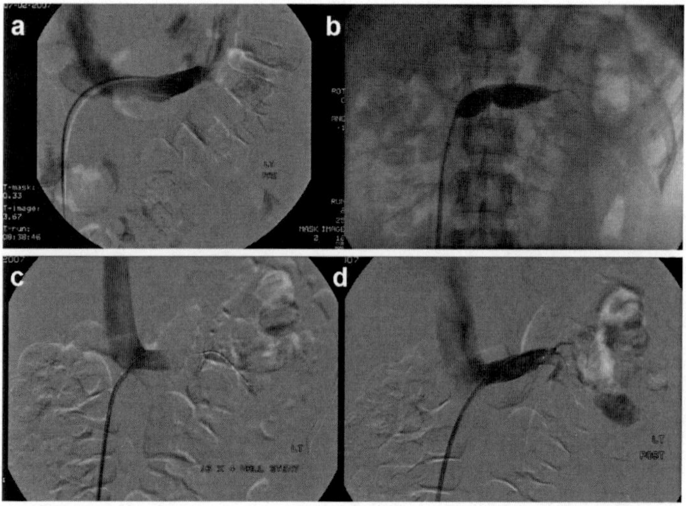

FIGURE 22.3 A 34-year-old female with 2 years of disabling pelvic pain. (**a**) Venogram confirming compression of the left renal vein by the superior mesenteric artery, with an associated renal vein to inferior vena cava pressure gradient of 4 mmHg. (**b**) Balloon angioplasty of left renal vein, revealing "waste" at site of compression, with 16×40 mm^2 balloon. (**c**) Deployment of 16×40 mm^2 Wallstent. (**d**) Completion venogram following placement and post-dilation to 16 mm

Equipment List

Sheaths

- 5–8 F standard short sheaths

Selective Catheters

- Berenstein
- Cobra

Guidecaths (6–8 F)

- Renal Double Curve
- LIMA
- Cobra

Wires

- 0.035″ angled glidewire
- 0.035″ Amplatz

Balloons

- 14–16 mm non-compliant balloons

Stents

- Wallstent
- Analogous self-expanding stent

Bibliography

1. Menard MT. Nutcracker Syndrome: When Should It Be Treated and How? *Perspectives in Vasc Surg and Endovasc Therapy* 2009 Jun;21(2):117–24.
   → *Recent comprehensive review on the subject.*
2. Scultetus AH, Villavicencio JL, Gillespie DL. The nutcracker syndrome: it's role in the pelvic venous disorders. *J Vasc Surg.* 2001;34:812–819.
   → *Good overview of the pathophysiology of pelvic venous disease.*
3. Reed NR, Kalra M, Bower TC, Vrtiska TJ, Ricotta JJ 2nd, Gloviczki P. Left renal vein transposition for nutcracker syndrome. *J Vasc Surg.* 2009;49:386–393.
   → *Largest and most contemporary series.*

4. Neste MG, Narasimham DL, Belcher KK. Endovascular stent placement as a treatment for renal venous hypertension. *J Vasc Interv Radiol*. 1996;7:859–861.
   → *First published description of endovascular treatment for renal vein stenosis.*
5. Chiesa R, Anzuini A, Marone EM, et al. Endovascular stenting for the nutcracker phenomenon. *J Endovasc Ther*. 2001;8: 652–655.
   → *Excellent review of endovascular therapy for nutcracker syndrome.*

Index

C.D. Owens and Y. Yeghiazarians (eds.), *Handbook of Endovascular Peripheral Interventions*, DOI 10.1007/978-1-4614-0839-0,

MIX
Papier aus verantwortungsvollen Quellen
Paper from responsible sources
FSC® C105338

Printed by Books on Demand, Germany